SURGERY - PROCEDURES, COMPLICATIONS, AND RESULTS

BARIATRIC SURGERY

FROM INDICATIONS TO POSTOPERATIVE CARE

CHRISTOS R. IAVAZZO
EDITOR

Nova Biomedical
New York

For permission to use material from this book please contact us:
Telephone 631-231-7269; Fax 631-231-8175
Web Site: http://www.novapublishers.com

Additional color graphics may be available in the e-book version of this book.

Library of Congress Cataloging-in-Publication Data

ISBN: 978-1-62618-995-9

Library of Congress Control Number: 2013939135

Published by Nova Science Publishers, Inc. † New York

Contents

Preface

This book aims to become a useful tool in the field of bariatric surgery providing the most up-to-date research on the field, including the recent data on surgical techniques, the current strategies for diagnosis, treatment, and follow-up, as well as extensive discussion of the possible complications. More specifically, the following issues are discussed in the chapters of the book:

The problem of obesity and related diseases, including type 2 diabetes mellitus is still growing. There are many factors responsible for modern-day epidemics such as obesity and T2DM. The crucial ones seem to be the environmental factors e.g. caloric availability, fat consumption, low physical activity as well as genes which may interact with the environment. Recent studies defined roles for gut peptides in the control of beta cell growth and survival. The role of gastrointestinal endocrinology knowledge for example of incretines in bariatric surgery is discussed.

Current topics in obesity research involve new adipokines linking obesity to related co-morbidities. Adipocytokines participate in regulation of the energy homeostasis, glucose and lipid metabolism, immunity as well as neuroendocrine and cardiovascular function. Adipokines participate in various metabolic processes including the regulation of appetite control, cardiovascular function, energy expenditure, insulin sensitivity and secretion, as well as inflammation. Adipocyte dysfunctions belong to the primary defects in obesity and may link obesity to several health problems including increased risk of insulin resistance, type 2 diabetes, fatty liver disease, hypertension, dyslipidemia, atherosclerosis, dementia, airway disease, and some types of cancers.

The anatomy of the relevant parts of the gastrointestinal tract and abdominal wall and their relevance to the bariatric procedures currently in common use are outlined. Laparoscopic port placement with anatomical considerations, the role of hiatus and intra-abdominal, the structure of the stomach wall and gastric motility, omental and bowel anatomy, as well as Roux-en-Y gastric bypass (RYGB)- limbs and mesenteric defects are discussed.

It is questioned to have or not to have the Ring Banded Roux-en-Y Gastric Bypass by mentioning that the evolution from the band to the silicone ring was observed in both vertical banded gastroplasty and banded gastric bypass. The silicone ring develops a pseudocapsule which leads to less adhesion and is much easier to remove than the band.

The book deals with postoperative complications after bariatric surgery in general including late, immediate, hepatobilliary complications, intestinal obstruction, gastrointestinal bleeding, functional and nutritional compaction. The knowledge of normal anatomy and the surgical technique is fundamental to achieve excellent prognosis in patients who have undergone bariatric surgery.

It also discusses in detail the hepatobiliary complications (including gallstone disease, pancreatitis, hepatic complications) associated with bariatric surgery and the potential strategies to prevent and manage these complications. Of these by far the most common is the formation of gallstones and its subsequent sequelae. Although the majority of the complications can be dealt with by general surgeons, successful management requires a broad understanding of the anatomical and physiological changes following surgery and there should be a low threshold for involving an appropriately experienced bariatric unit.

Moreover, an overview of the causes, clinical presentation, investigations and treatment of postoperative intestinal obstruction after bariatric procedures with a particular emphasis on Roux-en-Y gastric bypass (RYGB) is provided.

The risk of postoperative infection is presented in particular the risk of SSI, as shown in multiple studies of diverse populations of patients. Stratification of infection risk for obese surgical patients with different and specific tools (e.g., scores for obese patients) may be necessary. From the existing data, it is clear that there are at least four strategies that should be considered in order to decrease the risk of SSI when operating on obese patients. First, tight perioperative glucose control is key to minimizing episodes of hyperglycemia that are associated with a higher rate of SSI. Second, optimizing tissue oxygen tension through increased perioperative FIO_2 and appropriate resuscitation improves the perfusion of tissues and oxygen radical-mediated defense mechanisms against infection. Third, larger doses of prophylactic antibiotics maximize serum and tissue concentrations, providing a real (and expected) decrease in SSI. Fourth, performing laparoscopic operations whenever feasible certainly decreases the area at risk and has a demonstrated ability to reduce SSI. Obesity management strategies mainly target behavioural components of the disorder, but are only marginally effective. If infections contribute to human obesity, then entirely different prevention and treatment strategies and public health policies could be needed to address this subtype of the disorder.

Bariatric surgery is susceptible to the development of nutritional deficiencies, i.e. anemia, due to low food intake, the effects of gastric restriction and malabsorption which occurs. Anemic etiology may be due to deficiencies of iron, folate and/or vitamin B_{12}. Orientation concerning nutritional deficiencies that may result from bariatric surgery are essential to the multidisciplinary team in the post-op phase, in order to maintain the good health and quality of life of patients. Such issues are also discussed.

It also discusses how oral health is influenced by bariatric surgery. Bariatric patients are at an increased risk for dental caries due to a smaller stomach volume and the need for smaller, more frequent meals/snacks throughout the day. Bariatric patients are also at an increased risk for dehydration and lactose intolerance that also contribute to caries activity due to the occurrence of xerostomia and reduced exposure to anticariogenic factors in milk. The medical team needs to relate to potential dental problems after bariatric surgery, and to supply their patients with the appropriate information. Instruction regarding oral hygiene maintenance, healthy diet patterns and regular dental health monitoring by a dentist or dental hygienist are of paramount importance.

The need for nutritional education is discussed and advice on how to cut and chew food, along with other eating behavior habits must be given to patients early in the preoperative period to avoid food intolerance. There is a tendency in looking for easy-to-swallow foods instead of protein foods. This may lead the patient to an extensive loss of lean mass and to nutritional deficiencies. Nutritional support is indispensable so that this tool may be used successfully, with the aim to achieve a healthy weight loss and maintenance.

The number of bariatric operations performed each year is growing continuously, and it is to be assumed that this trend will continue in the coming years. In the past, not all of our procedures for treating obesity were well chosen. Some of them were not adequate for the patient needs, behaviour or metabolic disease. Over time, there has been growing need for re-operations to improve outcome. There is a growing number of patients who need revisionary surgery due to poor weight loss after the primary operation. Patients in need of redo bariatric surgery usually come to a reference metabolic centre. The development and improvement of diagnostic procedures and guidelines prior to redo surgery is still one of our main objectives. The problem of choosing the right revisionary procedure and discussing it with the patient is of highest importance. Bariatric surgery, as a rule, leads to massive weight loss and marked changes in body contour, which assumes bizarre shapes. This impacts the quality of life of the individuals affected by these deformities, known as dysmorphisms. Brachial dysmorphism is treated surgically by brachioplasty to restore a more aesthetic looking cylinder-shaped arm contour. The surgical technique and complications are discussed.

It is mentioned that body-contouring procedures after massive weight loss following bariatric surgery is increasing. Great "positive" thinking of these patients towards body-contouring procedures creates enormous expectations for improvement in quality of life similar to the expectations which motivated these patients toward bariatric surgery. The main points of patient satisfaction are: "body image" greatly improved, self-esteem recovery, improvement in life relationships, and sexual life resumption or improvement.

The role of bariatric surgery in gestational diabetes, hypertensive disorders during pregnancy, as well as neonate's development and birth weight are discussed. Moreover, the diet, monitoring and complications of such women during pregnancy are also discussed. A question is also raised whether conception should be postponed or not for at least 18 months after bariatric operation to avoid complications concerning both mother and fetus mainly associated with nutritional deficiencies due to the anatomical and physiological changes of such operations.

Bariatric surgery can lead to significantly weight reduction of obese women, so this method also acts as a treatment for the pelvic floor disorders that those women face by offering improvement in incontinence and quality of life. The role of bariatric surgery operations in the improvement of the pelvic floor disorders that many obese women are facing is presented.

Medicolegal problems are also discussed in this edition. An introduction on the reasons why bariatric surgery has a high incidence of medico-legal problems (new surgery, poor mentorship, vulnerable patient group is made, as well as a brief discussion regarding the legal principles, issues regarding consenting, technical issues e.g., Roux en O, follow up issues and emergency presentations following bariatric surgery.

This book aims to provide the current reliable essentials of clinical practice in the field, but also to maintain a long "shelf life" in order to be used as a cornerstone of diagnosis and management.

Iavazzo Christos, MD, MSc, PhD
Iaso Maternity Hospital, Athens, Greece

In: Bariatric Surgery
Editor: Christos R. Iavazzo

ISBN: 978-1-62618-995-9

Chapter I

Intestinal Peptides Involved in T2DM Pathophysiology

***Dominika Stygar*[1]*, Tomasz Sawczyn*[1]*, Iwona Karcz-Socha*[1]*, Krystyna Zwirska-Korczala*[1] *and W. Konrad Karcz*[2]**
[1]Department of Physiology in Zabrze, Silesian Medical University, Poland
[2]Department of Abdominal Surgery, Videosurgery Division, Bariatric and Metabolic Surgical Center, University of Freiburg, Germany

Abstract

Despite the vast progress in obesity and type 2 diabetes mellitus (T2DM) research, many questions still needs to be answered in these fields e. g.: why people with type 2 diabetes mellitus do not feel satiety despite the high glucose level in their blood. Is the glucose really the main factor for regulating appetite? The crucial factors responsible for modern-day epidemics of T2DM are caloric availability, fat consumption, low physical activity as well as genes which may interact with the environment. Gastrointestinal factors involved in the regulation of carbohydrate homeostasis and appetite may also be of essential importance. Gastrointestinal hormones called incretins, play a significant role in the pathophysiology of type 2 diabetes. In this chapter we present the achievements of modern surgery, which opened the possibility for surgical treatment of diabetes, and also created new opportunities for research on the role of incretin hormones in the pathophysiology of diabetes.

Introduction

Considering problems of obesity and type 2 diabetes mellitus (T2DM) from an evolutionary point of view, we may conclude that nowadays we face the situation when a Paleolithic man has fallen into the ‘food hedonism’ view is summarized by the notion that `Human biology is designed for Sone Age conditions [1]. Human adaptedness to the hunter-gatherer way of life does not seem to be favorable in modern times, when Homo sapiens need to put no effort into the processes of acquiring and preparing food. For the first time in the history of our species ‘the food comes to us’. The problem of obesity and related diseases, including type 2 diabetes mellitus is still growing. According to Wild et al. the prevalence of diabetes is epidemic, with more than 170 million people affected worldwide in the year 2000, and it is estimated that this number will exceed 366 million by 2030 [2]. The diabetes epidemic relates particularly to type 2 diabetes, and it takes place both in the developed nations and the developing ones [3]. In a research with healthy human subjects, fasting glucose level is homeostatically regulated by insulin and glucagon, that subsequently control the hepatic glucose release as well as peripheral glucose uptake. Jean Mayer [4], more than 50 years ago, proposed that changes in blood glucose concentrations or arteriovenous glucose differences are detected by glucoreceptors that affect energy intake. According to this theory, the increase in blood glucose concentrations results in elevated feeling of satiety whereas a decrease in blood glucose concentrations has the opposite effect. Basing on Mayer's glucostatic theory and taking into consideration the disturbances in the glucose homeostasis characteristic of people with T2DM, a few questions still remain unanswered e. g., why people with type 2 diabetes mellitus do not feel satiety despite the high glucose level in their blood. Is this really the main factor for regulating appetite? There are many factors responsible for modern-day epidemics such as obesity and T2DM. The crucial ones seem to be the environmental factors e. g. caloric availability, fat consumption, low physical activity as well as genes which may interact with the environment. Yet there is mounting evidence indicating that gastrointestinal factors involved in the regulation of carbohydrate homeostasis and appetite may also be of essential importance [5]. Type-2 diabetes is a heterogeneous disorder. It is a group of metabolic diseases characterized by hyperglycemia resulting from defects in insulin secretion and/or insulin action. Abnormal insulin secretion, associated with varying degrees of insulin resistance are typical for T2DM. Genetic and acquired factors lead to impairment of beta-cell function, tissue insulin sensitivity and diabetes. Moreover, deterioration of diabetes control and insulin secretory function occurs within years in type 2 diabetic patients despite insulin resistance remaining stable [6]. Thus, beta-cell dysfunction is central to the development of diabetes, possibly due to a combination of decreased beta-cell mass and insulin secretion defects. Recent studies defined roles for gut peptides in the control of beta cell growth and survival [7]. Many research groups around the world examined roles of gut peptides in the regulation of carbohydrate metabolism, however, the mechanisms behind the alternations in glucose homeostasis are still elusive. Better understanding of this phenomenon is needed to improve therapeutic and preventive strategies against the T2DM development.

Gastrointestinal Endocrinology and the Bariatric Surgery

The birth of gastrointestinal endocrinology dates back at the beginning of the 20th century. In 1902, William M. Bayliss and Ernest H. Starling published ‘The mechanism of pancreatic secretion’ [8]. The authors described the action of an unknown factor contained in the acid extracts of intestinal mucosa, as stimulant of the pancreas exocrine secretion and they named this factor secretin. Three years later, on the basis of experiments on the action of secretin on pancreatic exocrine function, Starling proposed the word `hormone' for chemical factors which influence the function of a distant organ via blood stream [9,10]. Starling had considered the possibility that the duodenum may secrete factors which stimulate not only exocrine but also endocrine activity of the pancreas. This assumption led to attempts to use the extract, which potentially contains a factor affecting the endocrine function of the pancreas, as a cure for diabetes. Researchers examined anti-diabetic action of secretin solution through injecting of the secretin extract intravenously, but the results were negative. Moore et al. [11] undertook similar attempts choosing an oral route of supply of duodenal mucosa extract, but excluding three positive cases, other patients were treated with the extract with negative results. Despite the negative results obtained in both cases, which resulted from a mismatched group, more than from an assumed hypothesis, it was the first attempt to treat diabetes by administering the intestinal peptides.

The discovery of insulin by Banting and Best in 1921 resulted in the systematic study on intestinal hormones influencing carbohydrate metabolism. Before the outbreak of World War II, scientists made a few interesting discoveries in this field. La Barre and Still [12] purified crude secretin into a fraction which is only secretagogue (stimulating the exocrine pancreas) and another which lowers the blood sugar level. It is also very important that they claimed that the latter effect is mediated via stimulation of insulin secretion [10]. In 1932, La Barre [13] used for the first time the name ‘incretin’ to describe substances extracted from the upper gut mucosa, which produces hypoglycemia and does not stimulate pancreatic exocrine secretion.

Significant acceleration on the study of intestinal hormones was noted with the development of peptide chemistry and the modern technique of purification and protein sequencing. The discovery of glucose-dependent insulinotropic polypeptide (GIP) by John C. Brown in 1970, and of several other groups GLP-1 (glucagon-like peptide 1) in 1985 resulted in innumerable reports that describe the body's carbohydrate metabolism and the role of incretin hormones in its regulation [14, 15]. A plethora of interesting information in this topic emerged with the development of bariatric surgery. In principle, bariatric procedures have lead to weight loss, and an unintentional, but extremely important benefit of these treatments is remission of type 2 diabetes mellitus. This phenomenon appears before weight loss, which suggests a direct effect of the surgical intervention on the mechanisms that involve changes in the gastrointestinal hormones that are engaged in the regulation of glucose metabolism [16, 17, 18]. This discovery made it possible to develop a metabolic surgery and opened new avenues for type 2 diabetes mellitus research.

Gastrointestinal Tract and the Energy Homeostasis

Energy balance is a homeostatic system, regulated through a neuro-hormonal method. The major source of energy in humans is the carbohydrates of which glucose plays a pivotal role for the metabolism of most cells. The gastrointestinal tract (GI) and associated visceral organs play a crucial sensing and signaling role in the control of energy homeostasis. Through its role in digestion, absorption, assimilation of ingested nutrients and releasing gut hormones, the intestine influences a number of physiological processes and acts on tissues, including exocrine glands and nervous system [19, 20, 21, 22]. The intestine responds dynamically to the changes of internal and external stimuli. This ability called enteroplasticity is regulated on a cellular, molecular and physiological level and is of major nutritional importance [23]. The mechanism of intestinal adaptation is associated with a diet and the manner whereby dietary manipulation modulates these processes is linked with cellular and molecular events [24]. Changes in the synthesis of glucose carriers and their subsequent insertion into membranes affects the absorption of sugar from the gastrointestinal lumen into the enterocytes using sodium-dependent D-glucose transporters (SGLT1), facultative fructose transporter (GLUT 5) or the glucose transporter type 2 (GLUT2) [24, 25, 26]. Sugar absorption in response to sugar-rich meals and insulin is regulated by GLUT2 in enterocyte plasma membranes. Rapid trafficking of GLUT2 to the apical membrane induced by glucose during the assimilation of a meal is also linked with paracrine and endocrine hormone releasing, especially insulin and GLP-2 [25, 26]. The hypothalamus is the integrating center of peripheral and central signals of energy balance. The information about sources of energy stored as fat as well as the actual availability of energy including this from the gut is consolidated here. In addition to stimulation of the hypothalamus through vagal nerve, it also occurs through peptides hormones. In response to nutrients GI releases more than 20 different regulatory peptides and is the largest endocrine organ in the body. These peptides have numerous targets (gastrointestinal exocrine glands, smooth muscle, afferent nerve terminals, brain) and are involved in short-and long-term control of energy balance [17, 20]. Long lasting positive energy balance and imbalance between the uptake of energy and energy output leads to a disturbance of the mechanisms through which gut hormones regulate the energy homeostasis (demand, supply, storage and utilization of energy rich substrates like carbohydrates and lipids). The role of the gut in energy balance has been developed recently, especially in the field of research on obesity and type II diabetes mellitus. Clinical and experimental studies conducted on animals and humans who underwent metabolic surgery provide a plethora of interesting information. Surgical intervention on the GI led to novel approaches to the pathophysiology of T2DM and the role of gut peptides in this disease, indicating possible roles of gut pathways also in the genetic etiology of diabetes. There is a considerable interest in the development of intestinal endocrinology and understanding the role of intestinal peptides in the pathophysiology of disorders involving imbalances in the control of ingestion and disposal of energy.

Incretins and Hindgut Hypothesis

The hindgut hypothesis suggests that the quick transit of nutrients to the distal bowel improves glucose metabolism by stimulating secretion of intestinal peptides. Observed "incretin effect', also found after oral administration of glucose, results in stimulating insulin secretion, more potently than intravenously administrated glucose, even when plasma glucose excursions are matched [27]. Thus, among the known and investigated intestinal peptides, it seems that two peptides, glucagon-like peptide-1 (GLP-1) and glucose-dependent insulinotropic polypeptide (GIP) play the most important role in the mechanism of the incretin effect. These so-called 'incretins' are secreted by intestinal L and K respectively.

Cells L also secrete peptide YY (PYY_{3-36}). PYY_{3-36} is known as short-term central satiety signal via Y2 receptors [28].

The L-cells are an open-type intestinal epithelial endocrine cells that directly contact luminal nutrients through their apical surface [29]. The density of L-cells increases along the length of the gastrointestinal tract, with the highest numbers being found in the distal ileum and colon [19]. Reimann et al. described in details the signaling mechanisms underlying the release of glucagon-like peptide 1 [30]. GLP-1 is a product of the proglucagon gene, spinning 10 kilobases and located on the long arm of chromosome 2, that encodes not only GLP-1 but also glucagon, GLP-2 and other proglucagon-derived peptides (PGDPs) [31]. GLP-1 is cleaved from the fragment of proglucagon molecule corresponding to amino acids 78-107/108. Posttranslational processing of proglucagon in enteroendocrine L-cells and the central nervous system (CNS) liberates proglucagon-derived peptides like GLP-1, GLP-2, gut-derived glucagon (glicentin), peptide tyrosine-tyrosine (PYY), oxyntomodulin, and intervening peptide-2. The mechanism that triggers the release of GLP-1 from L cells is related to the sweet taste receptors which are components of the glucose sensor in the gut lumenand plays key roles in the regulation of GLP-1 release and the incretin effect. Thus, the primary physiologic stimulus for GLP-1 secretion from intestinal L-cells is mainly a mixed meal which contains glucose, triacylglycerol (TG) as well as fructose and some proteins and peptons [19, 32]. Additionally, other substances like hormones and neurotransmitters such as bombesin, acetyl choline, GIP, CGRP, fatty acids and bile acids, which may enhance GLP-1 secretion by increasing cAMP concentrations or by triggering the release of Ca^{2+} from intracellular stores were identified [30]. GLP-1 has been shown to enhance insulin gene transcription and all the steps of insulin biosynthesis [33]. Moreover, GLP-1 upregulates the genes for the cellular machinery involved in insulin secretion, such as the glucokinase and GLUT-2 (also known as SLC2A2) genes [34]. GLP-1 inhibits glucagon secretion, which in turn results in inhibition of hepatic glucose production. GLP-1 stimulates β cell proliferation and inhibits its apoptosis. This incretin also enhances the differentiation of new β cells from pancreatic progenitor cells [35]. Furthermore GLP-1 reduces appetite and gastrointestinal motility, lowering postprandial glucose excursions [36]. In normoglycemic human subjects, plasma GLP-1 levels are between 5 and 15 $pmol \cdot l^{-1}$ in the basal state, rising from 20 up to 60 $pmol \cdot l^{-1}$ after oral glucose intake [37, 38, 39]. Postprandial GLP-1 release starts approximately 10 to 15 min after a meal ingestion. The plasma concentration of GLP-1 increases in the second hour after food intake, and then slowly declines to the baseline. When administered intravenously in normal subjects and in diabetic patients, the plasma half-life (t1/2) of exogenous GLP-1 is only about 1-2 minutes. Dipeptidyl peptidase-4 (DPP-4) enzyme is thought to be primarily responsible for the degradation of glucagon-like peptide-1 (GLP-1) and glucose-dependent insulinotropic peptide (GIP) [40] present in the blood [41], intestine [42], liver [43], brain and kidneys [44]. DPP-4 is a member of a family of ubiquitous atypical serine proteases with many physiological functions in nutrition, metabolism, the endocrine and immune systems, cancer growth, bone marrow mobilization and cell adhesion [40]. DPP-4 rapidly inactivates the GLP-1 and other incretines by cleaving two amino acid residues at the N-terminus, where the main degradation product is GLP-1-(9-36) amide. Degradation of GLP-1 begins one minute after its release due to the presence of dipeptidyl peptidase IV in the capillary blood vessels adjacent to L cells in the intestinal mucosa, which means that this peptide serves mainly as a paracrine signal in the gastrointestinal tract [45]. GLP-1 also acts on the nervous system, while its secretion is partly controlled by the nervous system. Described incretin is a typical peptide of the brain-gut axis, which may act as an endocrine and paracrine signal. It also plays a role as a neurotransmitter of the autonomic nervous system and a neurotrophic factor. The mechanisms involved in controlling and coordinating L cells and in the formation of a pulsatile secretion pattern of GLP-1 depend on the parasympathetic nervous system in vivo in a man [46]. Also peripheral cholinergic transmission dependent on vagal efferent inputs is involved in the regulation of GLP-1 release [47]. Possibly, the muscarinic (cholinergic) receptors M1 and M2, located in the intestinal L cells, are involved in the transmission in humans and rats [48]. However, adrenergic transmission may also play a role in the control of ileal L-cell activity, since beta- and alpha-adrenergic agonists have been shown to enhance GLP-1 release [49]. GLP-1 induces a vagovagal reflex resulting in an altered function of the pancreatic islet β cells and thereby causes insulin to be released from the pancreatic β-cell [50]. Circulating GLP-1 and CCK-8 reduce food intake by capsaicin-insensitive, nonvagal mechanisms. Vagal or capsaicin-sensitive neurons are not necessary to reduce food intake by circulating (endocrine) GLP-1, or cholecystokinin. Vagal participation in satiation by these peptides may be limited to paracrine effects exerted near the sites of their secretion [51]. The presence of chyme in the duodenum stimulates its endocrine cells to release glucose-dependent insulin-releasing polypeptide (GIP) and cholecystokinin. The enteric neurons are stimulated to secrete gastrin-releasing peptide and calcitonin gene-related peptide. These gastrointestinal peptides, organized in the functional endocrinal duodeno-ileal loop, stimulate the release, and contribute to the control of GLP-1 [52]. It suggests that the intramural enteric nervous system is involved in mediating the ‘upper gut signal’ [19]. The β-cell stimulation by GLP-1 in the portal vein increased the response to intraportal glucose. This effect can be inhibited by ganglionic blockade, and insulin release may be mediated via a non-muscarinic, neural reflex of hepatic origin (36) [45]. GLP-1 secretion is also associated with the activity of other hormones involved in regulating energy homeostasis. Increased postpriandal leptin plasma concentrations and the presence of leptin receptor in L cells, have been shown to be a signal for GLP-1 release in the second phase after meal ingestion [53]. The basal activity of the L cells is under the tonic suppressory effect of somatostatin and the secretion of GLP-1 is inhibited by somatostatin, motilin [53], and galanin [53]. At the same time, GLP-1 augments the release of somatostatin, suggesting the existence of a feedback mechanism between these two hormones [54]. L cells secrete also PYY, mostly in the ileum and colon, and very high level of its secretion is observed in the rectum. $PYY_{3\text{-}36}$ next to $PYY_{1\text{-}37}$ is the main form produced postprandially, contributing to approximately 63% of circulating PYY in the fed state and 37% in the fasting state. PYY, PP, and NPY are members of the neuropeptide family, circulating satiety factors of tertiary structure [28]. These peptides contain 36 amino acids as well as several tyrosine residues, and require C-terminal amidation for biologic activity. $PYY_{3\text{-}36}$, the major circulating form (11) of PYY is a truncated 34-amino acid form created by cleavage of the N-terminal Tyr-Pro residues by dipeptidyl peptidase IV (DPPIV). The administration of PYY increases the absorption of fluids and electrolytes from the ileum after a meal and inhibits pancreatic and gastric secretions, gallbladder contraction, and gastric emptying [28]. Moreover, PYY reduces cardiac output, causes vasoconstriction, and reduction in glomerular filtration rate, plasma renin, and aldosterone activity, however, the physiologic significance of these actions has not been established. Low circulating PYY levels are proved to be an etiological factor in the development of obesity [28]. The majority of intestinal K cells is present in the duodenum and proximal jejunum with smaller numbers also occurring throughout the entire small intestine [29]. GIP (gastric inhibitory polypeptide, glucose-dependent insulinotropic polypeptide), is a 42 amino acid active form, synthesized and secreted by K cells in intestinal epithelium. GIP as well as GLP-1 is released in response to nutrient ingestion. It enhances glucose dependent insulin secretion and promotes nutrient deposition [55]. The effects of GIP are mediated through their binding with specific receptors. They belong to the 7 transmembrane-domain G-protein-coupled receptor family. GIP receptors are expressed in the pancreatic islets, gut, adipose tissue, heart, pituitary, adrenal cortex and in several regions of the brain [32]. GIP and its receptor have also been identified in the rodent CNS, including neurons, Schwann cells and Oligodendrocytes [55].

Dipeptidyl peptidase-4, rapidly convert $GIP_{(1-42)}$ into bioinactive $GIP_{(3-42)}$ a few minutes after secretion from the gut K cell [56]. The DPP-IV enzyme is widely expressed in the vascular endothelium of the capillaries of the villi. The majority of GIP arriving in the portal circulation is already inactivated, which explains their short half-life. When administered intravenously in normal subjects and in diabetic patients, the plasma half-life ($t_{1/2}$) of exogenous GIP is about 5-7 minutes [31].

GIP exhibits potent incretin activity in rodents and human subjects and the primary action of GIP is the stimulation of glucose-dependent insulin secretion. GIP may also play a role in adipocyte biology. There is evidence that GIP also regulates fat metabolism in adipocytes, including enhanced insulin-stimulated incorporation of fatty acids into triglycerides, stimulation of lipoprotein lipase activity, stimulation of fatty acids synthesis [57, 58]. Due to these central effects on the control of appetite and food intake, GIP has been shown to cause weight gain via its effects on adipose tissue [59]. GIP has been shown to exert proliferative and antiapoptotic actions on islet β cells. GIP improved survival of rat INS-1 cells after serum or glucose deprivation or following exposure to wortmannin or streptozotocin [60, 61] Moreover, a 2-week infusion of GIP also down regulated Bax and increased Bcl-2 expression in pancreatic b cells of ZDF rats [62]. Although the insulinotropic actions of GIP are diminished in hyperglycemic rodents due to, partially, reduced levels of GIP receptor expression [63], much less is known about the chronic effects of diabetes on preservation of GIP-dependent pathways linked to cell growth and survival. GIP, but not other nutrient-stimulated duodenal endocrine peptides, might regulate secretion of the intestinal PGDPs, including tGLP-1, in response to nutrient ingestion in vivo in the rat. The importance of GIP for glucose homeostasis has been studied using peptide antagonists of GIP action or antisera directed against the GIP receptor in rats and mice. These experiments have demonstrated a predominant role for GIP in the regulation of postprandial glucose clearance. The chronic desensitization of the GIP receptor by hyperglycemia and decreased receptor expression in the islet may cause the ineffectiveness of GIP [64]. The administration of a GIP receptor antagonist reduced postprandial insulin release in conscious rats by 72% [65]. High glucose levels in the diabetic range increase the degree of ubiquitination of GIP receptor. The metabolic results states in GIP receptors ubiquitination in a ligand independent manner [64, 65]. In physiological conditions, smaller loads of rapidly absorbable nutrients would preferentially activate GIP, whereas ingestion of larger meal containing more complex nutrients would activate the distal incretin GLP-1 [31]. In contrast to studies with GLP-1, endogenous GIP does not appear to be important for control of fasting glucose [65, 66]. Placement of either fat or glucose directly into the duodenal lumen significantly increased plasma levels of GIP [67].

Although postprandial intestin endocrine cell stimulation is related to the secretion of other peptides, which also play an important role in regulating energy homeostasis of the body, shown above, GLP-1 and GIP seem to play the most important role in regulating the carbohydrates homeostasis. Results of studies in humans as well as studies in rodents (mice with double knock-out of the GIP and GLP-1 receptors, diabetic rats ZDF) consistently showed their role in glucose homeostasis maintenance and the additive effect of these two hormones in the incretin effect [19, 34].

Incretins and Its Role in T2DM Pathophysiology

The incretin effect is reduced or lost in obese type 2 diabetic mellitus patients (BMI 37 kg/m2). It has prompted speculations that abnormalities in the entero-insular axis may precede, and perhaps even predispose the development of diabetes. Moreover, evidence that the strengthening of incretin effect improves glucose tolerance in people with type 2 diabetes mellitus [68].

Several studies have reported significant reductions in GLP-1 levels after mixed meal ingestion in patients with type 2 diabetes [37, 69, 70]. Nevertheless, there are conflicting reports regarding meal-induced GLP-1 responses in D2M patients in comparison with the healthy control [37, 71]. The decreased response of GLP-1 in TD2M patients is related to BMI and the actual diabetic state [37]. The impaired secretion of GLP-1 seems to be a consequence of diabetes and develops as glucose intolerance progresses [72]. Different responses in GLP-1 secretion between type 2 diabetic patients and healthy participants may be predicted by such characteristics as age, body weight, fasting NEFA concentrations, fasting glucagon concentrations and insulin resistance. Different GLP-1 responses in patients with type 2 diabetes depend on the individual balance of the mentioned factors and the rate of gastric emptying [19]. A therapeutic strategy based on incretin hormones may restore beta cell responsiveness to glucose in T2DM. Also intensified treatment resulting in near normal glucose levels may lead to a partial restoration of incretin action of GLP-1 and GIP [73]. Continuous subcutaneous administration of native GLP-1 to type 2 patients lowers fasting and postprandial glucose levels, HbA1C and also results in weight loss [74].

GIP

In patients with type 2 diabetes the impairment of GIP secretion is more evident in the second and third hour after meal intake compared to the healthy glucose tolerant controls [37, 36]. Physiological as well as supraphysiological concentrations of human GIP, do not stimulate insulin secretion in type-2 diabetic patients as it was observed in normal subjects [74]. An intravenous infusion of GIP in patients with type 2 diabetes, under hyperglycemic conditions, elicited 46% of the insulin responses found in the healthy control subjects [75]. The loss of GIP activity is more evident during its continuous infusion than after an intravenous bolus administration of the peptide. The lack of glucose-lowering activity of GIP in type 2 diabetes may also be related to its stimulation of glucagon release [75]. The absence of GIP effect on glucagon secretion is due to the increased glucose concentrations. Glucagon secretion is stimulated by GIP only under the basal glucose concentrations, whereas insulin secretion is enhanced under the hyperglycemic conditions showing a role for GIP in the feedback control of glucose homeostasis [76]. Nevertheless, the reduced incretin effect in type-2 diabetic patients is most likely to be explained by the reduced insulinotropic effectiveness of GIP [74]. Meier et al. 2010 [75], suggested that the inability of GIP to augment insulin secretion during hyperglycemia is primarily due to the lack of glucose-potentiation of insulin release in patients with diabetes. Moreover, potentially unequal insulinotropic efficacy of GIP and GLP-1 in patients with type 2 diabetes is due to an additional mechanism of action rather than due to a specific defect in GIP signaling. On the basis of such reasoning, the reduction of the incretin effect in patients with diabetes may simply be an epi-phenomenon of chronic hyperglycemia, independent of any primary defect in GIP or GLP-1 action. Reducing hyperglycemia and enhancing β-cell function in general terms may therefore also improve the incretin effect, independently of specific interventions related to circulating levels of GIP or GLP-1 [75].

Peptide YY

The circulating levels of PYY_{3-36} increase within 15 minutes after a meal intake, with a highest level 60 min-120 min postpriandally, and then slowly declines to baseline for up to 6h [77, 78]. PYY reduces food intake and body weight. Circulating PYY_{3-36} concentrations are decreased in obese people in comparison to their non-obese counterparts [79, 80]. The PP-fold acts via the Y family of G protein-coupled receptors. Moreover, it is proved that low circulating levels of PYY play a role in the etiology of type 2 diabetes and associated obesity. It is also known, that females produce a larger PYY response to a meal than male participants [62]. Nevertheless, other studies show no significant differences in PYY plasma concentrations between lean and obese subjects [62, 81]. Intravenous infusion of PYY_{3-36} in diet-induced insulin-resistant mice improve insulin sensitivity, as assessed by hyperinsulinemic-euglycemic clamp [82].

Moreover, a 4-week subcutaneous infusion of PYY_{3-36} by osmotic pump in diabetic fatty Zucker rats also improved glycemic indices [83]. The pattern of PYY secretion may be a physiologic satiety signal, acting to terminate the meal and stimulating coordinated gastrointestinal responses to aid digestion and absorption. The release of PYY occurs before nutrients have reached the distal gastrointestinal tract and the predominant sites of PYY secretion, this implies that release of PYY occurs via a neural reflex, possibly through the vagus nerve.

The impaired postprandial PYY release may impair satiety and help maintain obesity, if not it acts as a primary driver of initial development of obesity. PYY_{3-36} modulates the activities of orexigenic neuropeptide Y (NPY) neurons and anorexigenic proopiomelanocortin (POMC) neurons in the hypothalamus to inhibit food intake. Reduced PYY signaling is a primary cause of obesity, it is certainly true that retained PYY sensitivity in the obese makes it an attractive therapeutic target [28]. Besides its known effects as a short-term regulator of energy homeostasis, PYY levels also reflect long-term changes in body composition. Batterham and colleagues proved the effects of PYY_{3-36} on satiety, food intake and body weight in animals and humans [84, 85]. They showed that PYY_{3-36} acts on the arcuate nucleus in the hypothalamus to reduce food intake and body weight inhibiting NPY neurons and stimulating POMC expressing neurons via Y2 receptors [84].

Moreover, peripherally administered PYY_{3-36} activates neurons in the area postrema and nucleus tractus solitaries, via regions of the brainstem, to reduce food intake by inducing an aversive response [86]. Boey et al. 2006 [87] showed that, fasting serum PYY_{3-36} levels in female patients with genetic predispositions to type 2 diabetes were lower when compared to the healthy counterparts. Association between PYY_{3-36} and insulin secretion with low circulating levels of PYY predisposing to high insulin secretion. Moreover, fasting serum PYY_{3-36} levels in type 2 diabetes melitius, were positively correlated with insulin sensitivity and adiponectin, which may predict adiposity and insulin sensitivity.

In Searching of the Missing Protein(s)

Described in the previous section incretins play a significant role in the pathophysiology of type 2 diabetes. Modern surgery opened the possibility of surgical treatment of diabetes, and also opened new opportunities for research on the role of incretin hormones in the pathophysiology of diabetes. Changes in gastrointestinal hormones have been analyzed for those bariatric procedures that alter food transit and also for those in which rearrangement of intestine is not related to the exclusion of part of the intestine with the passage of food, but with an earlier delivery of food to the hindgut through the transposition of ileum to proximal part of jejunum (Ileal transposition) [88].

In the latter case, the increase level of GLP-1 in plasma is could be explained by early stimulation of L cells. It is possible that after malabsorptive/restrictive operations like Roux-en- Y gastric bypass (RYGB), BPD (bilipancreatic diversion) or DJB (duodeno-jejunal bypass) expedited delivery of nutrient chyme to the distal intestine occurred, enhancing stimulation of L cells and GLP-1 releasing which results in glucose tolerance amelioration [89, 90, 91, 92]. However, the effect of improving glucose tolerance can be achieved only by bypassing a short segment of the proximal intestine. Rubino et al. in an experiment carried out on Goto-Kazaki diabetic rats indicated that the exclusion of a short segment of proximal intestine from the food passage resulted in improved glucose tolerance [16]. To confirm the effect obtained by using duodenal-jejunal bypass or gastrojejunostomy, after four weeks they conducted the second operation restoring duodenal transit which resulted in reestablished glucose intolerance. Despite the fact that the level of incretin in the experiment was not examined, this study suggests that the proximal small bowel contributes to the alterations of glucose metabolism in type 2 diabetes. These findings have led researchers to formulate the `foregut hypothesis' which holds that in normal condition stimulation of proximal intestine triggers the mechanism which involves at least two factors secreted by intestinal endocrine cells. One of them is the glucose dependent insulinotropic polypeptide (GIP) which increases insulin secretion, and the second one is an unknown factor which controls insulin action to prevent hypoglycemia [16]. Thus, the authors postulated the existence of another factor which is involved in the regulation of glucose homeostasis by acting antagonistically to the incretin hormones.

The imbalance between the mentioned factors (incretin and `anti-incretin'), caused by chronic stimulation with particular nutrients may play a significant role in causing insulin resistance and type 2 diabetes [16]. Unfortunately, the experiment described above does not show incretin levels data, making it more difficult to substantiate the interpretations, however, it entitles to seek new factors involved in glucose homeostasis maintenance. Extremely interesting is the fact that healthy Wistar rats that underwent duodenal-jejunal bypass (DJB) had impaired glucose tolerance [17, 93]. Although the mechanism responsible for the aggravation of glucose homeostasis in normal non-diabetic Wistar rats is still unknown, these findings indicate that the relevant factor could be hidden in the rearrangement part of the intestine [17, 93].

Diabetes Treatment and Incretins

The main goal of T2DM treatment is to reduce the risk of diabetic complications and premature death. Before 2007 combinations of the five medicines: biguanides, sulfonylureas, meglitinides, thiazolidinediones and alpha-glucosidase inhibitors were commonly used in the T2DM treatment. Apart from the oral therapy, the modification of the sedentary lifestyle and over nutrition was and is very important [94]. Hyperglycemia plays a key role in the pathogenesis of T2DM, inducting insulin resistance and β-cell failure [95]. Incretin mimetic and DPP-4 inhibitors are the new hypoglycemic agents in the management of T2DM [96]. These groups of medicines reduced successfully fasting and postprandial glucose concentrations and gyrated hemoglobin [96, 97]. Infusion of GLP-1 improves the glycemic control and influences the β-cell function as well as weight and cardiovascular risk factors [97]. GLP-1 prevents β-cell glucolipotoxicity [35], regulates cell proliferation in the pancreas [98], inhibits the cell apoptosis and improves glucose responsiveness of isolated human islets [99]. Exogenous infusion of GLP-1 improves left ventricular function in patients with chronic heart failure [100], myocardial infarction [101], and reduce the blood pressure [102]. The mechanism of the glycemic effects of DPP-4 inhibitors is still not clear. Inhibition of DPP-4 does not increase the "total' volume of circulating GLP-1 [103].

On the other hand, there are studies describing modest increase in GLP-1 in circulation (probably it depends on how specific assays were used) [104, 105]. It is possible that other mechanisms independent of GLP-1 decide about the efficiency of DPP-4 inhibitors in treatment of T2DM, for example pituitary adenylate cyclase-activating polypeptide [105, 106]. Currently, degradation-resistant GLP-1 receptor agonists and inhibitors of the enzyme DPP-4 are widely used in the treatment of T2DM. Exenatide and liraglutide are injectable drugs [97]. Exenatide has a 53% homology to human GLP-1. We have to use it twice daily, 5 μg per dose or the 10 μg. Nevertheless, nausea, vomiting, diarrhea and abdominal pain are the main side effects [107]. Liraglutide has 97% homology to native GLP-1 for one daily subcutaneous administration. Common side effects are nausea and gastrointestinal symptoms [108]. Action of GLP-1 agonists are characterized by the low risk of hypoglycemia [107, 108]. Sitagliptin, saxagliptin and vildagliptin, are oral agents that belong to DPP-4 inhibitors.

Application of DPP-4 inhibitors improves glycemic control by increasing GLP-1 longevity. The selective DPP-4 inhibitors e. g. sitagliptin, alogliptin, saxagliptin, and vildagliptin, applied in the treatment of Type 2 diabetes, increase the level of active incretin hormones, decrease level of circulating glucagon thus preserve or enhanc β-cell function [40]. GLP-1 has been the basis of two novel classes of glucose lowering agents, incretin mimetics like GLP-1 receptor agonists and inhibitors of protease dipeptidyl peptidase (DPP)-4 [40].

The analysis of the treatment with metformin type 2 diabetic patients has shown to enhance GLP-1 responses [19].

References

[1] Williams GC, Nesse RM (1991) The dawn of Darwinian medicine. *Q. Rev. Biol.,* 66:1–22.

[2] Wild S, Roglic G, Green A, Sicree R, King H (2004) Global prevalence of diabetes: estimates for the year 2000 and projections for 2030. *Diabetes Care,* 27:1047–1053.

[3] Zimmet P, Alberti KG, Shaw J (2001) Global and societal implications of the diabetes epidemic. *Nature,* 414:782–787.

[4] Mayer J (1955) Regulation of energy intake and the body weight. *Ann. NY Acad. Sci.,* 63:1543.

[5] Ferrannini E (1998) Insulin resistance versus insulin deficiency in non-insulin-dependent diabetes mellitus: problems and prospects. *Endocr. Rev.,* 19:477–490.

[6] Marchetti P, Dotta F, Lauro D, Purrello F (2008) An overview of pancreatic beta-cell defects in human type 2 diabetes: Implications for treatment. *Regul. Peptides,* 146:4–11.

[7] Drucker DJ (2003) Glucagon-Like Peptides: Regulators of Cell Proliferation, Differentiation, and Apoptosis. *Mol. Endocrinol.,* 17:161–171.

[8] Bayliss WM, Starling EH (1902) The mechanism of pancreatic secretion. *J. Physiol.,* 28:325– 353.

[9] Starling EH (1905) The Cronian Lectures on the chemical correlation of the functions of the body. *Lancet,* 2:339–583.

[10] Creutzfeld W (2005) The [pre-] history of the incretin concept. *Regul. Peptides,* 128:87–91.

[11] Moore B, Edie ES, Abram JH (1906) On the treatment of diabetes mellitus by acid extract of duodenal mucous membrane. *Biochem. J.,* 28–38.

[12] La Barre J, Still EU (1939) Studies of the physiology of secretin. *Am. J. Physiol.,* 91:649–653.

[13] La Barre J (1932) Sur les possibilités d'un traitment du diabéte par l' incrétine. *Bull. Acad. Med. Belg.,* 12:620–634.

[14] Mojsov S, Weir GC, Habener JF (1987) Insulinotropin: glucagon-like peptide-1 (7–36) co-encoded in the glucagon gene is a potent stimulator of insulin release in the perfused rat pancreas. *J. Clin. Invest.,* 79:616–619.

[15] Kreymann B, Williams G, Ghatei MA, Bloom SR (1987) Glucagon-likepeptide-1 7–36: a physiological incretin in man. *Lancet,* 2:1300–1304.

[16] Rubino F, Forgione A, Cummings DE, Vix M, Gnuli D, Mingrone G, Castagneto M, Marescaux J (2006) The mechanism of diabetes control after gastrointestinal bypass surgery reveals a role of the proximal small intestine in the pathophysiology of type 2 diabetes. *Ann. Surg.,* 244(5):741–9.

[17] Rubino F (2008) Is Type 2 Diabetes an Operable Intestinal Disease? A provocative yet reasonable hypothesis. *Diabets Care,* 31:290–296.

[18] Sánchez-Pernaute A, Herrera MA, Pérez-Aguirre ME, Talavera P, Cabrerizo L, Matía P, et al. (2010) Single anastomosis duodeno-ileal bypass with sleeve gastrectomy (SADI-S). One to three-year follow-up. *Obes. Surg.,* 20(12):1720–1726.

[19] Nauck M, Vardarli I, Deacon C, Holst JJ, Meier JJ (2011) Secretion of glucagon-like peptide-1 (GLP-1) in type 2 diabetes: what is up, what is down? *Diabetologia,* 54:10–18.

[20] Murphy KG, Bloom SR (2006) Gut hormones and the regulation of energy homeostasis. *Nature,* 444/7121:854–859.

[21] Kahn SE, Hull RL, Utzschneider KM (2006) Mechanisms linking obesity to insulin resistance and type 2 diabetes. *Nature,* 444/7121:840–846.

[22] Cahová M, Vavrínková H, Kazdová L (2007) Glucose-fatty acid interaction in skeletal muscle and adipose tissue in insulin resistance. *Physiol. Res.,* 56(1):1–15.

[23] Thomson AB, Wild G (1997) Adaptation of intestinal nutrient transport in health and disease. Part I. *Dig. Dis. Sci.,* 42(3):453–69.

[24] Thomson AB, Wild G (1997) Adaptation of intestinal nutrient transport in health and disease. Part II. *Dig. Dis. Sci.,* 42(3):470–88.

[25] Ait-Omar A, Monteiro-Sepulveda M, Poitou C, Le Gall M, Cotillard A, Gilet J, et al. (2011) GLUT2 accumulation in enterocyte apical and intracellular membranes: a study in morbidly obese human subjects and ob/ob and high fat-fed mice. *Diabetes,* 60(10):2598–2607.

[26] Kellett GL, Brot-Laroche E, Mace OJ, Leturque A (2008) Sugar absorption in the intestine: the role of GLUT2. *Annu. Rev. Nutr.,* 28:35–54.

[27] Creutzfeld W (1979) The incretin concept today. *Diabetologia,* 16:75–85.

[28] Wren A, Bloom S (2007) Gut hormones and appetite control. *Gastroenterology,* 132:2116–2130.

[29] Baggio L, Drucker JD (2007) Biology of Incretins: GLP-1 and GIP. *Gastroenterology,* 132:2131–2157.

[30] Reimann F, Ward P, Gribble F, (2006) Signaling Mechanisms Underlying the Release of Glucagon-Like Peptide 1. *Diabetes,* 55(2):78–85.

[31] Gautier JF, Fetita S, Sobngwi E., Salaün-Martin C (2005) Biological actions of the incretins GIP and GLP-1 and therapeutic erspectives in patients with type 2 diabetes. *Diabetes Metab.,* 31:233–242.

[32] Cordier-Bussat M, Bernard C, Levenez F, Klages N, Laser-Ritz B, Philippe J et al. (1998) Peptones stimulate both the secretion of the incretin hormone glucagon-like peptide 1 and the transcription of the proglucagon gene. *Diabetes,* 47:1038–45.

[33] Fehmann HC, Goke R, Goke B (1995) Cell and molecular biology of the incretin hormones glucagon-like peptide-1 and glucosedependent insulin releasing polypeptide. *Endocr. Rev.,* 16:390–410.

[34] Wang Y, Perfetti R, Greig NH, Holloway HW, DeOre KA, Montrose-Rafizadeh Ch et al. (1997) Glucagon-like peptide-1 can reverse the age-related decline in glucose tolerance in rats. *J. Clin. Invest.,*99:2883–2889.

[35] Buteau J, El-Assaad W, Rhodes CJ, Rosenberg L, Joly E, Prentki M (2004) Glucagon-like peptide-1 prevents beta cell glucolipotoxicity. *Diabetologia,* 47:806–815.

[36] Knop FK (2009) Resolution of type 2 diabetes following gastric bypass surgery: involvement of gut-derived glucagon and glucagonotropic signalling? *Diabetologia,* 52:2270–2276.

[37] Toft-Nielsen MB, Damholt MB, Madsbad S, Hilsted LM, Hughes TE, Michelsen BK, Holst JJ (2001) Determinants of the impaired secretion of glucagon-like peptide-1 in type 2 diabetic patients. *J. Clin. Endocrinol. Metab.,* 86:3717–3723.

[38] Kreymann B, Williams G, Ghatei MA, Bloom SR (1987) Glucagon-like peptide-1 [7-36]: a physiological incretin in man. *Lancet,* 2:1300–1304.

[39] Ørskov C, Rabenhøj L, Wettergren A, Kofod H, Holst JJ (1994) Tissue and plasma concentrations of amidated and glycineextended glucagon-like peptide 1 in humans. *Diabetes,* 43:535– 539.

[40] Kirby M, Yu DMT, O'Connor SP, Gorrell MD (2010) Inhibitor selectivity in the clinical application of dipeptidyl peptidase-4 inhibition. *Clinical Science,* 118:31–41.

[41] Ajami K, Abbott CA, McCaughan GW, Gorrell MD (2004) Dipeptidyl peptidase 9 has two forms, a broad tissue distribution, cytoplasmic localization and DPIV-like peptidase activity. *Biochim. Biophys. Acta.,* 1679:18–28.

[42] Maes MB, Dubois V, Brandt I, Lambeir AM, Van der Veken P, Augustyns K et al. (2007) Dipeptidyl peptidase 8/9-like activity in human leukocytes. *J. Leukocyte. Biol.,* 81:1252–1257.

[43] Schade J, Stephan M, Schmiedl A, Wagner L, Niestroj AJ et al. (2008) Regulation of expression and function of dipeptidyl peptidase 4 (DP4), DP8/9, and DP10 in allergic responses of the lung in rats. *J. Histochem. Cytochem.,* 56:147–155.

[44] Bjelke JR, Christensen J, Nielsen PF, Branner S, Kanstrup AB, Wagtmann N et al. (2006) Dipeptidyl peptidases 8 and 9: specificity and molecular characterization compared with dipeptidyl peptidase IV. *Biochem. J.,* 396:391–399.

[45] Hansen L, Deacon CF, Ørskov C, Holst JJ (1999) Glucagon-like peptide-1-(7–36) amide is transformed to glucagon-like peptide-1-(9–36)amide by dipeptidyl peptidase IV in the capillaries supplying the L-cells of the porcine intestine. *Endocrinology,* 140(11):5356– 5363.

[46] Balks HJ, Holst JJ, von zur Mühlen A, Brabant G (1997) Rapid oscillations in plasma glucagon-like peptide-1 (glp-1) in humans: cholinergic control of glp-1 secretion via muscarinic receptors. *J. Clin. Endocrinol. Metab.,* 82(3):786– 790.

[47] Anini Y, Hansotia T, Brubaker PL (2002) Muscarinic receptors control postprandial release of glucagon-like peptide-1: in vivo and in vitro studies in rats. *Endocrinology,* 143:2420–26

[48] Anini Y, Brubaker PL (2003) Muscarinic receptors control glucagon-like peptide-1 secretion by human endocrine L cells. *Endocrinology,* 144:3244–50.

[49] Claustre J, Brechet S, Plaisancie P et al. (1999) Stimulatory effect of beta-adrenergic agonists on ileal L cell secretion and modulation by alpha-adrenergic activation. *J. Endocrinol.,* 162:271–78.

[50] Nishizawa M, Nakabayashi H, Uchida K, Nakagawa A, Niijima A (1996) The hepatic vagal nerve is receptive to incretin glucagon-like peptide-1, but not to glucose-dependent insulinotropic polypeptide, in the portal vein. *J. Auton. Nerv. Syst.,* 61:149–154.

[51] Zhang J, Ritter RC (2012) Circulating GLP-1 and CCK-8 reduce food intake by capsaicin-insensitive, nonvagal mechanisms. *Am. J. Physiol. Regul. Integr. Comp. Physiol.,* 302:R264–R273.

[52] Hansen L, Holst JJ (2002) The effects of duodenal peptides on glucagon-like peptide-1 secretion from the ileum: A duodeno–ileal loop? *Regul. Peptides,* 110:39– 45.

[53] Herrmann-Rinke C, Horsch D, McGregor GP, Göke B (1996) Galanin is a potent inhibitor of glucagon-like peptide-1 secretion from rat ileum. *Peptides,* 17:571–76.

[54] Hansen L, Hartmann B, Minco H, Holst JJ (2004) Glucagon-like peptide-1 secretion is influenced by perfusate glucose concentration and by a feedback mechanism involving somatostatin in isolated perfused porcine ileum. *Regul. Pept.,* 118:11–18.

[55] Buhren BA, Gasis M, Thorens B, Müller HW, Bosse F (2009) Glucose-dependent insulinotropic polypeptide (GIP) and its receptor (GIPR): cellular localization, lesion-affected expression, and impaired regenerative axonal growth. *J. Neurosci. Res.,* 87(8):1858–70.

[56] Kieffer TJ, Huang Z, McIntosh CH, Buchan AM, Brown JC, Pederson RA (1995) Gastric inhibitory polypeptide release from a tumor-derived cell line. *Am. J. Physiol.,* 269:E316–E322.

[57] Yip RGC, Wolfe MM (2000) GIP biology and fat metabolism. *Life Sci.,* 66:91–103.

[58] Parthier C, Kleinschmidt M, Neumann P, Rudolph R, Manhart S, Schlenzig D et al. (2007) Crystal structure of the incretin-bound extracellular domain of a G protein-coupled receptor. *Proc. Natl. Acad. Sci. USA,* 104(35):13942–7.

[59] Meier JJ, Gallwitz B, Siepmann N, Holst JJ, Deacon CF, Schmidt WE, Nauck MA (2003) Gastric inhibitory polypeptide (GIP) dose-dependently stimulates glucagon secretion in healthy human subjects at euglycaemia. *Diabetologia,* 46:798–801.

[60] Ehses JA, Casilla VR, Doty T, Pospisilik JA, Winter KD, Demuth HU, Pederson RA, McIntosh CH (2003) Glucose-dependent insulinotropic polypeptide promotes beta-(INS-1) cell survival via cyclic adenosine monophosphate-mediated caspase-3 inhibition and regulation of p38 mitogen-activated protein kinase. *Endocrinology,* 144:4433–4445.

[61] Trumper A, Trumper K, Trusheim H, Arnold R, Goke B, Horsch D (2001) Glucose-dependent insulinotropic polypeptide is also a growth factor for beta (INS-1) cells by pleiotropic signalling. *Mol. Endocrinol.,* 15:1559–70.

[62] Kim SJ, Winter K, Nian C, Tsuneoka M, Koda Y, McIntosh CH (2005) Glucose-dependent insulinotropic polypeptide (GIP) stimulation of pancreatic beta-cell survival is dependent upon phosphatidylinositol 3-kinase (PI3-K)/protein kinase B (PKB) signaling, inactivation of the forkhead transcription factor Foxo1 and downregulation of bax expression. *J. Biol. Chem.,* 280:22297–22307.

[63] Lynn FC, Pamir N, Ng EH, McIntosh CH, Kieffer TJ, Pederson RA (2001) Defective glucose-dependent insulinotropic polypeptide receptor expression in diabetic fatty Zucker rats. *Diabetes,* 50:1004–1011.

[64] Kazakos K (2001) Incretin effect: GLP-1, GIP, DPP4. Diabetes *Res. Clin. Pract.,* 93:32–36.

[65] Tseng CC, Kieffer TJ, Jarboe LA, Usdin TB, Wolfe MM (1996) Postprandial stimulation of insulin release by glucose-dependent insulinotropic polypeptide (GIP). Effect of a specific glucose-dependent insulinotropic polypeptide receptor antagonist in the rat. *J. Clin. Invest.,* 98:2440–2445.

[66] Lewis JT, Dayanandan B, Habener JF, Kieffer TJ (2000) Glucose-dependent insulinotrophic peptide confers early phase insulin release to oral glucose in rats: demonstration by a receptor antagonist. *Endocrinology*, 141:3710–3716.

[67] Roberge JN, Brubaker PL (1993) Regulation of intestinal proglucagon-derived peptide secretion by glucose-dependent insulinotropic peptide in a novel enteroendocrine loop. *Endocrinology,* 133:233–40.

[68] Nauck M, Stöckmann F, Ebert R, Creutzfeldt W (1986) Reduced incretin effect in Type 2 (non-insulin-dependent) diabetes. *Diabetologia,* 29:46-52.

[69] Muscelli E, Mari A, Casolaro A, Camastra S, Seghieri G, Gastaldelli A, Holst JJ, Ferrannini E (2008) Separate impact of obesity and glucose tolerance on the incretin effect in normal subjects and type 2 diabetic patients. *Diabetes,* 57:1340–1348.

[70] Vilsbøll T, Krarup T, Deacon CF, Madsbad S, Holst JJ (2001) Reduced postprandial concentrations of intact biologically active glucagon-like peptide 1 in type 2 diabetic patients. *Diabetes,* 50:609–613.

[71] Vollmer K, Holst JJ, Baller B, Ellrichmann M, Nauck MA, Schmidt WE, Meier JJ (2008) Predictors of Incretin Concentrations in Subjects With Normal, Impaired, and Diabetic Glucose Tolerance. *Diabetes,* 57:678–687.

[72] Holst JJ, Vilsbřll T, Deacon CF (2009) The incretin system and its role in type 2 diabetes mellitus. *Mol. Cell Endocrinol.,* 297:127–136.

[73] Hojberg PV, Zander M, Vilsboll T, Knop FK, Krarup T, Volund A (2008). Near normalisation of blood glucose improves the potentiating effect of GLP-1 on glucose-induced insulin secretion in patients with T2DM. *Diabetologia,* 51:632–640.

[74] Nauck MA, Heimesaat MM, Ørskov C, Holst JJ, Ebert R, Creutzfeldt W (1993) Preserved incretin activity of glucagonlike peptide 1 [7-36 amide] but not of synthetic human gastric inhibitory polypeptide in patients with type-2 diabetes mellitus. *J. Clin. Invest.,* 91:301–307.

[75] Meier JJ, Nauck MA (2010) Is the diminished incretin effect in type 2 diabetes just an epi-phenomenon of impaired β-Cell function? *Diabetes,* 59:1117– 1125.

[76] Meier JJ, Hücking K, Holst JJ, Deacon CF, Schmiegel WH, Nauck MA (2001) Reduced insulinotropic effect of gastric inhibitory polypeptide in first-degree relatives of patients with type 2 diabetes. *Diabetes,* 50:2497–2504.

[77] Adrian TE, Ferri GL, Bacarese-Hamilton AJ, Fuessl HS, Polak JM, Bloom SR (1985) Human distribution and release of a putative new gut hormone, peptide YY. *Gastroenterology,* 89:1070–1077.

[78] Le Roux CW, Batterham RL, Aylwin SJ, Patterson M, Borg CM, Wynne KJ et al. (2006) Attenuated peptide YY release in obese subjects is associated with reduced satiety. *Endocrinology,* 147:3–8.

[79] Roth CL, Enriori PJ, Harz K, Woelfle J, Cowley MA, Reinehr T (2005) Peptide YY is a regulator of energy homeostasis in obese children before and after weight loss. *J. Clin. Endocrinol. Metab.,* 90:6386–6391.

[80] Alvarez BM, Borque M, Martinez-Sarmiento J, Aparicio E, Hernandez C, Cabrerizo L, Fernandez-Represa JA (2002) Peptide YY secretion in morbidly obese patients before and after vertical banded gastroplasty. *Obes. Surg.,* 12:324–327.

[81] Stock S, Leichner P, Wong ACK, Ghatei MA, KieVer TJ, Bloom SR, Chanoine,J, (2005) Ghrelin, Peptide YY, Glucose-dependent insulinotropic polypeptide, and hunger

responses to a mixed meal in anorexic, obese, and control female adolescents. *J. Clin. Endocrinol. Metab.,* 90:2161–2168.

[82] Van den Hoek AM, Heijboer AC, Corssmit EPM, Voshol PJ, Romijn JA, Havekes LM, Pijl H (2004) PYY3-36 reinforces insulin action on glucose disposal in mice fed a high-fat diet. *Diabetes,* 53:1949–1952.

[83] Pittner R, Moore C, Bhavsar S, Gedulin B, Smith P, Jodka C, Parkes D, Peterniti J, Srivastava V, Young A (2004) Effects of PYY [3-36] in rodent models of diabetes and obesity. *Int. J. Obesity,* 28:963–971.

[84] Batterham RL, Cowley MA, Small CJ, Herzog H, Cohen MA, Dakin CL et al. (2002) Gut hormone PYY(3-36) physiologically inhibits food intake. *Nature,* 418:650–654.

[85] Batterham RL, Cohen MA, Ellis SM, Le Roux CW, Withers DJ et al. (2003) Inhibition of food intake in obese subjects by peptide YY3-36. *N. Engl. J. Med.,* 349:941–948.

[86] Halatchev IG, Cone RD (2005) Peripheral administration of PYY(3–36) produces conditioned taste aversion in mice. *Cell Metab.,* 1:159–168.

[87] Boey D, Heilbronn L, Sainsbury A, Laybutt R, Kriketos A, Herzog H, Campbell LV (2006) Low serum PYY is linked to insulin resistance in first-degree relatives of subjects with type 2 diabetes. *Neuropeptides,* 40:317–324.

[88] Wang TT, Hu SY, Gao HD, Zhang GY, Liu CZ, Feng JB, Frezza EE (2008) Ileal Transposition Controls Diabetes as Well as Modified Duodenal Jejunal Bypass With Better Lipid Lowering in a Nonobese Rat Model of Type II Diabetes by Increasing GLP-1. *Ann. Surg.,* 247(6):968–75.

[89] Cummings DE, Overduin J, Foster-Schubert KE (2004) Gastric bypass for obesity: mechanisms of weight loss and diabetes resolution. *J. Clin. Endocrinol. Metab.,* 89:2608–2615.

[90] Mason EE (2005) The mechanism of surgical treatment of type 2 diabetes. *Obes Surg.,* 15:459–461.

[91] Patriti A, Facchiano E, Sanna A, Gulla L, Donini A (2004) The enteroinsular axis and the recovery from type 2 diabetes after bariatric surgery. *Obes Surg.,* 14:840–848.

[92] Mason EE (1999) Ileal transposition and enteroglucagon/GLP1 in obesity (and diabetic?) surgery. Obes Surg 9:223–228.

[93] Reimann F (2010) Molecular mechanism underlying nutrient detection by incretin-secreting cells. *Int. Dairy J.,* 20(4):236–242.

[94] Nathen DM, Buse JB, Davidson MB, Heine RJ, Holman RR, Sherwin R, Zinman B (2006) Management of hiperglycaemia in type 2 diabetes: a consensus algorithm for the indication and adjustment of therapy, a consensus statement from the American Diabetes Association and the European Association for the Study of Diabetes. *Diabetologia,* 49:1711-1721.

[95] DeFronzo RA (2009) Banting lecture. From the triumvirate to the ominous octet: a new paradigm for the treatment of type 2 diabetes mellitus. *Diabetes,* 58:773–795.

[96] Nauck M, Smith U (2009) Incretin-based therapy: how do incretin mimetics and DPP-4 inhibitors fit into treatment algorithms for type 2 diabetic patients? *Best Pract. Res. Cl. En.,* 23:513-523.

[97] Drucker DJ, Nauck MA (2006) The incretin system: glucagon-like peptide-1 receptor agonists and dipeptidyl peptidase-4 inhibitors in type 2 diabetes. *Lancet,* 368:1696–1705.

[98] Brubaker PL, Drucker DJ (2004) Minireview: glucagon-like peptides regulate cell proliferation and apoptosis in the pancreas, gut, and central nervous system. *Endocrinology,* 145:2653–2659.

[99] Farilla L, Bulotta A, Hirshberg B (2003) Glucagon like peptide 1 inhibits cell apoptosis and improves glucose responsiveness of freshly isolated human islets. *Endocrinology,* 144:5149–5158.

[100] Nikolaidis LA, Mankad S, Sokos GG, Miske G, Shah A, Elahi D et al. (2004) Effects of glucagon-like peptide 1 in patients with acute myocardial infarction and left ventricular disfunction after successful reperfusion. *Circulation,* 109: 962–965.

[101] Sokos GG, Nikolaidis LA, Mankad S, Elahi D, Shannor RP (2006) Glucagon-like peptide 1 infusion improves left ventricular ejection fraction and functional status in patients with chronic heart failure. *J. Card. Fail.,* 12: 694–699.

[102] Gutzwiller JP, Tschopp S, Bock A, Zehnder C, Huber AR, Kreyenbuehl M et al. (2004) Glucagon-like peptide 1 induces natriuresis in healthy subjects and in insulin-resistant obese men. *J. Clin. Endocrinol. Metab.,* 89:3055–3061.

[103] El-Ouaghlidi A, Rehring E, Holst JJ, Schweizer A, Foley J, Holmes D et al. (2007) The dipeptidyl peptidase 4 inhibitor vildagliptin does not reduce glucose-induced glucagon-like peptide 1 and gastric inhibitory polypeptide secretion. *J. Clin. Endocrinol. Metab.,* 92:4165–4171.

[104] Green BD, Flatt PR, Bailey CJ (2006) Dipeptidyl peptidase IV (DPP IV) inhibitors: a newly emerging drug class for the treatment of type 2 diabetes. *Diab. Vasc. Dis. Res.,* 3:159–165.

[105] Nauck MA, El-Ouaghlidi A (2005) The therapeutic actions of DPP-IV inhibition are not mediated by glucagon-like peptide 1. *Diabetologia,* 48: 608–611.

[106] Ahren B, Hughes TE (2005) Inhibition of dipeptidyl peptidase-4 augments insulin secretion in response to exogenously administered glucagon-like peptide 1, glucose-dependent insulinotropic polypeptide, pituitary adenylate cyclase-activating polypeptide, and gastrin-releasing peptide in mice. *Endocrinology,* 146:2055–2059.

[107] Drucker DJ, Buse JB, Taylor K Kendall DM, Trautmann M, Zhuang D, Porter L, DURATION-1 Study Group (2008) Exenatide once weekly versus twice daily for the treatment of type 2 diabetes: a randomized, open-label, non-inferiority study. *Lancet,* 372:1240–1250.

[108] Nauck MA, Hompesch M, Filipczak R, Le TDT, Zdravkovic M, Gumprecht J (2006) Five weeks of treatment with the GLP-1 analogue liraglutide improves glycaemic control and lowers body weight in subjects with type 2 diabetes. *Exp. Clin. Endocrinol. Diabetes,* 114:417–423.

In: Bariatric Surgery
Editor: Christos R. Iavazzo
ISBN: 978-1-62618-995-9

Chapter II

Adipokines and Ghrelin Influenced Glucose Metabolism

***Tomasz Sawczyn*[1], *Dominika Stygar*[1], *Iwona Karcz-Socha*[1], *Krystyna Zwirska-Korczala*[1] *and W. Konrad Karcz*[2]**
[1]Department of Physiology in Zabrze, Silesian Medical University, Poland
[2]Department of Abdominal Surgery, Videosurgery Division, Bariatric and Metabolic Surgical Center, University of Freiburg, Germany

Abstract

Adipose-derived secreted factors called adipocytokines or adipokines are considered to be strongly involved in the pathogenesis of type 2 diabetes mellitus and obesity complications. Adipocytokines play important roles in insulin resistance, participate in regulation of the energy homeostasis, glucose and lipid metabolism. Adipokines dysfunctions belong to the primary defects in obesity and may link obesity to several health problems including increased risk of insulin resistance, type 2 diabetes, hypertension and dyslipidemia. The current research in field of obesity strongly involve new adipokines linking obesity to related co-morbidities. In this chapter, we focus on the role of adipokines in glucose metabolism and its connections with T2DM.

Introduction

Early diagnosis of type 2 diabetes mellitus is a crucial factor in avoiding common diabetic complications. Morbidity and mortality among T2DM patients are mostly connected with a complicated course of the disease. Beside hyperglycemia, adipokines can be viewed as other factors in the pathogenesis of diabetic complications [1]. According to current studies, adipocytokines play important roles in the pathogenesis of diabetes mellitus, insulin resistance, and are also associated with metabolic conditions such as hypertension and dyslipidemia [2]. The adipose tissue, by changes in production of adipokines, can contribute to insulin resistance in the liver and muscle [3, 4]. Adipocytokines participate in regulation of the energy homeostasis, glucose and lipid metabolism, immunity as well as neuroendocrine and cardiovascular function. Adipokines participate in various metabolic processes including the regulation of appetite control, cardiovascular function, energy expenditure, insulin sensitivity and secretion, as well as inflammation [2, 5-8]. Adipocyte dysfunctions belong to the primary defects in obesity and may link obesity to several health problems including increased risk of insulin resistance, type 2 diabetes, fatty liver disease, hypertension, dyslipidemia, atherosclerosis, dementia, airway disease, and some types of cancers [5, 6]. Adipose tissue secretes pro-inflammatory cytokines and adipokines like TNFα, transforming growth factor β (TGFβ) and interferon-c, C-reactive protein (CRP), interleukins (IL)-1, -6, -8, -10, plasminogen activator inhibitor-1 (PAI-1), fibrinogen, haptoglobin, angiopoietin-related proteins, metallothionein, complement factor 3, serum amyloid A (SAA) protein, anandamide, and 2-AG as well as chemoattractant cytokines, such as monocyte chemotactic protein-1 (MCP-1), progranulin and macrophage inflammatory protein-1a [1, 3, 5, 6, 8]. The current topics in obesity research involve new adipokines linking obesity to related co-morbidities.

Leptin

Leptin seems to play a pivotal role in the mechanism of proper control of metabolic homeostasis, in which various molecules build an integrated network of functional interactions. In the 1950s, the Jackson Laboratory identified two strains of mutant mice that eat excessively and become profoundly obese. In 1994, Zhang et al. successfully identified and cloned the *ob* gene and demonstrated that it is expressed selectively in adipose tissue [9, 10]. Subsequently the peptide hormone coded by *ob* gene was termed leptin, mutation of which caused obesity in the *ob/ob* mouse. It was only a matter of time until the receptor for leptin would be cloned. Indeed, not long thereafter, Tartaglia et al. cloned this protein, the expression of which was demonstrated in the hypothalamus and other tissues, and the db mutation was localized to this gene locus [11, 12]. Animals in leptin synthesis failure and non-functional leptin receptor exhibit not only hyperphagia and obesity but also insulin resistance and type 2 diabetes mellitus as well [9, 13]. The discoveries noted above have given scientists a large research capacity in a field of neuroscience, pharmacology, and even metabolic surgery (metabolic operations undertaken on fa/fa rats with non-functional leptin receptor). Over the past few decades, the synthesis, regulation and effects of leptin have been extensively investigated in a field of its pleiotropic role in human physiology and also in the pathophysiology of metabolic disorders like metabolic syndrome, type 2 diabetes mellitus and many others. In our considerations, we will focus only on the role of leptin in glucose homeostasis, including its neural component of activity.

As noted above, leptin receptors (LepRb) have been found in the hypothalamus. The hypothalamus is a part of central nervous system CNS which governs appetite regulation and energy homeostasis. Via complex neuronal networks, the hypothalamus integrates the signals from the gastrointestinal tract and adipose tissues and produces reactions responsible for the regulation of food intake and energy metabolism [14]. Afferent signals, such as the hormones insulin and leptin, convey information to the brain regarding long-term energy stores, while information regarding short-term energy availability is conveyed by nutrient signals like glucose and free fatty acids as well as hormones like grehlin (see below). Neurons within the arcuate nucleus of the hypothalamus (ARC) play a key role in leptin's metabolic actions [15-18]. The molecular mechanism underlying leptin's metabolic effect is based on IRS-PI3K pathway activation in the hypothalamus. Pharmacological inhibition of PI3K activity in the brain blocks the satiety caused by leptin action [19]. In the ARC, two populations of leptin responsive neurons have been found: neuropeptide Y/agouti-related-peptide (NPY/AgRP) and pro-opiomelanocortin neurons (POMC). Leptin inhibits the firing rate of NPY/AgRP neurons, while at the same time depolarizing POMC [20, 21]. AgRP stimulates appetite by acting as an antagonist of anorexigenic amelanocyte-stimulating hormone (α-MSH) at melanocortin–receptors (MC-Rs), while POMC neurons produce several neuropeptides, including α-MSH, which inhibit food-intake, increase energy expenditure and promote weight loss [22, 23, 24]. With respect to the functions noted above, in the condition of reduced leptin signaling (e. g. fasting or induced weight loss) POMC neurons are inhibited while NPY/AgRP neurons are stimulated. This leads to promotion of positive energy balance and the recovery of weight loss [18]. Moreover, leptin action in POMC neurons normalizes glucose and glucagon levels and improves hepatic insulin sensitivity [25]. It is noteworthy that feeding behaviors are stimulated not only by releasing NPY, but also by reducing melanocortin signaling through the release of endogenous melanocortin-3/4 receptor agonist [26]. The discovery of coordinated function of the two neuronal subpopulations shows both their crucial role in the central regulation of energy homeostasis and the pivotal role of leptin.

Besides its well established role in energy homeostasis, leptin plays an important role in glucose homeostasis as well. Several observations indicate that leptin regulates glucose metabolism independent of its effect on energy balance. The simplest proof is the presence of insulin resistance and type 2 diabetes mellitus in mice with genetic leptin deficiency (*ob/ob*) or leptin receptor deficiency (*db/db* mouse or *fa/fa* rat). Rossetti et al. observed that acute intravenous leptin infusion enhanced insulin's ability to suppress hepatic glucose production without affecting peripheral insulin action [27]. A similar effect was obtained by intracerebroventricular (ICV) leptin administration. Acute ICV infusion of leptin inhibits the action of insulin on the gene expression of phosphoenolpyruvate carboxykinasein (PEPCK) in the liver and results in marked changes in the intrahepatic partitioning of glucose fluxes with increased gluconeogenesis and decreased glycogenolysis [28]. German et al. determined that continuous infusion of leptin directly into the brain normalizes blood glucose levels in STZ-induced diabetic rats. In this model, in which the rats have beta cells damaged by streptozotocin treatment, this effect cannot be explained by recovery of pancreatic beta cells. Moreover, the authors indicated that this effect also cannot be explained by reduced food intake and increased urinary glucose losses. They postulate that leptin action in the brain potently suppressed hepatic glucose production while increasing tissue glucose uptake despite persistent, severe insulin deficiency [29]. Interestingly, this effect was also observed at the level of isolated cells and organs. Decreased activities of gluconeogenic enzymes like glucose 6-phosphatase and PEPCK were found in correlation with increased activities of glycolytic enzymes like glucokinase and pyruvate kinase in isolated hepatocytes from *fa/fa* rats. Basal lactate/pyruvate-dependent gluconeogenesis in these hepatocytes is reduced by 60% compared to lean rats [30].

Isolated perfused livers of lean rats were used to investigate the role of leptin in direct action on liver glucose metabolism. This allowed examination of direct hepatic leptin action independent of its other effects that may also affect hepatic glucose metabolism [31]. Using this approach in studies of postprandial glycogenolysis, Halaas et al. [31] pointed out that recombinant mouse leptin suppressed epinephrine-stimulated glucose production. The authors postulated that certain metabolic changes found in the *db/db* mouse and the *fa/fa*rat, which are leptin-resistant as a result of mutations of the OB gene receptor, can also be explained by impaired leptin action at the level of the liver [31].

Taken together, these results reveal an extensive and integrated role of leptin in the regulation of not only energy homeostasis but of glucose homeostasis as well, and the central nervous system is involved in both central and peripheral leptin effects [18].

Adiponectin

Adiponectin, also known as Acrp30, AdipoQ or gelatin-binding protein, is one of the most important substances secreted by adipose tissue. Its protective effects against metabolic syndrome and type II diabetes have been reported and adiponectin is currently considered as a potential therapeutic target or biological marker in the disorders mentioned above and many others including atherosclerosis, thrombosis, coronary heart disease (CHD) and infertility [32-34]. A growing body of evidence suggests that adiponectin affects energy balance through its regulating role in tissue insulin sensitivity as well as GLUT4 translocation, glucose uptake and fatty acids oxidation [35,36]. Adiponectin has also been implicated in direct energy balance regulation by increasing thermogenesis [37]. In this part of our paper, we focus on the dependence between alterations of the adiponectin level and the effect on glucose homeostasis.

Adiponectin is an adipokine occurring in the plasma in three different molecular weight isoforms: a trimer (low molecular weight), a hexamer (trimer-dimer) of medium molecular weight, and a larger molecular weight form (High Molecular Weight - HMW) [38]. It can be assumed that different isoforms might play different roles. Indeed, there are several studies confirming this hypothesis. Pajvani et al. 2004 [39] found that increases in the ratio of plasma HMW adiponectin levels to total adiponectin levels correlate with improvement in insulin sensitivity during thiazolidinedione treatment in both mice and human diabetic patients, whereas increases in total serum adiponectin levels do not show positive correlation with improvement in insulin sensitivity during treatment with the medication at the individual level. Moreover, reduced levels of HMW adiponectin were reported to be associated with upper body fat distribution, insulin resistance, impaired lipid oxidation, and dyslipidemia affecting multiple lipoprotein subclasses [40]. Similarly, Fisher et al. 2005 showed that serum high molecular weight complex (HMW) of adiponectin correlates better with glucose tolerance than total serum adiponectin [41]. It is noteworthy that levels of total adiponectin, HMW adiponectin, LMW adiponectin, and the HMW-to-total adiponectin ratio all correlated significantly with the crucial features of central obesity and the insulin-stimulated glucose disposal rate, as measured by hyperinsulinemic-euglycemic clamp [40]. However, the HMW rather than total adiponectin, seems to be the more active form of the protein. Furthermore, rare mutations: G84R and G90S, in the collagen domain are closely associated with type 2 diabetes mellitus (T2DM), and hypoadiponectynemia. Subjects with either of these two mutations did not form HMW adiponectin multimers [42-44].

As we mentioned above, adiponectin plays a pivotal role in energy homeostasis, hence is one of most important substances in the integrated network of functional interactions between the factors involved in the pathogenesis of metabolic syndrome and type 2 diabetes mellitus. Reduced adiponectin levels are characteristic for insulin resistant individuals, and can be caused by interactions of genetic factors themselves and environmental factors like lifestyle changes that cause obesity, such as a high-fat diet and sedentary lifestyle [45].

The adiponectin gene (ADIPOQ) is located on the 3q27 chromosome. It has been reported that many single nucleotide polymorphisms (SNPs) in the ADIPOQ gene, are associated with a variety of disorders. Most of the disorders are part of metabolic syndromes e. g. impaired glucose tolerance, type 2 diabetes, obesity, and dyslipidemia [46]. An approximately doubled risk for developing type 2 diabetes mellitus has been found in Japanese individuals who had two alleles of SNP 276 (G/G genotype) [43]. In the study of the Indian population, a positive association was found between SNP45 T >G genotype and type 2 diabetes. Therefore, SNP45T >G in the adiponectin gene may be one of the risk factors for type 2 diabetes [46]. Also, studies undertaken on different ethnic groups showed similar associations of the adiponectin gene with susceptibility to type 2 diabetes mellitus [43, 47-49].

In times in which high-caloric foods are readily available, this "genetic ballast" seems to be really "cumbersome". In this context, the lifestyle should be considered as the second factor causing obesity, insulin resistance, type 2 diabetes mellitus and hypoadiponectynemy. It has been shown that levels of adiponectin are changed in the pathogenesis of these diseases. Adiponectin has been shown to directly and indirectly affect insulin sensitivity through modulation of the insulin signaling pathway and modulation of the molecules involved in glucose and lipid metabolism [35, 50- 52]. It has been reported that an acute increase in the level of circulating adiponectin in the plasma of diabetic mice causes a transient decrease in the basal glucose level by inhibiting the expression of hepatic gluconeogenic enzymes and the rate of endogenous glucose production [53]. Further experiments on insulin resistance in vivo made on adiponectin transgenic mice and adiponectin-deficient mice provide consistent data, and the reported discrepancies were most likely due to differences in genetic background [54, 55]. The proposed mechanism underlying the insulin-sensitizing action of adiponectin is based on stimulation of AMP-activated protein kinase (AMPK) phosphorylation [52]. Adenosine monophosphate-activated protein kinase (AMPK) is an evolutionally well-conserved heterotrimeric serine/threonine kinase [56]. AMPK regulates cellular and systemic energy homeostasis [56]. High expression of AMPK increases food intake and body weight; whereas dominant negative AMPK expression in the hypothalamus leads to reduction of food intake and body weight [57]. This effect was abolished by the use of dominant-negative AMPK, indicating that stimulation of glucose utilization by adiponectin occurs via activation of AMPK. [52]. It is noteworthy that activation of AMPK increases glucose uptake in muscle cells and provokes catabolic transformations that generate ATP, while switching off anabolic cellular processes (e. g. glycogen synthesis) [58]. Current evidence suggests that many effects of adiponectin are mediated through AMPK stimulation. It has been demonstrated that AMP-kinase activation promotes depletion of cellular glycogen stores and reduces glycogen synthesis in L6 rat skeletal muscle [36, 59]. Ceddia et al. 2005 also showed that globular adiponectin increases GLUT4 translocation and glucose uptake in L6 rat skeletal muscle, independent of insulin action involving AMPK [36]. Administration of physiological doses of adiponectin reduced triglyceride accumulation in skeletal muscle and liver by enhancing fatty acid combustion and energy dissipation in skeletal muscle [60, 61]. It has been demonstrated that adiponectin increases fatty acid oxidation in the liver and skeletal muscle, and this process is associated with enhanced insulin sensitivity *via* PPARα and AMPK stimulation [62-65]. Adiponectin can stimulate cellular molecules involved in energy homeostasis through binding to membrane receptors. Two different proteins have been localized as adiponectin receptors: AdipoR1 and AdipoR2 [66]. AdipoRs are ubiquitously expressed in liver, muscle, heart, adipose tissue, osteoblasts, pancreas and brain of humans, rodents and various other mammals. AdipoR1 is quite ubiquitous, including an abundant expression in skeletal muscle, whereas AdipoR2 is most abundantly expressed in the liver [45]. Expression or suppression of both AdipoR1 and AdipoR2 receptors confirms the hypothesis that after globular or full length adiponectin binding, they mediate increased AMPK, PPARα ligand activates, fatty acids oxidation, and glucose uptake [62]. Thus, with respect to the molecular mechanism underlying the insulin-sensitizing action of adiponectin, not only the adiponectin level is important for this phenomenon, but also AdipoRs expression. Indeed, obesity decreases not only plasma adiponectin levels but also AdipoR1/R2 expression, which leads to reduction of adiponectin sensitivity and insulin resistance [66]. It has been also reported that expression of adiponectin receptors in the skeletal muscle of patients with type 2 diabetes mellitus decreased [67]. In addition, Adiporl mRNA and Adipo R2 mRNA expression was positively correlated with in-vivo C-peptide concentration and triglyceride concentration, respectively [68].

Taken together, these results reveal an extensive and integrated network of functional interactions between adiponectin and other molecules involved in glucose and lipid homeostasis. This opens up many opportunities for therapeutic strategy in the treatment of insulin resistance, type 2 diabetes mellitus, metabolic syndrome and cardiovascular disease.

Visfatin

Visfatin, was previously known as a pre-B cell colony-enhancing factor (PBEF), and its function in the immune system was indicated as a growth factor for early B cells [69]. It was identified in 2004 as an adipokine [70] and named visfatin, which suggested that it would be predominantly produced and secreted in visceral fat tissue. However, the name turned out to beslightly misleading. Subsequent studies have identified visfatin as a nicotinamide phosphoribosyltransferase (NAMPT) capable of producing nicotinamide mononucleotide (NMN), a precursor for the metabolic co-factor NADC [71]. Moreover, it has been shown that visfatin/PBEF/NAMPT is produced not only in human leukocytes and adipocytes but also hepatocytes and muscle [72, 73].

The discovery by Fukuhara et al. [70] that plasma concentration of visfatin correlates strongly with the amount of visceral fat in human subjects and visfatin had insulin-mimetic effect in rodent models of insulin resistance and obesity *in vivo*, caused a flurry of research on its relationship to type 2 diabetes mellitus, insulin secretion and sensitivity and also to other adipokines (i. e. adiponectin). However, despite significant interest, relatively little data was published which could clearly indicate the biological function of visfatin in metabolic disorders.

Fukuhara et al. [70] showed that visfatin exerted an insulino-mimetic effect *in vitro* and lowered the plasma glucose level in mice. They also suggested that visfatin binds to and activates the insulin receptor. Recent data show that the NAD biosynthetic activity of NAMPT/Visfatin is crucial for the regulation of glucose metabolism. Revollo et al. [74] found that heterozygous mice (Nampt$^{+/-}$) and islets have defects in NMN/NAD biosynthesis and glucose intolerance, mainly caused by insulin secretion deficiency. This impaired beta cell function can be ameliorated by administration of nicotinamide mononucleotide (NMN), the product of visfatin on NAD biosynthesis [74]. Thus, NAD biosynthesis could be physiologically more important than the insulin-mimetic activity of visfatin for the regulation of glucose metabolism through its role in amelioration of islet dysfunction. Caton et al. investigated NAMPT/Visfatin activity on beta cells *in vitro* with induced inflammation and *in vivo* on mice fed a fructose-rich diet (FRD) causing impaired insulin secretion and elevated islet expression of IL1β [75]. They found that NMN restored insulin secretion in cultured islet cells, and this effect was partially blocked by inhibition of sirtuin 1. Furthermore, administration of exogenous NMN to FRD-fed mice alleviates inflammation-induced islet dysfunction. Thus, the onset of beta cells failure in FRD-fed mice may occur *via* lowered secretion of extracellular NAMPT [75]. Nevertheless, Brown and co-authors suggest that visfatin can regulate insulin secretion and insulin receptor phosphorylation as well as the expression of a number of genes associated with beta cell function in mice [76]. They found 12 of the 84 genes tested were significantly up or down-regulated by treatment with visfatin, including insulin and sytaxin 4, which enhance glucose-stimulated insulin secretion [76]. Moreover, the specific visfatin inhibitor FK866 blocks not only increasing visfatin-induced insulin secretion but also activation of the ERK1/2 insulin receptor. Both visfatin and NMN induced ERK1/2 activation. These data suggest that visfatin has a role in multiple aspects of islets biology, including a role in the regulation of insulin secretion and receptor signaling.

Taken together, the above data show that visfatin may be a compensatory mechanism or its role in pathophysiology of diabetes is partial.

Vaspin

Visceral adipose tissue-derived serpin (vaspin) has gained interest in obesity research after the observation that its expression in white adipose tissue (WATs) ameliorates certain aberrations seen in the diabetic/obesity metabolic syndrome by sensitizing insulin action in a rat model of obesity [77]. Elevated vaspin serum concentrations have been associated with obesity, impaired insulin sensitivity, and fitness level in human subjects [78]. Administration of vaspin to obese mice restores the mRNA of various genes expressed in WATs to normal levels. The mRNA were mostly related to the metabolic syndrome including glucose transporter-4, leptin, resistin, and adiponectin, improving glucose tolerance and insulin sensitivity [77].

Wada 2008 suggests vaspin and its analogues as a new perspective for drug development [79]. Moreover, central vaspin administration leads to reduced food intake and has sustained blood glucose-lowering effects [80]. Vaspin was identified for first time by Hida as a serpin A12 member of the serine protease inhibitor family [2, 77], which has been found to be expressed in visceral adipose tissue of Otsuka Long-Evans Tokushima Fatty (OLETF) rats, an animal model of abdominal obesity and type 2 diabetes mellitus [77]. In OLETF rats, vaspin serum levels were reduced in parallel with aging and the development of severe hyperglycemia, a process which could be reversed by insulin or pioglitazone treatment [1, 77]. Kempf and her co-workers investigated the association of vaspin single nucleotide polymorphisms (SNPs) with type 2 diabetes mellitus and obesity [81]. Recently, a significant association of vaspin SNP rs2236242 with type 2 diabetes has been reported in 2,759 participants of the KORA F3 study. The authors found that the AA genotype is associated with an increased diabetes risk and this association seems to be independent of obesity. Kempf and her team suggested a link between the novel adipokine vaspin and glucose metabolism [81]. Expression of vaspin mRNA has been detected in human white adipose tissue [82], stomach [80], liver, pancreas [83] as well as in the hypothalamus and cerebrospinal fluid of *db/db* and C57BL/6 mice [80]. In addition, in mice and humans, the skin has been shown to express relatively high vaspin mRNA levels [84]. Lean human subjects (BMI < 25) had a vaspin mRNA expression almost undetectable in both visceral and subcutaneous (SC), which is in accordance with the hardly detectable vaspin expression in young OLETF rats [77]. This revealed that vaspin mRNA expression can be inducible by increased body fat and metabolic abnormalities, which develop in older OLETF rats [77]. Vaspin mRNA expressions in visceral adipose tissue were more frequently detected in overweight or obese patients with type 2 diabetes. Moreover, increased body fat is the strongest predictor for decreased insulin sensitivity, and the strongest determinant of SC vaspin gene expression. It has been proved that visceral vaspin expression is significantly correlated with BMI, percentage of body fat, and 2 hours OGTT plasma glucose [82], whereas subcutaneous vaspin expression has shown a significant correlation with waist-to-hip ratio (WHR) and fasting plasma insulin concentration [82]. Further analysis revealed vaspin mRNA expression in preadipocytes and mature adipocytes of human omental adipose tissue and the stromal vascular fraction (SVF) as well [85]. The details of the mechanisms of vaspin action in glucose metabolism and insulin sensitivity are still not fully understood. Recent data indicate that vaspin inhibits a protease which plays a role in the degradation of a hormone or molecule with direct or indirect glucose-lowering effects [1].

Vaspin serum concentrations were significantly higher in lean healthy women compared to men [78]. Of note, the significant gender differences in circulating vaspin levels starts to develop during pubertal progression in girls [83]. In lean individuals with normal glucose tolerance, vaspin serum concentration increased with age [78, 83]. In adolescents, that concentration has been shown to increase in parallel with worsening insulin resistance and was acutely down-regulated following glucose provocation in insulin-resistant young subjects independent of obesity [83]. Körner et al. also showed that, regardless of gender, age and BMI, lower circulating vaspin level was associated with better insulin sensitivity, higher systolic blood pressure and impaired endothelial function. In overweight women with polycystic ovary syndrome,metformin decreased the vaspin serum levels concomitantly with improvement in insulin sensitivity and a decrease in insulin resistance following 6 months of metformin therapy [86]. The lowering effects of metformin on the circulating vaspin level have been confirmed in drug-naïve patients with type 2 diabetes [1]. Interesting correlations of circulating vaspin with age, gender, and BMI are attenuated in obese patients with metabolic diseases and cardiovascular complications [2, 87]. Changes in serum vaspin concentrations observed after Roux en-Y gastric bypass (RYBG) were significantly correlated with the weight loss. Those changes in plasma vaspin levels were also associated with the decrease of circulating insulin levels and the improvement of HOMA, independent of the reduction in BMI. Handisurya (2010) remarked that the up-regulation of circulating vaspin levels in obesity associated with insulin resistance, represents an endogenous compensatory mechanism to preserve glycemic control [87]. Circulating vaspin significantly correlates with leptin serum concentrations, which indicates that vaspin closely reflects body fat mass [1]. In contrast, several studies found no association between circulating vaspin levels and insulin sensitivity in non-metabolic patients like non-diabetic subjects, patients on chronic hemodialysis, first-degree relatives of D2M patients or hypothyroid patients [88, 89, 23 90, 91].

Apelin

Apelin (APJ endogenous ligand) is a peptide growth factor that binds the APJ receptor with high affinity. It's mRNA encodes preproproteins, consisted of 77 amino acid residues, which is proteolytically processed to several active molecular forms, such as apelin-36, -17, -13, and the pyroglutamated form of apelin-13. Apelin-13 contains the part of the molecule which was demonstrated to be an endogenous ligand for the G protein-coupled receptor, APJ [92]. Analyses have shown that the C-terminal part of this polypeptide is the bioactive region of the apelin, and it is found to be conserved between frogs and mammals [93]. Apelin with a length of 36 amino acids was originally isolated from bovine stomach tissue extracts. It is a major component in the lung, testis, and uterus. The aa form of apelin13 was detected in the mammary gland, apelin17 aa and apelin12 aa were detected in different tissues [94,95]. High expression of apelin mRNA was detected in the mammary gland of rats during pregnancy and lactation, reaching a maximal level around parturition. Apelin and APJ mRNA are associated with functional effects in both the central nervous system and peripheral tissues [96]. This adipokin is abundantly secreted especially in bovine colostrum and has been detected in bovine milk [97]. Developmental studies of mice and frogs have shown that APJ receptor is highly expressed in endothelial precursor cells and nascent vascular structures in embryos of those species. Apelin is a potent angiogenic factor and acts as a mitogenic, chemotactic and anti-apoptotic agent, and the expression of the apelin gene increases under conditions of hypoxia [93]. The sequencing of the human, bovine, rat, and mouse preproapelin has shown that there is a high sequence homology among the four species and has a 100% sequence identity for the last C-terminal amino acids [92, 98]. Apelin-13 binds with high affinity and selectivity to human cardiac tissue. Moreover, a wide distribution of the APJ receptor in the human vasculature highlights the properties of a novel potent vasoconstrictor in the human vasculature. Apelin ligand is coexpressed with APJ in frog vascular tissues and in developing blood vessels of the perinatal mouse retina [93, 99]. Apelin has been shown to be involved in the regulation of cardiovascular and fluid homeostasis, food intake, cell proliferation, and angiogenesis [100]. Apelin receptor is expressed in insulin-responsive tissues like adipose tissue, skeletal muscles, heart and in the liver [101]. Adipose tissue has been shown to produce and secrete apelin and thus considered as adipokine, which seems to be involved in obesity and carbohydrate metabolism [102].

In mice, apelin inhibited glucose-stimulated insulin secretion in pancreatic islets [103], suggesting a connection with glucose homeostasis. Dray and colleagues have shown that both short and long-term apelin treatment of high-fat diet (HFD) obese and insulin-resistant mice improves insulin sensitivity, thus altering glucose metabolism mainly by an increase in glucose uptake in skeletal muscle [101, 104]. Administration of apelin to mice with generalized apelin deficiency (APKO) and *db/db* mice resulted in improved insulin sensitivity, proving that apelin is necessary for the maintenance of insulin sensitivity in vivo. The effects of apelin on glucose uptake and Akt phosphorylation are in part mediated by a Gi- and AMPK-dependent pathway [105]. Long-term apelin treatment of mice deficient in apelin signaling has reversed the changes in increased FFA, glycerol, and leptin concentrations as well as abdominal adiposity [106]. Apelin administration inhibits isoproterenol-induced lipolysis in cultured adipocytes as well [106]. After 4 weeks of chronic apelin treatment, insulin-resistant and high-fat diet (HFD)-induced obese mice had significantly lower plasma levels of glycemia, and were protected from hyperinsulinemia compared to control HFD phosphate-buffered saline (PBS)-treated mice. Moreover, the apelin-treated mice had lower plasma concentrations of triglycerides (TG) and reduced adiposity, whereas plasma fatty acids (FA) levels remained unchanged. Indirect calorimetry measurements on HFD apelin-treated obese and insulin-resistant mice showed lower respiratory exchange ratio values (RER), which is characteristic for a better use of lipids. With a rise in energy expenditure and promoting complete lipid use in soleus muscle of insulin-resistant mice, apelin treatment contributes to insulin sensitivity improvement [104]. A plethora of FFAs or hyperglycemic conditions lead to increased production of reactive oxygen species (ROS), and, thus reduced mitochondrial biogenesis, causing mitochondrial dysfunction. Subsequently, mitochondrial dysfunction observed in muscle and liver tissues drives decreased β-oxidation and ATP production, resulting in insulin resistance, diabetes, and cardiovascular disease [107]. AMP-activated protein kinase (AMPK) stimulates metabolic processes such as glucose transport and FA oxidation, in order to supply cellular ATP and, thus mitochondria of skeletal muscles and liver can adapt to energy demand [107, 108]. 4-week treatment of insulin resistant, obese mice with apelin13 provoked an increase in mitochondrial biogenesis and a reduction in the adverse alterations in the ultrastructure of both intra-myofibrillar and subsarcolemmal mitochondria of soleus muscle, which are usually present in T2DM [104]. Apelin increases AMPK and acetyl CoA carboxylase phosphorylation in muscle of insulin-resistant mice [104]. These biological changes in the mitochondria of skeletal muscle were connected with increased mitochondrial DNA and higher expression of peroxisome proliferator-activated receptor γ co-activator 1α (PGC1α). It was also connected with nuclear respiratory factor-1 (NRF-1) and mitochondrial transcription factor A (TFAM), which increased mitochondrial oxidative phosphorylation and mitochondrial biogenesis [109].

In humans, insulin and tumor necrosis factor-α (TNFα) have been shown to be main regulating factors of apelin expression and secretion in adipose tissue [96, 110]. Circulating apelin levels and its expression in adipose tissue are significantly higher in morbidly obese patients [111], type 2 diabetes mellitus subjects [112] and obese patients with impaired glucose level (IFG) [110]. That is why it can be involved in the pathophysiology of obesity [113]. Fasting plasma apelin levels have correlated positively with HOMA-IR, BMI, TC, LDL-C, FBG and fasting plasma insulin. HOMA-IR, BMI, and TC were independent related factors influencing plasma apelin levels [112]. Furthermore, non-obese subjects, patients with type 2 diabetes or with impaired glucose tolerance also showed higher levels of apelin than control subjects [112]. The hypocaloric diet associated with weight loss in women with moderate obesity resulted in a reduction of plasma apelin levels [114]. In morbidly obese patients with diabetes 2 mellitus or with impaired fasting glucose, bariatric surgery led to a significant decrease in apelin levels [113]. On the other hand, no significant change in the concentration of apelin was found in the group of morbidly obese patients with NFG [113]. These findings show that weight loss is not crucial for the reduction in apelin levels. Moreover, the combination of insulin-sensitizing medications such as metformin and rosiglitazone improves the glycemic profile and allows an increase in plasma apelin levels in patients with diabetes 2 mellitus [115]. As a whole, these findings point out that the increased levels of apelin may, in a first phase of metabolic disease, be a compensatory delay mechanism of the insulin resistance and may play a role in the pathogenesis of type 2 diabetes mellitus [104, 113].

Ghrelin

Ghrelin was described by Kojima, and Hosoda for the first time in 1999 as a 28-amino-acid peptide hormone isolated from the cells of the gastric mucosa of rats, and secreted primarily by the epithelial cells of the fundus of the stomach in humans [116-118]. Ghrelin is a powerful orexigenic peptide that was identified secondary to its effect on the growth hormone (GH) release from somatotroph cells of the anterior pituitary [119]. Ghrelin stimulates the appetite via secretion in the hypothalamic neurons via orexigenic hormones neuropeptide Y (NPY) /AgRP [120] and in hypothalamic arcuate nucleus (ARC) via ghrelin receptor GHS-R1a [121, 122]. Adenosine monophosphate-activated protein kinase (AMPK) is an evolutionally well-conserved heterotrimeric serine/threonine kinase [56]. AMPK regulates cellular and systemic energy homeostasis [56]. High expression of AMPK increases food intake and body weight; whereas dominant negative AMPK expression in the hypothalamus leads to a reduction of food intake and body weight [123]. Hypothalamic AMPK activity may be stimulated via central (intracerebroventricular) and peripheral (intraperitoneal) ghrelin administration [124, 125]. The main ways of AMPK activation in the hypothalamus by ghrelin's signalling pathways has been described through the identification of the endocannabinoid system [124, 125] and calmodulin kinase kinase 2 (CaMKK2) [126]. The fatty acid pathway, hypothalamic mitochondrial respiration, and uncoupling protein 2 have been considered as downstream targets of AMPK and mediators of ghrelin's appetite stimulating effect [127]. Plasma ghrelin levels were reduced in obese subjects compared to lean controls, and also negatively correlated with percentage of body fat, fasting insulin and leptin concentrations [128]. Diet-induced obesity (DIO) causes ghrelin resistance by reducing NPY/AgRP responsiveness to plasma ghrelin and suppressing the neuroendocrine ghrelin axis to limit further food intake [129].

Very diverse changes in serum ghrelin levels after bariatric surgery have been reported so far. Postoperative decreases in ghrelin serum concentrations were observed following procedures that isolated or removed the fundus of the stomach. Reduced production of ghrelin after gastric bypass may be responsible for weight loss [130]. The RYGB mediates weight loss and improves glucose tolerance via a few mechanisms, including impairment in ghrelin secretion in the long-limb variants of RYGB [131]. Postoperative reduction in ghrelin and gastric inhibitory polypeptide (GIP) levels are opposite to the increases caused by diet-induced weight loss. These changes are thought to contribute to the greater efficacy of gastric bypass [132]. By contrast, other reports showed that serum ghrelin levels increased or remained unchanged after RYGB, adjustable gastric banding (AGB), vertical banded gastroplasty (VBG), and biliopancreatic diversion with Roux-en-Y gastric bypass (BPD-RYGBP) in a period from 6 months to 2 years after surgery. Plausibly, acute reductions of plasma ghrelin are associated with short-term follow-up of one year or less [133]. Varying data on serum ghrelin concentrations may be explained by a negative energy mode of the patients after surgery, differed laboratory procedures among the study sites, and different bariatric procedures [133].

References

[1] Blüher M (2012) Vaspin in obesity and diabetes: pathophysiological and clinical significance. *Endocrine,* 41:176–182.

[2] Gülçelik NE, Usman A, Gürlek A (2009) Role of adipocytokines in predicting the development of diabetes and its late complications. *Endocrine,* 36, 397–403.

[3] Hotamisligil GS (1999)Mechanisms of TNF-alpha-induced insulin resistance. *Exp. Clin. Endocrinol. Diabetes,* 107:119–125.

[4] Guilherme A, Virbasius JV, Puri V, Czech MP (2008) Adipocyte dysfunctions linking obesity to insulin resistance and type 2 diabetes. *Natl. Rev. Mol. Cell Biol.,* 9:367–377.

[5] Blüher M (2009) Adipose tissue dysfunction in obesity. *Exp. Clin. Endocrinol. Diabetes,* 117: 241–250.

[6] Bays HE (2009) ''Sick fat,'' metabolic disease, and atherosclerosis. *Am. J. Med.,* 122:S26–S37.

[7] Kralisch S, Blüher M, Paschke R, Stumvoll M, Fasshauer M (2007) Adipokines and adipocyte targets in the future management of obesity and the metabolic syndrome. *Mini. Rev. Med. Chem.,* 7:39–45.

[8] Van Gaal LF, Mertens IL, DeBlock CE (2006) Mechanisms linking obesity with cardiovascular disease. *Nature,* 444:875–880.

[9] Zhang Y, Proenca R, Maffei M, Barone M, Leopold L, Friedman JM (1994) Positional cloning of the mouse obese gene and its human homologue. *Nature,* 372:425-432.

[10] Cammisoto P, Bendayan M (2012) A review on gastric leptin: the exocrine secretion of gastric hormone. *Ant. Cell Biol.,* 45(1): 1-16.

[11] Lee GH, Proenca R, Montez JM, Carroll KM, Darvishzadeh JG, Lee JI, Friedman JM (1996) Abnormal splicing of the leptin receptor in *diabetic* mice. *Nature,* 379: 632–635.

[12] Tartaglia LA, Dembski M, Weng X, Deng N, Culpepper J, Devos R, Richards GJ, Campfield LA, Clark FT, Deeds J, Muir C, Sanker S, Morlarty A, Moore KJ, Smutko JS, Mays GG, Woolf EA, Monroe CA, Tepper RI (1995) Identification and expression cloning of a leptin receptor, OB-R. *Cell,* 83: 1263–1271.

[13] Takaya K, Ogawa Y, Hiraoka J, Hosoda K, Yamori Y, Nakao K, Koletsky RJ (1996) Nonsense mutation of leptin receptor in the obese spontaneously hypertensive Koletsky rat. *Nat. Genet.,* 14: 130–131.

[14] Druce M, Bloom SR (2006) The regulation of appetite. *Arch. Dis. Child.,* 91:183–187.

[15] Bjørbæk C (2009) Central leptin receptor action and resistance in obesity. *J. Investig. Med.,* 57: 789–794.

[16] Satoh N, Ogawa Y, Katsuura G, Hayase M, Tsuji T, Imagawa K, Yoshimasa Y, Nishi S, Hosoda K, Nakao K (1997) The arcuate nucleus as a primary site of satiety effect of leptin in rats. *Neurosci. Lett.,* 224: 149–152.
[17] Morton GJ, Niswender KD, Rhodes CJ, Myers MG, Jr., Blevins JE, Baskin GD, Schwartz MW (2003) Arcuate nucleus-specific leptin receptor gene therapy attenuates the obesity phenotype of Koletsky (fa(k)/fa(k)) rats. *Endocrinology*, 144: 2016–2024.
[18] Morton GJ, Schwartz MW (2011) Leptin and the central nervous system control of glucose metabolism. *Physiol. Rev.,* 91:389-411.
[19] Niswender KD, Morrison CD, Clegg DJ, Olson R, Baskin DG, Myers MG Jr, Seeley RJ, Schwartz MW (2003) Insulin activation of phosphatidylinositol 3-kinase in the hypothalamic arcuate nucleus: a key mediator of insulin-induced anorexia. *Diabetes,* 52: 227–231.
[20] Van den Top M, Lee K, Whyment AD, Blanks AM, Spanswick D (2004)Orexigen-sensitive NPY/AgRP pacemaker neurons in the hypothalamic arcuate nucleus. *Nat. Neurosci.,* 7: 493–494.
[21] Cowley MA, Smart JL, Rubinstein M, Cerdan MG, Diano S, Horvath TL, Cone RD, Low MJ (2001) Leptin activates anorexigenicPOMC neurons through a neural network in the arcuate nucleus. *Nature,* 411: 480–484.
[22] Wilson BD, Bagnol D, Kaelin CB, Ollmann MM, Gantz I, Watson SJ, Barsh GS (1999) Physiological and anatomical circuitry between Agouti-related protein and leptin signaling. *Endocrinology,* 140: 2387–2397.
[23] Cone RD (2005) Anatomy and regulation of the central melanocortin system. *Nat. Neurosci.,* 8: 571–578.
[24] Fan W, Boston BA, Kesterson RA, Hruby VJ, Cone RD (1997) Role of melanocortinergic neurons in feeding and the agouti obesity syndrome. *Nature,* 385: 165–168.
[25] Berglund ED, Vianna CR, Donato J Jr., Kim MH, Chuang J, Lee CE, Lauzon DA, Lin P, Brule LJ, Scott MM, Coppari R, Elmquist JK (2012) Direct leptin action on POMC neurons regulates glucose homeostasis and hepatic insulin sensitivity in mice. *J. Clin. Ivest.,* 122(3): 1000-1009.
[26] Ollmann MM, Wilson BD, Yang YK, Kerns JA, Chen Y, Gantz I, Barsh GS (1997) Antagonism of central melanocortin receptors in vitro and in vivo by agouti-related protein. *Science,* 278: 135–138.
[27] Rossetti L, Massillon D, Barzilai N, Vuguin P, Chen W, Hawkins M, Wu J, Wang J (1997) Short term effects of leptin on hepaticgluconeogenesis and in vivo insulin action. *J. Biol. Chem.,* 272: 27758–27763.
[28] Liu L, Karkanias GB, Morales JC , Hawkins M, Barzilai N, Wang J, Rossetti L (1998) Intracerebroventricular Leptin Regulates Hepatic but Not Peripheral Glucose Fluxes. *J. Biol. Chem.,* 273 (47): 31160–31167.
[29] German JP, Thaler JP, Wisse BE, Shinsuke oh-I, Sarruf DA, Fischer JD, Matsen ME, Taborsky GJ Jr., Schwartz MW, Morton GJ (2011)Leptin activates a novel CNS mechanism for insulin-independentnormalization of severe diabetic hyperglycemia. *Endocrinology,* 2: 394–404.
[30] Sanchez-Gutierrez J, Sanchez-Arias J, Lechuga CG, Valle JC, Samper B, Feliu JE (1994) Decreased responsiveness of basal gluconeogenesis to insulin action in hepatocytes isolated from genetically obese (fa/fa) Zucker rats. *Endocrinology,* 134:1868-1873.

[31] Nemecz M, Preininger K, Englisch R, Rinsinn CF,Schneider B, Waldhäusl W, RodenM (1999) Acute Effect of Leptin on Hepatic Glycogenolysis and Gluconeogenesis in Perfused Rat Liver. *Hepatology,* 29: 166-172.
[32] Ekmekci H, Ekmekci OB (2006) The role of adiponectin in atherosclerosis and thrombosis. *Clin. Appl. Thromb. Hemost.,* 12(2): 163-168.
[33] Bersinger RA, Wunder DM (2010) Adiponectin isoforms distribution in serum and in follicular fluid of women undergoing treatment by ICSI. *Acta. Obestet. Gynecol. Scand.,* 89(6): 782-788.
[34] Empana JP (2008) Adiponectin isoforms and cardiovascular disease: the epidemiological evidence has just begun. *European Heart Journal,* 29:1221-1223.
[35] Kadowaki, T, Yamauchi T (2005) Adiponectin and adiponectin receptors. *Endocr. Rev.,* 26:439–451.
[36] Ceddia RB, Somwar R, Maida A, Fang X, Bikopoulos G, Sweeney G (2005) Globular adiponectin increases GLUT4 translocation and glucose uptake but reduces glycogen synthesis in rat skeletal muscle cells. *Diabetologia,* 48: 132-139.
[37] Spranger J, Verma S, Göhring I, Bobbert T, Seifert J, Sindler AL, Pfeiffer A, Hileman SM, Tschöp M, Banks WA (2006) Adiponectin does not cross the blood-brain barrier but modifies cytokine expression of brain endothelial cells. *Diabetes,* 55: 141-147.
[38] Pajvani UB, Du X, Combs TP, Berg AH, Rajala MW, Schulthess T, Engel J, Brownlee M, Scherer PE (2003) Structure–function studies of the adipocyte-secreted hormone Acrp30/adiponectin. Implications for metabolic regulation and bioactivity. *J. Biol. Chem.,* 278: 9073–9085.
[39] Pajvani UB, Howkins M, Combs TP, Rajala MW, Doebber T, Berger JP, Wagner JA, Wu M, Knopps A, Xiang AH, Utzschmeider KM, Khan SE, Olefsky JM, Buchanan TA, Scherer PE (2004) Complex distribution, not absolute amount of adiponectin, correlates with thiazolidinedione-mediated improvement in insulin sensitivity. *J. Biol. Chem.,* 279:12152–12162.
[40] Castro LC, Luo N, Wallace P, Klein RL, Garvey WT (2006) Adiponectin Multimeric Complexes and the Metabolic Syndrome Trait Cluster. *Diabetes*, 55: 249-259.
[41] Fisher M, Trujillo ME, Hanif W, Barnett AH, McTernan PG, Scherer PE, Kumar S (2005) Serum high molecular weight complex of adiponectin correlates better with glucose tolerance than total serum adiponectin in Indo-Asian males. *Diabetologia,* 48: 1084–1087.
[42] Waki H, Yamauchi T, Kamon J, Ito Y, Uchida S, Kita S, Hara K, Hada Y, Vasseur F, Fraguel P, Kimura S, Nagai R, Kadowaki T (2003) Impaired multimerization of human adiponectin mutants associated with diabetes: molecular structure and multimer formation of adiponectin. *J. Biol. Chem.,* 278:40352–40363.
[43] Hara K, Boutin P, Mori Y, Tobe K, Diana C, Yasuda K, Yamauchi T, Otabe S, Okada T, Eto K, Kadowaki H, Hagura R, Akanuma Y, Yazaki Y, Nagai R, Taniyama M, Matsubara K, Yoda M, Nakano Y, Kimura S, Tomita M, Kimura S, Ito C, Fraguel P, Kadowaki T (2002) Genetic variation in the gene encoding adiponectin is associated with an increased risk of type 2 diabetes in the Japanese population. *Diabetes,* 51:536–540.
[44] Tasanen K, Eble JA, Aumailley M, Schumann H, Batge J, Tu H, Bruckner P, Bruckner-Tuderman L (2000) Collagen XVII is destabilized by a glycine substitution mutation in the cell adhesion domain Col15. *J. Biol. Chem.,* 275:3093–3099.

[45] Kadowaki T, Yamauchi T, Kubota N, Hara K, Kueki K, Tobe K (2006) Adiponectin and adiponectin receptors in insulin resistance, diabetes, and metabolic syndrome. *J. Clin. Invest.,* 116: 1784- 1792.

[46] Biswas D, Vettriselvi V,• Choudhury J, Jothimalar R (2011) Adiponectin Gene Polymorphism and its Association with Type 2 Diabetes Mellitus. *Ind. J. Clin. Biochem.,* 26(2):172–177.

[47] Nakatani K, Noma K, Nishioka J, Kasai Y, Marioka K, Katsuki A, Hori Y, Yano Y, Sumida Y, Wada Hideo, Nobori T (2005) Adiponectin gene variation associates with the increasing risk of Type 2 diabetes in non-diabetic Japanese subjects. *Int. J. Mol. Med.,* 15:173–7.

[48] Gable DR, Matin J, Whittall R, Cakmak H, Li KW, Cooper J, Miller GJ, Humpries SE (2007) Common adiponectin gene variants show different effects on risk of cardiovascular disease and Type 2 diabetes in European subjects. *Ann. Hum. Genet.,* 71(4):453–66.

[49] González-Sánchez JL, Zabena CA, Martinez-Larrad MT, Fernández-Pérez C, Pérez-Barba M, Laakso M, Serrano-Ríos M (2005) An SNP in the adiponectin gene is associated with decreased serum adiponectin levels and risk for impaired glucose tolerance. *Obes. Res.,* 13:807–12.

[50] Matsuzawa Y (1997) Pathophysiology and molecular mechanisms of visceral fat syndrome: the Japanese experience. *Diabetes Metab. Rev.,*13:3–13.

[51] National Cholesterol Education Program (2001) Executive Summary of the Third Report of the National Cholesterol Education Program (NCEP) Expert Panel on Detection, Evaluation, and Treatment of High Blood Cholesterol in Adults (Adult Treatment Panel III). *JAMA,* 285:2486–2497.

[52] Yamauchi T, Kamon J, Minokoshi Y, Ito Y, Waki H, Uchida S, Yamashita S, Noda M, Kita S, Ueki K, Eto K, Akanuma Y, Fraguel P, Faufelle F, Ferre P, Carling D, Kimura S, Nagai R, Kahn BB, Kadowaki T (2002) Adiponectin stimulates glucose utilization and fatty-acid oxidation by activating AMP-activated protein kinase. *Nat. Med.,* 8:1288–1295.

[53] Berg AH, Combs TP, Du X, Brownlee M, Scherer PE (2001) The adipocyte-secreted protein Acrp30 enhances hepatic insulin action. *Nat. Med.,* **7**:947–953.

[54] Kubota N, Terauchi Y, Yamauchi T, Kubota T, Moroi M, Matsui J, Eto K, Yamashita T, Kamon J, Satoh H, Yano W, Froguel P, Nagai R, Kimura S, Kadowaki T, Noda T (2002) Disruption of adiponectin causes insulin resistance and neointimal formation. *J. Biol. Chem.,*277:25863–25866.

[55] Nawrocki, A. R (2006) Mice lacking adiponectin show decreased hepatic insulin sensitivity and reduced responsiveness to peroxisome proliferator-activated receptor gamma agonists. *J. Biol. Chem.,*281:2654–2660.

[56] Kola B, Boscaro M, Rutter GA, Grossman AB, Korbonits M (2006) Expanding role of AMPK in endocrinology. *Trends Endocrinol. Metab.,* 17:205–215.

[57] Minokoshi Y, Alquier T, Furukawa N, Kim YB, Lee A, Xue B et al. (2004) AMP-kinase regulates food intake by responding to hormonal and nutrient signals in the hypothalamus. *Nature,* 428:569–574.

[58] Hardie DG (2004) AMP-activated protein kinase: a key system mediating metabolic responses to exercise. *Med. Sci. Sports Exerc.,* 36:28–34.

[59] Wojtaszewski JF, Jorgensen SB, Hellsten Y, Hardie DG, Richter EA (2002) Glycogen-dependent effects of 5 aminoimidazole- 4-carboxamide (AICA)-riboside on AMP-activated protein kinase and glycogen synthase activities in rat skeletal muscle. *Diabetes,* 51:284–292.

[60] Yamauchi T, Kamon J, Waki H, Terauchi Y, Kubota N, Hara K, Mori Y, Abe M, Tanaka J, Ohsumi J, Ide T, Murakami K, Tsuboyama-KN, Ezaki O, Akanuma Y, Gavrilova O, Vinson C, Reitman ML, Kagechika H, Shudo K, Yoda M, Nakano Y, Tobe K, Nagai R, Kimura S, Tomita M, Froguel P, Kadowaki T (2001) Replenishment of the fat-derived hormone adiponectin reverses insulin resistance associated with both lipoatrophy and obesity. *Nat. Med.,* 7:941–946.

[61] *Fruebis J, Tsao TS, Javorschi S, Reed DE, Erickson MR, Yen FT, Bihain BE, Lodish HF (2001) Proteolytic cleavage product of 30-kDa adipocyte complement-related protein increases fatty acid oxidation in muscle and causes weight loss in mice. Proc. Natl. Acad. Sci. USA,98:*2005–*2010.*

[62] Yamauchi T, Kamon J, Ito Y et al. (2003) Cloning of adiponectin receptors that mediate antidiabetic metabolic effects. *Nature,* 423:762–769.

[63] Fruebis J, Tsao TS, Javorschi S et al. (2001) Proteolytic cleavage product of 30-kDa adipocyte complement-related protein increases fatty acid oxidation in muscle and causes weight loss in mice. *Proc. Natl. Acad. Sci. USA,* 98:2005–2010.

[64] Tomas E, Tsao TS, Saha AK et al. (2002) Enhanced muscle fat oxidation and glucose transport by ACRP30 globular domain: acetyl-CoA carboxylase inhibition and AMP-activated protein kinase activation. *Proc. Natl. Acad. Sci. USA,* 99:16309–16313.

[65] Yoon MJ, Lee GY, Chung JJ, Ahn JH, Hong SH, Kim JB (2006) Adiponectin Increases Fatty Acid Oxidation in Skeletal Muscle Cells by Sequential Activation of AMP-Activated Protein Kinase, p38 Mitogen-Activated Protein Kinase, and Peroxisome Proliferator–Activated Receptor α. *Diabetes,* 55: 2563-2570.

[66] Tsuchida A et al. (2004) Insulin/Foxo1 pathway regulates expression levels of adiponectin receptors and adiponectin sensitivity. *J. Biol. Chem.,*279:30817–30822.

[67] Civitarese AE et al. (2004) Adiponectin receptors gene expression and insulin sensitivity in non-diabetic Mexican Americans with or without a family history of type 2 diabetes. Diabetologia. 47:816–820.

[68] Harald S et al. (2004) Expression of adiponectin receptor mRNA in human skeletal muscle cells is related to in vivo parameters of glucose and lipid metabolism. *Diabetes,*53:2195–2201.

[69] Samal B, Sun Y, Stearns G, Xie C, Suggs S, McNiece I (1994) Cloning and characterization of the cDNA encoding a novel human pre-B-cell colony-enhancing factor. *Mol. Cell Biol.,* 14:1431–1437.

[70] Fukuhara A, Matsuda M, Nishizawa M, Segawa K, Tanaka M, Kishimoto K, Matsuki Y, Murakami M, Ichisaka T, Murakami H, Watanabe E, Takagi T, Akiyoshi M, Ohtsubo T, Kihara S, Yamashita S, Makishima M, Funahashi T, Yamanaka S, Hiramatsu R, Matsuzawa Y, Shimomura I (2005) Visfatin: aprotein secreted by visceral fat that mimics the effects of insulin. *Science,* 307:426–430.

[71] Kim MK, Lee JH, Kim H, Park SJ, Kim SH, Kang GB, Lee YS, Kim JB, Kim KK, Suh SW et al. (2006) Crystal structure of visfatin/pre-B cell colony-enhancing factor 1/nicotinamide phosphoribosyltransferase, free and in complex with the anti-cancer agent FK-866. *Journal of MolecularBiology,* 362: 66–77.

[72] Garten A, Petzold S, Barnikol-Oettler A, Körner A, Thasler WE, Kratzsch J, Kiess W, Gebhardt R (2010) Nicotinamide phosphoribosyltransferase (NAMPT/ PBEF/visfatin) is constitutively released from human hepatocytes. *Biochem. Biophys. Res. Commun.*, 391(1):376-81.

[73] Costford SR, Bajpeyi S, Pasarica M, Albarado DC, Thomas SC, Xie H, Church T, Jubrias SA, Conley KE, Smith SR (2010) Skeletal muscle nampt is induced by exercise in humans. *Am. J. Physiol. Endocrinol. Metab.*, 98: E117-E126.

[74] Revollo JR, Korner A, Mills KF, Satoh A, Wang T, Garten A, Dasgupta B, Sasaki Y, Wolberger C, Townsend RR et al. (2007) Nampt/PBEF/Visfatin regulates insulin secretion in beta cells as a systemic NAD biosynthetic enzyme. *Cell Metab.*, 6(5):363-375.

[75] Caton PW, Kieswich J, Yaqoob MM, Holness MJ, Sugden MC (2011) Nicotinamide mononucleotide protects against pro-inflammatory cytokine-mediated impairment of mouse islet function. *Diabetologia,* 54: 3083-3092.

[76] Brown JE, Onyango DJ, Ramanjaneya M, Conner AC, Patel ST, Dunmore SJ, Randeva HS (2010) Visfatin regulates insulin secretion, insulin receptor signalling and mRNA expression of diabetes-related genes in mouse pancreatic beta-cells. *J. Mol. Endocrinol.*, 44(3):171-8.

[77] Hida K, Wada J, Eguchi J, Zhang H, Baba M, Seida A et al. (2005)Visceral adipose tissue-derived serine protease inhibitor: a unique insulin-sensitizing adipocytokine in obesity. *Proc. Natl. Acad. Sci. USA,* 102:10610–10615.

[78] Youn BS, Klöting N, Kratzsch J, Lee N, Park JW, Song ES et al. (2008) Serum vaspin concentrations in human obesity and type 2 diabetes. *Diabetes,* 57:372–377.

[79] Wada J (2008) Vaspin and insulin resistance. *Rinsho. Byori.*, 56:705–711.

[80] Klöting N, Kovacs P, Kern M, Heiker JT, Fasshauer M, Schön MR et al. (2011) Central vaspin administration acutely reduces food intake and has sustained blood glucose-lowering effects. *Diabetologia,* 54:1819–1823

[81] Kempf K, Rose B, Illig T, Rathmann W, Strassburger K, Thorand B et al. (2010) Vaspin (SERPINA12) genotypes and risk of type 2 diabetes: results from the MONICA/KORA studies. *Exp. Clin. Endocrinol. Diabetes,* 118:184–189.

[82] Klöting N, Berndt J, Kralisch S, Kovacs P, Fasshauer M, Schön M et al. (2006) Vaspin gene expression in human adipose tissue: association with obesity and type 2 diabetes. *Biochem. Biophys. Res. Commun.,* 339:430–436.

[83] Körner A, Neef M, Friebe D, Erbs S, Kratzsch J, Dittrich K et al. (2011) Vaspin is related to gender, puberty and deteriorating insulin sensitivity in children. *Int. J. Obes. Lond.,* 35:578–586.

[84] Meyer-Hoffert U (2009) Reddish, scaly, and itchy: how proteases and their inhibitors contribute to inflammatory skin diseases. *Arch. Immunol. Ther. Exp.,* 57:345–354.

[85] Fain JN, Buehrer B, Bahouth SW, Tichansky DS, Madan AK (2008) Comparison of messenger RNA distribution for 60 proteins in fat cells vs the nonfat cells of human omental adipose tissue. *Metabolism,* 57:1005–1015.

[86] Tan BL, Heutling D, Chen J, Farhatullah S, Adya R, Keay SD, Kennedy SR, Lehnert H, Randeva HS (2008) Metformin decreases the adipokine vaspin in overweight women with polycystic ovary syndrome concomitant with improvement in insulin sensitivity and a decrease in insulin resistance. *Diabetes,* 57:1501–1507.

[87] Handisurya A, Riedl M, Vila G, Maier C, Clodi M, Prikoszovich T et al. (2010) Serum vaspin concentrations in relation to insulin sensitivity following RYGB-induced weight loss. *Obes. Surg.,* 20:198–203.

[88] von Loeffelholz C, Möhlig M, Arafat AM, Isken F, Spranger J, Mai K, Randeva HS, Pfeiffer AF, Weickert MO (2010) Circulating vaspin is unrelated to insulin sensitivity in a cohort of nondiabetic humans. *Eur. J. Endocrinol.,* 162:507–513.

[89] Seeger J, Ziegelmeier M, Bachmann A, Lössner U, Kratzsch J, Blüher M et al. (2008) Serum levels of the adipokine vaspin in relation to metabolic and renal parameters. *J. Clin. Endocrinol. Metab.,* 93:247–251.

[90] Akbarzadeh S, Nabipour I, Jafari SM, Movahed A, Motamed N, Assadi M, et al.

[91] (2012) Serum visfatin and vaspin levels in normoglycemic first-degree relatives of Iranian patients with type 2 diabetes mellitus. *Diabetes Res. Clin. Pract.,* 95(1):132–8.

[92] Cinar SN, Gülçelik NE, Aydín K, Akín S, Usman A, Gürlek A (2011) Serum vaspin levels in hypothyroid patients. *Eur. J. Endocrinol.,* 165: 563–569.

[93] Lee DK, Cheng R, Nguyen T, Fan T, Kariyawasam AP, Liu Y et al. (2000) Characterization of apelin, the ligand for the APJ receptor. *J. Neurochem.,* 74, 34–41.

[94] Cox CM, D'Agostino SL, Miller MK, Heimark RL, Krieget PA (2006) Apelin, the ligand for the endothelial G-protein-coupled receptor, APJ, is a potent angiogenic factor required for normal vascular development of the frog embryo. *Dev. Biol.,* 296:177–189.

[95] Kawamata Y, Habata Y, Fukusumi S, Hosoya M, Fujii R, Hinuma S et al. (2001) Molecular properties of apelin: tissue distribution and receptor binding. *Biochim. Biophys. Acta.,* 1538:162–171.

[96] Masri B, Knibiehler B, Audigier Y (2005) Apelin signalling: a promising pathway from cloning to pharmacology. *Cell Signal.,* 17:415–26.

[97] Carpéné C, Dray C, Attané C, Valet P, Portillo MP, Churruca I et al. (2007) Expanding role for the apelin/APJ system in physiopathology. *J. Physiol. Biochem.,* 63:359–373.

[98] Habata Y, Fujii R, Hosoya M, Fukusumi S, Kawamata Y, Hinuma S et al. (1999) Apelin, the natural ligand of the orphan receptor APJ, is abundantly secreted in the colostrums. *Biochim. Biophys. Acta.,* 1452:25–35.

[99] Tatemoto K, Hosoya M, Habata Y, Fujii R, Kakegawa T, Zou MX et al. (1998) Isolation and characterization of a novel endogenous peptide ligand for the human APJ receptor. *Biochem. Biophys. Res. Commun.,* 251:471–476.

[100] Saint-Geniez M, Masri B, Malecaze F, Knibiehler B, Audigier Y (2002) Expression of the murine msr/apj receptor and its ligand apelin is upregulated during formation of the retinal vessels. *Mech. Dev.,* 110:183–186.

[101] Castan-Laurell I, Dray C, Attané C, Duparc T, Knauf C, Valet Ph (2011) Apelin, diabetes, and obesity. *Endocrine,* 40:1–9.

[102] Dray C, Knauf C, Daviaud D, Waget A, Boucher J, Buléon M (2008) Apelin stimulates glucose utilization in normal and obese insulin-resistant mice. *Cell Metab.,* 8:437–445.

[103] Rayalam S, Della-Fera MA, Krieg PA, Cox CM, Robins A, Baile CA (2008) A putative role for apelin in the etiology of obesity. *Biochem. Biophys. Res. Commun.,* 368:815–9.

[104] Sörhede Winzell M, Magnusson C, Ahrén B (2005) The apj receptor is expressed in pancreatic islets and its ligand, apelin, inhibits insulin secretion in mice. *Regul. Pept.,* 131:12–7.

[105] Attané C, Foussal C, Le Gonidec S, Benani A, Daviaud D, Wanecq E et al. (2012) Apelin treatment increases complete fatty acid oxidation, mitochondrial oxidative capacity, and biogenesis in muscle of insulin-resistant mice. *Diabetes,* 61:310–320.

[106] Yue P, Jin H, Aillaud M, Deng AC, Azuma J, Tomoko A (2010) Apelin is necessary for the maintenance of insulin sensitivity. *Am. J. Physiol. Endocrinol. Metab.,* 298:E59–E67.

[107] Yue P, Jin H, Xu S, Aillaud M, Deng AC, Azuma J et al. (2011) Apelin decreases lipolysis via Gq, Gi, and AMPK- dependent mechanisms. *Endocrinology,* 152:59–68.

[108] Kim JA, Wei Y, Sowerset JR (2008) Role of mitochondrial dysfunction in insulin resistance. *Circ. Res.,* 102:401–414.

[109] Hegarty BD, Turner N, Cooney GJ, Kraegen EW (2009) Insulin resistance and fuel homeostasis: the role of AMP-activated protein kinase. *Acta. Physiol.,* (Oxf.) 196:129–145.

[110] Scarpulla RC (2008) Transcriptional paradigms in mammalian mitochondrial biogenesis and function. Physiol Rev 88:611–638.

[111] Boucher J, Masri B, Daviaud D, Gesta S, Guigne C, Mazzucotelli A et al. (2005) Apelin, a newly identified adipokine up-regulated by insulin and obesity. *Endocrinology,* 146:1764–1771.

[112] Heinonen MV, Purhonen AK, Miettinen P, Paakkonen M, Pirinen E, Alhava E, et al. (2005) Apelin, orexin-A and leptin plasma levels in morbid obesity and effect of gastric banding. *Regul. Peptides,* 130:7–13.

[113] Li L, Yang G, Li Q, Tang Y, Yang M, Yang H, Li K (2006) Changes and relations of circulating visfatin, apelin, and resistin levels in normal, impaired glucose tolerance, and type 2 diabetic subjects. *Exp. Clin. Endocr. Diab.,* 114:544–548.

[114] Soriguer F, Garrido-Sanchez L, Garcia-Serrano S, Garcia-Almeida JM, Garcia-Arnes J, Tinahones FJ et al. (2009) Apelin Levels Are Increased in Morbidly Obese Subjects with Type 2 Diabetes Mellitus. *Obes. Surg.,* 19:1574–1580.

[115] Castan-Laurell I, Vitkova M, Daviaud D, Dray D, Kovacikova M, Kovacova Z et al. (2008) Effect of hypocaloric-induced weight loss in obese women on plasma apelin and adipose tissue expression of apelin and AP. *Eur. J. Endocrinol.,* 158:905–910.

[116] Kadoglou NP, Tsanikidis H, Kapelouzou A, Vrabas I, Vitta I, Karayannacos PE, et al. (2010) Effects of rosiglitazone and metformin treatment on apelin, visfatin, and ghrelin levels in patients with type 2 diabetes mellitus. *Metabolism,* 59:373–379.

[117] Kojima M, Hosoda H, Date Y, Nakazato M, Matsuo H, Kangawa K (1999) Ghrelin is a growth-hormone-releasing acylated peptide from stomach. *Nature,* 402: 656-660.

[118] Domonvilelle CC, Bjorkqvist M, Sandvik AK, Bakke I, Zhao CM, Chen D et al. (2001) A-like cells in the rat stomach contain ghrelin and do not operate under gastrin control. *Regulat. Peptides,* 99: 141-150.

[119] Ianelli A, Dainese R, Piche T (2008) Laparoscopic sleeve gastrectomy for morbid obesity. *World J. Gastroenterol.,* 14:821–7.

[120] Korbonits M, Grossman AB (2004) Ghrelin: update on a novel hormonal system. *Eur. J. Endocrinol.,* 1:S67–S70.

[121] Seoane LM, Lopez M, Tovar S, Casanueva FF, Senaris R, Dieguez C (2003) Agouti-related peptide, neuropeptide Y, and somatostatin-producing neurons are targets for ghrelin actions in the rat hypothalamus. *Endocrinology,* 144:544–551.

[122] Cowley MA, Smith RG, Diano S, Tschop M, Pronchuk N, Grove KL et al. (2003) The distribution and mechanism of action of ghrelin in the CNS demonstrates a novel hypothalamic circuit regulating energy homeostasis. *Neuron,* 37:649–661.

[123] Egecioglu E, Stenstrom B, Pinnock SB, Tung LY, Dornonville dlC, Lindqvist A et al. (2008) Hypothalamic gene expression following ghrelin therapy to gastrectomized rodents. *Regul. Pept.,* 146:176–182.

[124] Minokoshi Y, Alquier T, Furukawa N, Kim YB, Lee A, Xue B et al. (2004) AMP-kinase regulates food intake by responding to hormonal and nutrient signals in the hypothalamus. *Nature,* 428:569–574.

[125] Kola B, Hubina E, Tucci SA, Kirkham TC, Garcia EA, Mitchell SE et al. (2005) Cannabinoids and ghrelin have both central and peripheral metabolic and cardiac effects via AMP-activated protein kinase. *J. Biol. Chem.,* 280:25196–25201.

[126] Kola B, Farkas I, Christ-Crain M, Wittmann G, Lolli F, Amin F et al. (2008) The orexigenic effect of ghrelin is mediated through central activation of the endogenous cannabinoid system. *PLoS One,* 3(3): e1797.

[127] Anderson KA, Ribar TJ, Lin F, Noeldner PK, Green MF, Muehlbauer MJ et al. (2008) Hypothalamic CaMKK2 contributes to the regulation of energy balance. *Cell Metab.,* 7:377–388.

[128] Kola B, Korbonits M (2009) Shedding light on the intricate puzzle of ghrelin's effects on appetite regulation. *J. Endocrinol.,* 202:191–198.

[129] Tschop M, Weyer C, Tataranni PA, Devanarayan V, Ravussin E, Heiman ML (2001) Circulating ghrelin levels are decreased in human obesity. *Diabetes,* 50:707–709.

[130] Briggs DI, Enriori PJ, Lemus MB, Cowley MA, Andrews ZB (2010) Diet-induced obesity causes ghrelin resistance in arcuate NPY/AgRP neurons. *Endocrinology,* 151:4745–4755.

[131] Geloneze B, Tambascia MA, Pilla VF, Geloneze SR, Repetto EM, Pareja JC (2003) Ghrelin: a gut hormone: effect of gastric bypass surgery. *Obes. Surg.,* 13:17–22.

[132] Cummings DE, Overduin J, Foster-Schubert KE (2004) Gastric bypass for obesity: mechanisms of weight loss and diabetes resolution. *J. Clin. Endocrinol. Metab.,* 89:2608 –15.

[133] Blackburn GL (2005) Solutions in weight control: lessons from gastric *surgery Am. J. Clin. Nutr.,*82:248S–52S.

[134] Tymitz K, Engel A, McDonough S, Hendy MP, Kerlakian G (2010) Changes in Ghrelin Levels Following Bariatric Surgery: Review of the Literature. *Obes. Surg.,* 21:125–130.

In: Bariatric Surgery
Editor: Christos R. Iavazzo
ISBN: 978-1-62618-995-9

Chapter III

Surgical Anatomy and Bariatric Surgery

Khaled Hamdan[1] and Omar Khan[2]
[1]Brighton and Sussex University Hospitals, Brighton, England, UK
[2]Department of Upper GI Surgery, St George's Healthcare NHS Trust, London, UK

Abstract

Bariatric surgery is technically demanding surgery and knowledge of the normal anatomy of the gastrointestinal tract and the alterations after bariatric surgery are important for all those involved in bariatric surgery and also for those who may be involved with dealing with complications that require surgical intervention. This chapter outlines the anatomical parts that are relevant to bariatric surgery including the abdominal wall, hiatus, stomach duodenum and small intestine. It also describes the relevance of the anatomical features of each part to the operative steps of procedures such as gastric bypass, gastric banding and sleeve gastrectomy. Detailed knowledge of the anatomical alterations particularly after gastric bypass surgery is also important in understanding and surgically dealing with certain complications such as internal herniation through mesenteric defects which is dealt with some details in this chapter.

Introduction

Bariatric surgery is technically demanding surgery requiring meticulous attention to detail. This is particularly true of laparoscopic procedures which now make up the overwhelming majority of cases internationally [1]. Sound knowledge of the normal anatomy of the gastrointestinal tract and the anatomical alterations after bariatric surgery are important for all those involved in bariatric surgery and also for those who may be involved with dealing with complications that require surgical intervention. This chapter outlines the anatomy of the relevant anatomical parts of the gastrointestinal tract and abdominal wall and their relevance to the bariatric procedures currently in common use.

Laparoscopic Port Placement: Anatomical Considerations

Detailed knowledge of the anatomy of the anterior abdominal wall is essential in order to correctly place the ports and avoid injury to important structures in the anterior abdominal wall and abdominal cavity. This knowledge of the anatomy should be coupled with a thorough understanding of the general principles that apply to entering the peritoneal cavity which include:

1) The ports must be placed in such a way as to prevent significant hemorrhage of the abdominal wall
2) The ports must be placed in a suitable position to allow manipulation of the appropriate viscera depending on the type of bariatric procedure. It is important to appreciate that due to the weight of the abdominal wall fat, the position of the umbilicus may not always be where it is expected and therefore this cannot be relied upon as a useful landmark.
3) The ports act as rigid portal which can restrict the freedom of movement of instruments- this is of particular importance in bariatric surgery due to the thickness of the abdominal wall.

With regards to gaining access to the peritoneal cavity several techniques have described. These include the closed Veress needle technique and the use of specially designed optical trocars such as Visiport© and Endopath Excel© which, in combination of a laparoscope, provide direct examination of the abdominal layers as they are traversed. Although the traditional open Hasson technique is still being used by some surgeons this technique is cumbersome in obese patients due to the thickness of the abdominal wall fat. Regardless of the method of entry, it is important to ensure that the patient is in the supine position without tilt, rotation or Trendelenburg positioning to avoid distortion of the abdominal wall topography and disorientation related to the intra-abdominal anatomy.

The umbilicus is a typical site of insertion for both the Veress needle and open Hasson technique. Alternatively, many prefer the Palmer's point for inserting the veress needle or optical ports as this has been found to be a safe and quick method for gaining entry into the abdominal cavity [2-4]. Palmer's point is located in the left subcostal margin between the mid-clavicular and anterior axillary lines (Figure 1).

Access through this site is facilitated by the fact that the abdominal wall layers are tethered against the lower rib cage. It is important to note that the Veress needle or optical trocar should be inserted perpendicular to the abdominal wall in order to avoid damage to the superior epigastric vessels which usually run medial to Palmer's point. Once pneumperitoneum is established the insertion of the rest of the trocars should be done under direct vision to avoid injury to intra-abdominal structures.

The anticipated use of these ports should be carefully considered by the surgeon and considerable experience is often required to ensure that the ports are positioned and angled in such way to maximise the freedom of movement for each port and to avoid frustration particularly in the early stages of performing bariatric procedures.

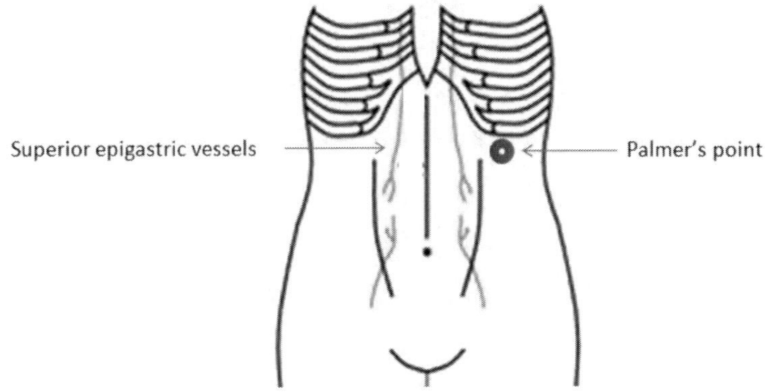

Figure 1. Schematic drawing showing the correct site of insertion of veress needle or optical trocar at Palmer's point and the relationship of the epigastric vessels.

Despite taking the above precautions there is an appreciable risk of injury irrespective of the technique used to gain entry the peritoneal cavity. The pattern of access injury varies with the site and technique chosen and immediate recognition of these injuries is important to reduce morbidity and mortality [5]. Typical injuries from using the umbilicus as a site of entry include damage to major vascular structures and bowel laceration particularly the transverse colon [6]. Delayed diagnosis of these injuries often results in exsanguination, abscess formation, peritonitis and death [7]. Access at Palmer's point can lead to damage to the left lobe if the liver or the spleen. Injury to omental or epigastric vessels can cause troublesome hemorrhage which, due to vasoconstriction, may not declare itself until after the surgery is over.

The Hiatus and Intra-Abdominal Esophagus

Dissection in the vicinity of the hiatus is a prerequisite for most bariatric procedures including gastric bypass, gastric band insertion and sleeve gastrectomy and therefore thorough knowledge of the anatomy of this rather complex region is required.

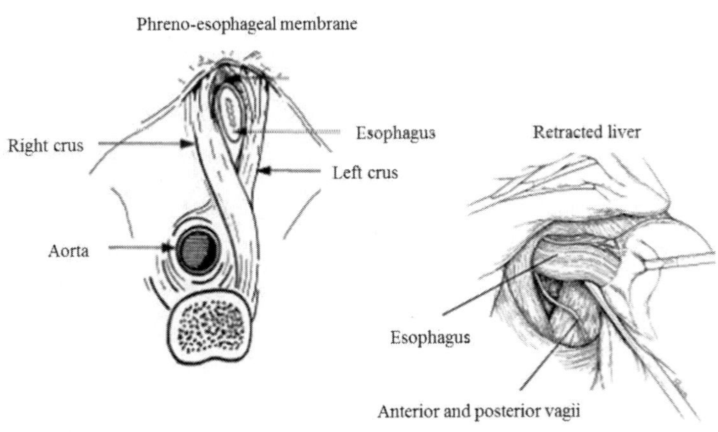

Figure 2. Schematic drawings showing the anatomical relations of the abdominal esophagus.

The oesophagus passes through the diaphragmatic hiatus and extends downwards and to the left to end at the gastro-esophageal junction which, in the absence of hiatus hernia, lies below the diaphragm. The intra-abdominal esophagus is about 0. 5-3 cm in length and is partially covered by peritoneum anteriorly and laterally on the left side. The anterior vagal nerve and the phreno-esophageal ligament lie anteriorly and the decussation of the left and right crura, the posterior vagal nerve and abdominal aorta lie posteriorly. To the right there are the right crus, caudate lobe and, more postero-laterally, the inferior vena cava while on the left there are the right crus and fundus of the stomach (Figure 2). The phrenic vessels course on the surface of the diaphragm close to the hiatus and if care is not taken during liver retraction and instrumentation these vessels can cause much unwanted bleeding. The Left phrenic vessels usually pass behind the esophagus but occasionally the vein passes anterior to it to terminate in the inferior vena cava.

The Stomach

Central to all bariatric procedures is the safe dissection, and if required, mobilisation and transaction of the stomach and therefore it is important to be familiar with the detailed anatomy of this part of the gastrointestinal tract. The stomach is described as having a lesser and a greater curvature which divide the stomach into an anterior and posterior surface. The lesser curvaturecontinues from the right border of the oesophagus and terminates at the pylorus.

The lesser omentum is attached to the lesser curvature. The incisura angularis is a prominent notch on the distal part of the lesser curvature. The left border of the oesophagus joins the stomach at an acute angle called the angle of His or the incisura cardiaca. From here the greater curvature arches over the fundus of the stomach and descends downwards and to the right to end at the pylorus. The sulcus intermedius is a slight groove on the greater curvature which lies roughly about 2-3 cm from the pylorus (Figure 3). The stomach is divided into 4 distinct parts. As the esophagus descends through the hiatus it opens into the stomach at the cardiac orifice which immediately leads to the cardia. The part of the stomach that lies above a line that passes horizontally across the cardia is known as the fundus. The body of the stomach lies between this line and the line joining the sulcus intermedius and incisura cardiaca. Distal to this lies the pyloric antrum which terminates at the gastroduodenal junction or the pyloric ring.

The pyloric ring represents the transition point between the thick wall of the stomach and the thin wall of the first part of the duodenum. It can be easily palpated with the fingers or by sweeping a grasper over it during laparoscopic surgery. Identification of the pyloric ring may be further aided by the presence of the pre-pyloric vein of Mayo which course over its anterior surface to drain into the right gastric vein.

A step common to most bariatric procedures involves dissection in the region of the fundus and cardia. This usually begins at the angle of His and requires gentle retraction of the fundus inferiorly and to the right and division of the peritoneum at the angle of His and fundus. This reveals Belsey's or sub-hiatal fat pad which overlies and often obscures the angle of His. This fat pad usually contains an artery, often referred to as Belsey's artery, which forms a collateral channel between the left gastric and left inferior phrenic artery.

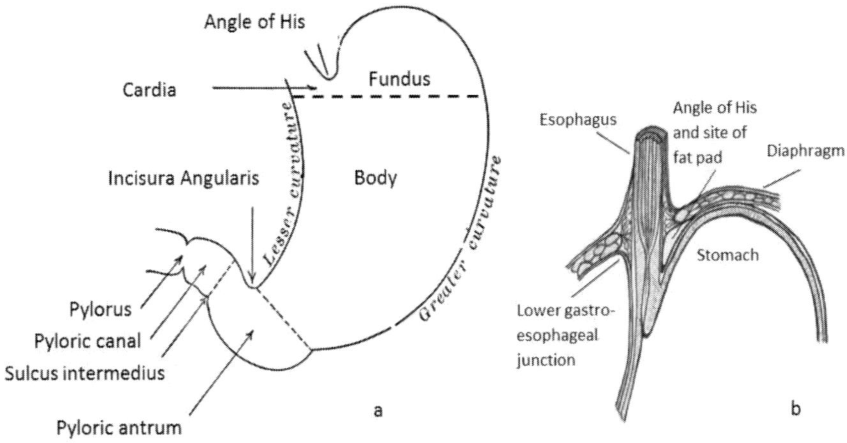

Figure 3. Schematic drawings showing the important anatomical parts of the stomach (a) and the detailed anatomy of the esophago-gastric region (b).

This artery runs transversely across the gastro-esophageal junction and dissection of the fat pad therefore requires meticulous hemostasis to avoid bleeding. Some surgeons prefer to excise Belsey's fat pad in order to improve visualisation of the angle of His and facilitate subsequent dissection. In the case of laparoscopic adjustable gastric banding excision of the fat pad may help achieve better exposure of the wall of the fundus thus allowing for more accurate placement of the sutures during gastric wall plication over the band. Furthermore, some surgeons believe that this step may minimise the risk of postoperative acute obstruction after gastric banding while others argue that this manoeuvre is associated with a higher incidence of oesophageal injury [8].

Structure of the Stomach Wall and Gastric Motility

The stomach wall is composed of 4 distinct layers namely the adventia or serosa, the muscularis externa, the submucosa and mucosa. The adventitia is a mesothelial layer that represents the visceral peritoneal covering of the stomach. Both anterior and posterior layers of the stomach unite to form the lesser omentum to the right and the greater omentum to the left. The posterior surface of the stomach is covered by peritoneum except over a small area close to the cardiac orifice which lies in opposition with the diaphragm and the upper part of the suprarenal gland. The muscularis externa, mainly composed of smooth muscle fibres, is further subdivided into an outer longitudinal, middle circular and inner oblique layer. The submucosa contains elastin fibres, vessels, lymphatics and Meissner's nerve plexus. The mucosa is the inner most layer of the wall of the stomach and is subdivided into muscularis mucosa, lamina propria and epithelial layer. The thickest part of the stomach wall is in the antrum- this has implication in terms of the choice of stapler used during sleeve gastrectomy.

Gastric motility is mainly controlled by both neural and hormonal mechanisms. The contractile waves of the stomach wall are initiated by a pacemaker that is located in the longitudinal muscle in the area of the cardia and fundus [9]. Gastric distension activates stretch receptors which in turn initiate depolarisation waves at a rate of 3/minute.

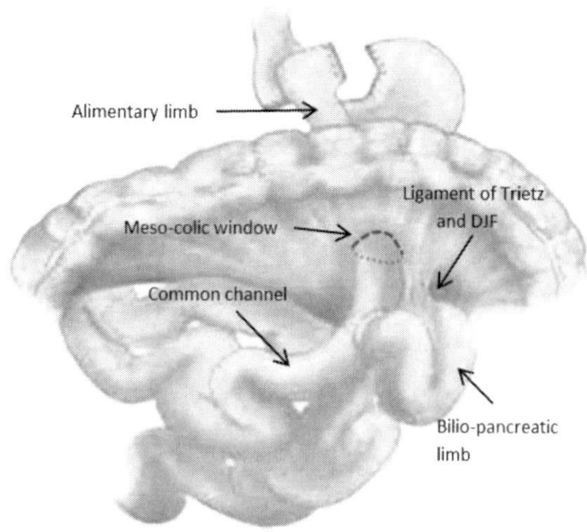

Figure 4. Anatomical landmarks in RYGB.

These waves propagate from the fundus through the body to the antrum. The force of contraction of these waves increases from the fundus with its thin muscular layer to reach a maximum at the pylorus. The function of these contractile waves is churn and mix food in the pyloric antrum and empty some of the chyme into the duodenum. Stomach emptying is augmented by vagal stimulation and various hormones such as gastrin,GIP and cholecystokinin. Sympathetic stimulation on the other hand leads to a reduction in gastric contractility and emptying. The anterior and posterior vagal trunks course distally to pass through the hiatus of the diaphragm each splitting into two branches at the level of the cardia. The anterior vagal trunk branches into the hepatic and anterior gastric nerves. The hepatic branch passes to the right in the lesser omentum giving off a branch that turns downward to supply the pylorus and first part of the duodenum.

The anterior gastric branch descends along the lesser curvature to supply the anterior gastric wall. From the posterior vagal trunk arise the celiac branch which passes to the celiac plexus and the posterior gastric branch that supplies branches to the posterior gastric wall. The anterior and posterior gastric branches course distally 0. 5-1. 0cm from the lesser curvature giving off branches to the stomach walls in what is commonly referred to as thenerves of Latarjetor “Crow’s foot”. .

The Lesser Omentum

The hepatogastric or lesser omentum extends from the infero-posterior surface of the liver and portahepatis to the lesser curvature of the stomach. The hepato-duodenal ligament which forms the free edge of the lesser omentum extends from the liver to the first part of the duodenum and it contains the hepatic triad which is composed of the hepatic artery, portal vein and common bile duct. Behind this free edge is the epiploic foramen of Winslow which leads into the lesser sac.

Visually, the lesser omentum is divided into a proximal denser portion, the pas condensa, and a transparent portion, the pars flacida. This latter part is the site of dissection in the pars flacida technique that is used in laparoscopic adjustable gastric banding. Embedded in the lesser omentum are the left and right gastric vessels, lymph nodes, branches of the vagal nerves including the hepatic division and the anterior and posterior gastric branches (nerves of Latarjet) and,in 25% of individuals, an accessory left hepatic artery (see below).

The most important structure in the lesser omentumto be aware of in bariatric surgery is the left gastric artery which is the smallest branch of the celiac axis. The artery first runs superiorly then turns anteriorly to approach the gastro-oesophageal junction where it gives off branches to the distal esophagus.

The main trunk of the artery courses inferiorly in the lesser omentum to run parallel to the lesser curvature where it terminates by forming anastomoses with branches of the right gastric artery. In a quarter of cases the left gastric artery gives rise to an accessoray left hepatic artery which replaces the main left hepatic artery in 10% of people. The posterior gastric vessels which are branches of the splenic vessels are reported to be present in as many as 70% of individuals. These vessels supply the proximal part of the posterior surface of the stomach and their hidden and often inconsistent location may lead to dangerous bleeding during the dissection of this area.

In the case of laparoscopic gastric banding the pars flacida part of the lesser omentum is incised to reveal the caudate lobe and the right crus. The inferior vena cava can also be seen to lie behind the caudate lobe and to the right of the right crus and great care should be taken not to damage it. It is often not necessary to extend pars flacida incision proximally into the pars condensa particularly if a large aberrant or replaced hepatic artery is to be divided. However, in some cases this artery and the accompanying hepatic branch of the anterior vagal nerve may be divided in order to achieve better views of the right crus. Sacrificing this nerve has not been shown to result in serious consequences although there are reports of increased incidence of cholecystolethiasis after its division [10-12].

Once a window in the lesser omentum is created the right crus is identified and a retrogastric tunnel is created starting at the anterior surface of the right crus at its lower limit. A useful landmark for initiating the dissection is a small transverse fat pad on the anterior aspect of the right crus. This useful landmark often contains a small venous tributary that runs across the junction between the two crura. Once a small window is created posterior dissection is then continued with utmost care to avoid unwanted bleeding or damage to the posterior wall of the stomach. The dissection should be minimal and the grasper is gently advanced in the direction of the angle of His. Inaccurate angulation of the grasper can lead to serious bleeding from the spleen or to inadvertent dissection into the substance of the left crus or the left pleural space.

In the case of RYGB dissection should remain close to the lesser curvature of the stomach in the perigastric plane. A suitable point to start this dissection is the level of the second visible vessel about 5cm from the gastro-oesophageal junction. It is worth noting that the lesser omentum at this level may be quite thick and meticulous dissection close to the stomach wall is important to prevent bleeding from the often thin walled veins. Extending this dissection proximally should be avoided to reduce the risk of damaging the left gastric artery and subsequent devascularisation of the stomach pouch. In addition, excessive dissection or transection of the lesser omentum to facilitate access to the lesser sac may at least theoretically exacerbate symptoms of dumping syndrome after RYGB by causing damage to the anterior vagus nerve and its branches [13]. Dissection in the perigastric plane is facilitated by getting the assistant to grasp the stomach wall close to the area being dissected and attempting to roll the lesser curvature laterally while dissection progresses. From here the dissection is continued into the lesser sac where posterior adhesions may be encountered. Once this part of the stomach is transected with a linear stapler dissection is continued proximally towards the angle of His where further posterior adhesions and the distal extent of the fat pad are often encountered. From the anatomical point of view it is important to appreciate that at this level the posterior wall of the fundus is often lax which can lead to excessively large gastric pouch. This is simply avoided by careful inspection of the posterior wall of the stomach and by applying left and downward traction on the fundus before proceeding with dividing the stomach. It is also important to appreciate that the area behind the gastric pouch contains fatty tissue which is adherent to the posterior wall. This often needs to be cleared for 1-2 cm proximal to the staple line to facilitate the formation of the gastro-jejunal anastomosis but care should be taken not to damage the left gastric artery which is in the immediate vicinity.

The Greater Omentum

The anterior and posterior peritoneal layers of the stomach unite at the greater curvature to form the gastrosplenic (lienogastric) and gastrocolic ligaments. The gastrocolic ligament extends to the right to the first part of the duodenum and inferiorly to continue as the greater omentum. The short gastric arteries which are branches of the splenic artery or one of its divisions run in the gastrosplenic ligament to supply the fundus of the stomach. Within the wall the fundus rich submucosal anastomoses exist between these arteries and the left gastric and gastroepiploic. This means that the short gastric arteries can be divided with impunity without compromising the blood supply to the fundus. Traction on the gastrosplenic ligament and division of the short gastric vessels is required during sleeve gastrectomy and utmost care should be taken here to avoid bleeding. In addition excessive traction on the fundus during mobilisation of the angle of His and fundus should be avoided to prevent tearing of the delicate capsule of the spleen.

Division of the short gastric vessels and the gastro-colic ligament along the greater curvature to a point about 5-6 cm proximal to the pylorus provides wide access to the lesser sac and posterior surface of the stomach during sleeve gastrectomy. Here the transverse mesocolon and its blood vessels, namely the middle colic artery,can be damaged and a segment of the transverse colon may be devascularised if the correct plane is not adhered to. To avoid this upward lift on the stomach and downward traction on the transverse mesocolon is required. Elevating or reflecting the stomach often reveals filmy gastro-pancreatic adhesions which need to be divided in order to free the posterior wall of the stomach.

The Small Bowel

For procedures that have a malabsorbtive component, notably the RGBY and the duodenal switch, a great deal of care and attention is required when handling and measuring the small bowl. The length of the small intestine is extremely variable ranging from 10 to 30 feet and averaging about 22 feet. The first part of the duodenum continues from the pylorus with the common bile duct, portal vein, gastroduodenal artery and IVC passing posteriorly. The second part of the duodenum lies anterior to the right kidney and IVC and posterior to the transverse colon. The common bile and pancreatic ducts open into the left side of this part of the duodenum. The third part of the duodenum passes horizontally to the left anterior to the IVC and posterior to the superior mesenteric vein and artery. The fourth part of duodenum crosses the spine and the aorta and ends at the duodeno-jejunal flexure to the left of the aorta. The proximal part of the small bowel is referred to as the jejunum and the remainder is the ileum. The jejunum commences at the duodeno-jejunal flexure (DJF) and it is differentiated from the ileum by virtue of its origin at the DJF and by its larger diameter and thicker wall which is caused its thick mucosal folds (valvulaeconniventes). The DJF is fixed by a suspensory ligament (of Trietz). Accurate identification of the ligament of Trietz is essential before proceeding with bowel division and the formation of entero-enterostomy in patients undergoing RYGB. This requires reflection of the often fat laden omentum over the transverse colon which itself is retracted cephalad into the upper abdomen by the assistant (Figure 4). The length of mesentery measured from the mesenteric border of the intestine to the root of the mesentery does not normally exceed 20-25cm. Its origin from the posterior abdominal wall commences at the DJF and extends downwards and to the left for about 15 cm. The mesentery contains the superior mesenteric vessels, lymphatic channels, lymph nodes and autonomic nerve fibres. The mesentery of jejunum has fewer vascular arcades and longer and infrequent terminal branches compared to the ileum which in contrast has more arcades and shorter and more numerous terminal vessels. In patients with extreme central obesity the jejunal mesentery is often foreshortened and this may limit the ability of the surgeon to pull the alimentary limb up to the level of the gastric pouch without undue tension. In this situation the retrocolic route is the preferred technique for passing the alimentary limb posteriorly into the lesser sac and the gastric pouch during RYGB. This is best done by creating an opening in the anteriorly retracted mesocolon to the left of the middle colic vessels. If the middle colic vessels cannot be identified a useful landmark for making the opening is approximately 2-3 cm anterior and to the left of the ligament of Trietz (Figure 4). The blood supply of the small intestines is derived from branches of the superior mesenteric artery. The vasa recta are the terminal branches from the arches of the arcades that pass towards the mesenteric border of the small intestine to supply the bowel wall. An important feature of these vessels is that they do not anastomose or form collateral circulation. While this configuration ensures excellent blood supply to the metabolically active small intestine it means that division of these vasa recta will increase the likelihood of causing ischemia of the affected part of the bowel wall. It is therefore important to accurately identify these vessels and ensure that the mesentery is divided parallel and not across these vessels during RYGB.

RYGB- Limbs and Mesenteric Defects

The procedure of RYGB results in the development of several mesenteric which can potentially lead to the development of internal hernias (Figure 5).

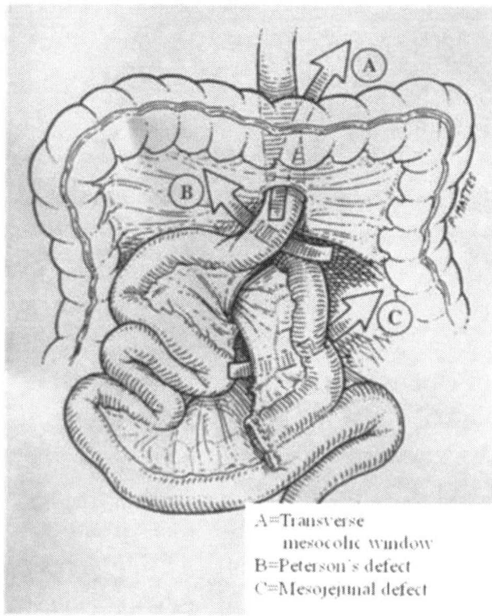

Figure 5. Mesenteric defects after RYGB.

Closure of these defects at the time of surgery may have a role in preventing the development of internal herniation which is considered to be the most common cause of intestinal obstruction after laparoscopic RYGB [14]. Understanding the origin and anatomical location of these defects is also important for the general surgeon who may be involved in managing patients presenting with intestinal obstruction or intermittent abdominal pain secondary to internal herniation.

The following is a brief description of how these mesenteric defects form. The procedure of RYGB involves the formation of 3 "limbs" – the Roux or alimentary limb which is anastomosed to the stomach pouch, the bilio-pancreatic (BP) limb which is anastomosed to the Roux limb and the common channel (CC) which continues to the terminal ileum and caecum. The first step involves the division of the jejunum and its mesentery some distance (50-100 cm) from the ligament of Trietz. This results in two free mesenteric edges; the proximal mesenteric edge which belongs to the BP limb and the distal mesenteric edge which belongs to the Roux limb.

The next step is forming the jejuno-jejunal anastomosis which involves joining the distal end of the BP limb to a point 70-150 cm from the proximal end of the Roux limb. This effectively brings the free mesenteric edge of the BP to lie against the flat surface of Roux limb mesentery thus creating a defect which is commonly referred to as the meso-jejunal mesenteric defect.

Once the gastric pouch is formed the gastro-jejunal anastomosis is constructed by pulling up the Roux limb either anterior to the transverse colon (the antecolic route) or through an opening in the mesocolon (the retrocolic route). In either case the free mesenteric edge of the Roux limb comes to lie against the transverse mesocolon thus creating a defect known as Peterson's window. In the case of using the retrocolic route the opening through the mesocolon results in another defect, the mesocolic defect, which is considered to be the most common site for internal herniation after RYGB.

References

[1] Reoch J, Mottillo S, Shimony A, Filion KB, Christou NV, Joseph L, Poirier P, Eisenberg MJ. Safety of laparoscopic vs open bariatric surgery: a systematic review and meta-analysis. *Arch. Surg.,* 2011 Nov;146(11):1314-22.

[2] Altun H, Banli O, Karakoyun R, Boyuk A, Okuducu M, Onur E, Memisoglu K. Direct trocar insertion technique for initial access in morbid obesity surgery: technique and results. SurgLaparoscEndoscPercutan Tech. 2010 Aug;20(4):228-30.

[3] Berch BR, Torquati A, Lutfi RE, Richards WO. Experience with the optical access trocar for safe and rapid entry in the performance of laparoscopic gastric bypass. *Surg. Endosc,* 2006 Aug;20(8):1238-41.

[4] Schwartz ML, Drew RL, Andersen JN. Induction of pneumoperitoneum in morbidly obese patients. *Obes.* Surg., 2003 Aug;13(4):601-4.

[5] Vilos GA, Ternamian A, Dempster J, Laberge PY, The Society of Obstetricians and Gynaecologists of Canada. Laparoscopic entry: a review of techniques, technologies, and complications. *J. Obstet. Gynaecol. Can.,* 2007 May;29(5):433-65.

[6] Podnos YD, Jimenez JC, Wilson SE, Stevens CM, Nguyen NT. Complications after laparoscopic gastric bypass: a review of 3464 cases. *Arch. Surg.,* 2003 Sep;138(9):957-61.

[7] Ahmad G, O'Flynn H, Duffy JM, Phillips K, Watson A. Laparoscopic entry techniques. *Cochrane Database Syst. Rev.,* 2012 Feb 15;2.

[8] Shen R, Ren CJ. Removal of peri-gastric fat prevents acute obstruction after Lap-Band surgery. *Obes. Surg.,* 2004 Feb;14(2):224-9.

[9] Rhee PL, Lee JY, Son HJ, Kim JJ, Rhee JC, Kim S, Koh SD, Hwang SJ, Sanders KM, Ward SM. Analysis of pacemaker activity in the human stomach. *J. Physiol.,* 2011 Dec 15;589(Pt 24):6105-18.

[10] Purdy M, Nykopp TK, Kainulainen S, Pääkkönen M. Division of the hepatic branch of the anterior vagus nerve in fundoplication: effects on gallbladder function. *Surg. Endosc.,* 2009 Sep;23(9):2143-6.

[11] Tomita R, Fujisaki S, Koshinaga T, Kusafuka T. Clinical assessments in patients ten years after pylorus-preserving gastrectomy with or without preserving both pyloric and hepatic branches of the vagal nerve for early gastric cancer. *Hepatogastroenterology,* 2010 Jul-Aug;57(101):984-8.

[12] Morton JM, Bowers SP, Lucktong TA, Mattar S, Bradshaw WA, Behrns KE, Koruda MJ, Herbst CA, McCartney W, Halkar RK, Smith CD, Farrell TM. Gallbladder function before and after fundoplication. *J. Gastrointest. Surg.,* 2002 Nov-Dec;6(6):806-10; discussion 810-11.

[13] Frantzides CT, Carlson MA, Shostrom VK, Roberts J, Stavropoulos G, Ayiomamitis G, Frantzides A. A survey of dumping symptomatology after gastric bypass with or without lesser omental transection. *Obes. Surg.,* 2011 Feb;21(2):186-93.

[14] Ballem N, Parikh R, Berber E, Siperstein A: Laparoscopic versus open ventral hernia repairs: 5-year recurrence rates. *Surg. Endosc.,* 2008; 22:1935-1940.

In: Bariatric Surgery
Editor: Christos R. Iavazzo
ISBN: 978-1-62618-995-9

Chapter IV

To Have or Not to Have the Ring Banded Roux-en-Y Gastric Bypass

W. Konrad Karcz
Department of Abdominal Surgery, Videosurgery Division,
Bariatric and Metabolic Surgical Center, University of Freiburg, Germany

Introduction

The evolution from the band to the silicone ring was observed in both vertical banded gastroplasty and banded gastric bypass. The silicone ring develops a pseudocapsule which leads to less adhesion and is much easier to remove than the band. A modification of the proximal gastric bypass by Fobi and Capella prevents dilation of the gastro-enteral anastomosis and of the adjacent small bowel with increased postoperative weight loss and significantly improved long-term weight maintenance.

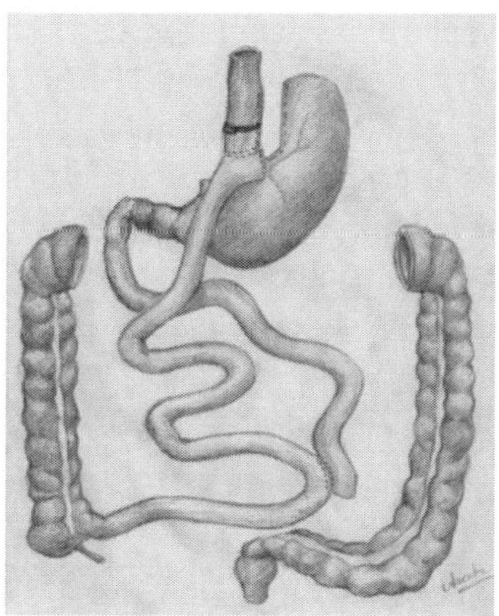

Figure 1. Schedule® of Banded Roux-en-Y Gastric Bypass (LBRYGB).

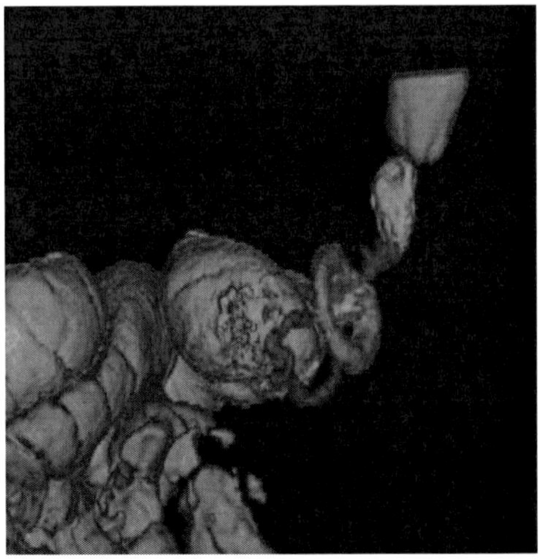

Figure 2. 3D volume rendering reconstruction of abdominal MSCT of a LBRYGB. Manual and semi-automatic segmentation techniques are applied to show the pouch (cyan), the Roux-limb (orange), the esophagus and intestine (blue), and the staple sutures (red).

We are currently waiting for results of multi-centre, prospective randomized studies that compare the banded to the conventional gastric bypass. Safety and feasibility are demonstrated by Fobi et al. in their published series of 50 consecutive patients with an in-creased excess weight loss of more than 70% and no increase of postoperative complications.

It is interesting that Fobi's modification of the gastric bypass is becoming more popular each year (Figure 1, 2). Need we be hesitant with regard to Silastic rings? How much we can profit from implantation and what do we have to risk? There are on the market several new products which could be implanted on the Stomach Pouch. All modern devices are made from silicone which made the implant safe and easy to remove.

Complications

There are many possible complications after proximal gastric bypass operations, only few of which are seen in combination with a Silastic rings. The incidence of regurgitation and the quality of eating is closely related to the ring size. Stubbs et al. reported that in 18 %, major restriction in the quality of eating occurred in a group of patients treated with a 5. 5 cm ring, whereas in groups with 6. 0 cm and 6. 5 cm rings only 8% and 4% respectively had similar problems. 29% of the patients Regurgitation occurred more than three times a week in 29% in the first group with 5. 5 cm and in only 14 % in the last one. The risk of developing chronic regurgitation is related to two independent factors, namely the lower esophageal sphincter function and the size of the silicone ring placed around the gastric pouch. The smaller the ring, the more frequent the chronic regurgitation. Hypotonia of the lower esophageal sphincter (the normal value 14-34 mmHg) increases the risk of chronic regurgitation. The chance is seven times greater compared to patients with normal lower esophagus sphincter pressure. Both LES hypotonia and a small band diameter increase the risk of frequent regurgitation. Patients with low LES pressure ought to receive alternative bariatric procedures, such as the Conventional RYGB or the BPD. Band erosion or migration into the gastric lumen after a Banded Gastric Bypass seem to be rather rare late complications. Most authors reported an incidence of around 0. 5%. Studies with larger patient collectives report a band erosion rate of 1. 63% (48 of 2,949 Patients). The incidence of erosion was lower (0. 92%) in primary operations. The following clinical symptoms appeared along with the pathology: weight regain (37. 5%), stenosis or obstruction (35. 4%), pain (18. 75%), bleeding (14. 58%). 89. 5% of patients lost the ring. In a 10-year observation of banded gastric bypass patients, Barroso found: 26 stenoses, 9 erosions, 2 spontaneous eliminations, 3 slippages, and two openings of the ring. The other very large group observed in the Elias Study presented 125 band's explantations in 138 medical, band-related events. Bands can be removed spontaneously through migration, per endoscopy, per laparoscopy or rarely by laparotomy. Some possible causes of band erosion are cited, like: constricting band, suturing the band to the stomach, imbricating the band with the stomach, and infection. Fobi proposed the mechanism of Band Errosion (BE), with the first step usually being an inflammation between the gastric wall and the band leading to band extrusion into the pouch lumen through stitch abscess formation and extrusion of the stitch. Afterwards, a dense fibrous reaction appears around the banded pouch.

Removal of the ring is combined with significant weight gain. Appreciable weight regain occurred in 43. 75% patients who underwent band removal, with an average of 14% excessive weight loss (EWL) regained. Primary replacement of the band is not recommended. As therapy guidelines, Fobi proposed: for asymptomatic patients the treatment can be waiting for spontaneous extrusion of the band and protone pump inhibitors (PPI) or H2-blockers. The management of choice is endoscopic removal of the band. If endoscopic removal is not feasible, which is especially the case when materials other than a silastic ring, such as non-absorbable sutures, were used, the band can be removed by a laparoscopic operation with intraoperative endoscopy. After laparoscopically performed RYGB, the erosion of non-dissolvable materials, such as Peri-Strips or silk sutures into the gastric pouch may occur. The most common presenting symptoms are abdominal pain, nausea, vomiting, dysphagia, and melena. The management of choice is therapeutic endoscopy which usually allows adequate management of most upper GI symptoms. Yu et al. show that the use of Vicryl sutures and Seamguard avoids foreign material erosion. In summary, the introduction of the silastic ring has reduced band-related complications. General bypass complications are comparable with those of the banded bypass. There are no ring-related lethal complications.

Ring Implantation Manual

All silicone rings can be introduced laparoscopicaly. The GaBP®Ring (Bariatric Solutions GmbH) (a pre-manufactured set with a prosthetic auto-locking band and a radiopaque marker made of implant-grade silicone rubber) seems to be the most useful and the smallest implant. It is placed around the pouch loosely about 2. 0 to 2. 5 cm from the end point of the pouch and 4 cm from the His angle. The preparation of the small curvature could be done with Maryland or scorpion forceps close to the stomach wall. Each silicone band develops a pseudocapsule that leads to less adhesion and is much easier to remove than other materials. The ring size ought to be 6. 0 to 6. 5 cm in circumference, which has a much better outcome in terms of quality of eating and ring migration. The pouch size is usually estimated at 10 to 25 ml. The ring is always fixed with non- resorbable sutures.

Mechanism of Action

Besides its restrictive role, it contributes to the reduction of undesirable side-effects, like dumping syndrome and foul flatulence. The banded bypass causes satiety and reduces caloric intake by delaying gastric emptying and inducing the satiation sensation even with low food intake. The silicone ring controls the diameter and area of the gastroenterostomy.

Redo Surgery with the Ring

The Redo-surgery made by Fobi on VBG patients with preservation of the band or the ring as a restriction lead to the development of the banded gastric bypass technique. If an insufficient loss of weight or even a regain of weight occurs and in case of insufficient restriction, a re-operation might be necessary. The precise diameter and anastomosis area estimation allows the surgeon to choose the better redo surgery strategy and to select the best operative option for his patients. It is proven that GE anastomosis dilatation is responsible for gaining weight. If the patient is able to tolerate the restriction amplification, there are still several surgical options. (Figure 3, 4). Endoscopic suturing with f. i. Stomafix or Anubis (STORZ GmbH) to tighten dilated gastric pouch is technically feasible and safe and may lead to weight loss for certain patients. Another logical therapy option is implantation of the GaBP Ring as a redo procedure which converts the conventional to the banded bypass. An analogous procedure with additional LA Gastric Banding to the Roux-en-Y GB was also proposed Bessler et al. . We therefore advise using rings of at least 6. 5 cm length and 7. 0 cm in Redo operations. The easy conversion between those two operations and better weight reduction results will probably influence the number of banded bypass procedures.

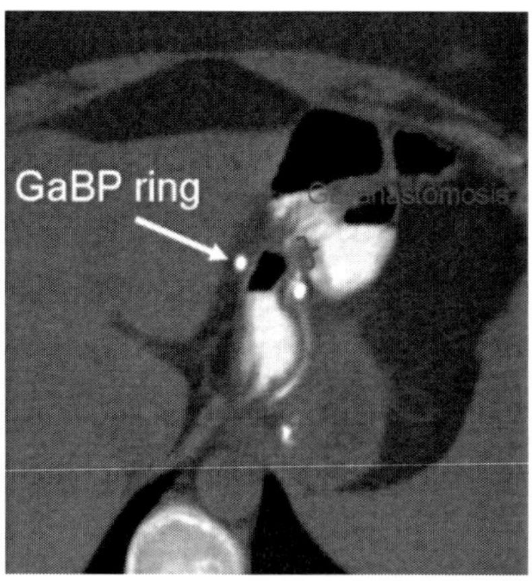

Figure 3. CT-Scan of abdominal cavity after LBRYGB with GE anastomosis stenosis after LBRYGB, the ring did not influence stenosis.

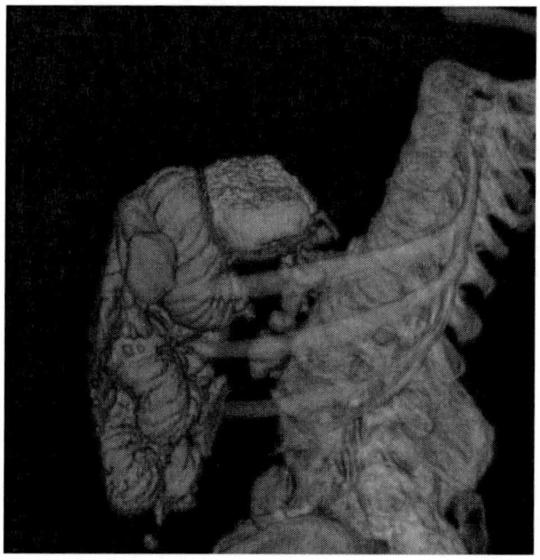

Figure 4. 3D volume rendering reconstruction of abdominal MSCT showing a dilatation of the stomach pouch (51cm^3) and GE anastomosis (Diameter 3. 4cm, area 10. 1cm^2). Manual and semi-automatic segmentation techniques are applied to show the pouch (green), the Roux-limb (orange), and the staple sutures (red).

Weight Loss Differences

The influence of the silastic ring on the percentage of excess weight loss within the first year was significant: between 81. 3 and 73. 5. EWL. After two years, the percentage ranged around 80%, and at 5 years follow-up a EWL of about 75% could be found. Only a slight weight regain of 2. 5% or 5% is observed between the second and fifth postoperative year, whereas a weight regain by LCRYGB of over 10% in the same period is reported. The EWL after conventional GB reached 58. 2% after five years in the best series. Bessler performed the first prospective study that directly compared the two operation methods. After the second or third postoperative year, the patient seems to adapt to the surgery and to suffer from its side-effects in lower intensity, which brings a tendency for some recovery of lost weight. But weight gain is very slight compared to the conventional gastric bypass.

References

[1] Fobi MAL. Placement of the GaBP Ring system in the Banded Gastric Bypass Operation. *Obes. Surg.,* 2005; 8: 1196 - 1201.

[2] Bessler M, Daud A, Kim, DiGiorgi M. Prospective randomized trial of banded versus nonbanded gastric bypass for the super obese: early results. Surg Obes Relat Dis. 2007 Jul-Aug;3 (4): 480-4; discussion 484-5. Epub 2007 Jun 4.

[3] Stubbs et al.: What ring size should be used in association with Vertical Gastric Bypass? *Obes. Surg. Obes. Surg.,* 2006; 16: 1298-1303. .

[4] Fobi MAL, Lee H, Igwe D et al. Band erosion: Incidence, Etiology, Management and Outcome after Banded Vertical Gastric Bypass. *Obes. Surg.,* 2001; 11: 699-707.

[5] Barroso FL, Leite Ma, Almeida Azet al. Problems with the silicone rings in the Fobi/ Campella Operations. *Oral. Presentation.,* 2007 IFSO Congress, Porto, Portugal.
[6] Elias OA, Garrido AB, Berti LV, Oliveira MR, Suguitani NB. Complications related to the ring after 7000 Roux-en-Y gastric bypass with silicone ring for the obesity treatment. *Oral. Presentation.,* 2007 IFSO Congress, Porto, Portugal.
[7] Karcz W, Küsters S, Koter E, et al. Redo Bariatric Surgery Influenced By 3D Volume Rendering Reconstruction of Abdominal MSCT. Submitted to Obesity Surgery June 2008.

In: Bariatric Surgery
Editor: Christos R. Iavazzo
ISBN: 978-1-62618-995-9

Chapter V

Postoperative Complications after Bariatric Surgery

***Ioannis D. Gkegkes*[1] *and Christos Iavazzo*[2]**
[1]Department of Surgery, Korinthos General Hospital, Korinthos, Greece
[2]Iaso Maternity Hospital, Athens, Greece

Abstract

There is a variety of complications that could arise following any of the bariatric surgical procedures that necessitate a more careful understanding of the specific anatomy of the operation performed (Table 1). According to the type of procedure performed, postoperative complications after surgical treatment of morbid obesity can be divided in immediate and in delayed.

Immediate Complications

Pulmonary embolism, anastomotic leak and bleeding are the most common immediate complications that are generally treated with by the operating team. Laboratory values and clinical data, such as an increased C-reactive protein and the tachycardia level, could be most of the times the only objective signs.

According to Assessment of Bariatric Surgery study, 4. 3% is the incidence of major adverse events in early postoperative period. [1] Even though these encouraging reports, bariatric surgery is associated with a number of complications that can be characterized as potentially fatal. Shock secondary to hemorrhage, sepsis from an anastomotic dehiscence and cardiopulmonary complications in high-risk comorbid population are some of the most serious consequences. According to national studies, 0. 34% is the estimated incidence of death following bariatric surgery, due to increased risk for thromboembolic events. [2,3] Therefore mechanical as well as pharmacological measures for deep vein thrombosis are normally practiced with the intention to reduce this specific risk. [4, 5]

Table 1. Main postoperative complications after bariatric surgery

Mechanism of action	Type of operation	Type of postoperative complications
Restrictive	Vertical banded gastroplasty	-band slippage -erosion of the band -port access site problems
	Adjustable gastric banding	
Largely Restrictive/Mildly Malabsorptive	Roux-en-Y gastric bypass	-incisional hernias -vomiting -bowel obstruction -gastrointestinal hemorrhage -malabsorption
Mildly Restrictive/ Largely Malabsorptive	Biliopancreatic diversion	-incisional hernias -bowel obstruction -malabsorption
	Duodenal switch	

Moreover one of the most grave complication in the surgical treatment of morbid obesity is gastrointestinal leak, which the procedure performed, could be ranging from 1%, for gastric banding, to 2%, for gastric bypass and sleeve gastrectomy. [6-8] Anastomotic sites and staple lines can be in the majority of times the origin of leaks while iatrogenic bowel injuries are less frequently responsible. [5] Conservative management is the indication only for leaks that can be controlled by a surgical drain, in a hemodynamically stable patients, while in contrary situations, a more aggressive approach that include surgical exploration should be indicated. Furthermore, in 1–4% of bariatric surgeries could be complicated by episodes of early bleeding, taking into consideration both intraluminal and intraperitoneal events. [5] Volume resuscitation, transfusion of blood products and close clinical observation could be in the majority of the cases essential for early recognition of hemodynamic instability that imposes urgent surgical intervention. [9-11]

Late Complications

Late Complications after Restrictive Procedures

Laparoscopic adjustable gastric banding (LAGB) is one of the most popular bariatric operations probably due to the fact that it is a relatively simple procedure with extremely low rates of early morbidity and mortality (30-day) compared with other procedures such as Roux-en-Y gastric bypass (RYGB). [12, 13] Nevertheless, the rate of reoperation as well as the incidence of late complications could reach 10–20 per cent. Additionally, band slippage and erosion are the two major complications of LAGB. Up to 15–20 per cent of patients could occur the band slippage, which is more often takes place distally. [14, 15] Patients' history reveals frequently acid reflux, regurgitation or sense of dysphagia as well as an obstructive symptomatology with the presence of upper abdominal pain, occurring some time after the procedure.

In addition, a distal migration or abnormal orientation of the band can be evident in a plain abdominal X-ray and more particularly on oblique views. Furthermore, in contrast study of the upper gastrointestinal, is more likely to show evidence of malposition of the band as well as a dilatation in the proximal pouch combined with obstruction. Generally, a well-positioned gastric band rests below the gastro-oesophageal junction with an inclination of about 45° according to the spine. [16]

Slipped band could presented in a relative horizontal position, a dilatation of gastric pouch proximal to band, combined with little contrast passing through it. These radiological findings pose the differential diagnosis between band slippage and the less severe problem of pouch dilatation, condition with which patients often tend to present less acutely with , decreased satiety, acid reflux symptoms and occasionally pain located at the left upper quadrant but no obstructive symptoms.

The first step in the management of band slippage is the without delay deflation. It can be achieved by locating the port with two fingers while at the same time advancing a non-coring (Huber needle) or else a spinal needle until it hits the steel plate at the back of the port. [12] The needle is immediately withdrawn, when fluid is withdrawn and the band is completely deflated. This procedure can also be conducted under ultrasound guidance or fluoroscopy. If the success of this procedure has as result the symptomatic relief, it is reasonable to do nothing proposing a review by a bariatric surgeon.

On the other hand, if this procedure is unsuccessful, the most appropriate is to consider also the possibility of the rare but serious complication of gastric necrosis which requires urgent exploratory laparoscopy or laparotomy. [17] The band should be removed completely, if there is absence of an experienced surgeon. The procedure requires cautiously the division of the fibrotic scars over the band, eviting gastric or esophageal tissue injury. An alternative but also technically challenging procedure is to unbuckle the band and leave it at the site for later adjustment by a bariatric surgeon. [12, 18, 19]

The erosion of gastric band takes place in up to 4 per cent of patients with LAGB and is presented usually as a late complication caused by ischemia due to pressure on the gastric wall. [20, 21] Patients with band erosion may be asymptomatic or with non-specific abdominal pain, weight loss gastrointestinal bleeding as well as abdominal sepsis. Gastrointestinal endoscopy shows partial- or full-thickness erosion, and barium swallow may evidentiate the flow of contrast around the part of the band that has eroded into the stomach. [22]

Contrast-enhanced computed tomography (CT) should be requested, if clinical symptoms suggest an intra-abdominal abscess. Endoscopic band removal is the treatment of choice for gastric band erosion. Though, when there is extensive erosion and necrosis of the stomach wall, laparoscopic or laparotomic removal of the affected stomach should be reconsidered. [23]

A rare (less than 0·5 per cent) but also well reported late complication after LAGB is considered megaoesophagus. [24] Progressive dysphagia, regurgitation and often retrosternal chest pain are some of the symptoms that patients typically mention. The diagnosis is made by means of endoscopy or an upper gastrointestinal contrast study. When the megaoesophagus is often caused by proximal migration of the gastric band thus mimicking achalasia, necessitates the removal of the band in most cases.

Other late complications after vertical sleeve gastrectomy (VSG) include gastrocutaneous fistula and tube stricture (<1 per cent). [25] The management of these types of complications requires specialist bariatric surgery and probably may include stent insertion and conversion to RYGB.

Hepatobiliary Complications

The formation of cholesterol gallstones can be the consequence of rapid weight loss. 13 to 36 per cent of patients develop gallstones within a period of 6 months after the surgical operation. [26, 27] In general, cholecystectomy is performed only if the patient is symptomatic. [28, 29] In patients who have previously undergone a bypass procedure, intraoperative cholangiography is advisable, as a result of the difficulty in reaching the biliary tract by endoscopic retrograde cholangiopancreatography (ERCP). New endoscopic techniques such as the transgastric approach and double balloon enteroscopy can be applied in order to access the biliary tree in occasions where the performance of standard ERCP is technically difficult (such as after previous RYGB). [30] The removal of common bile duct (CBD) stones can be achieved, in the absence of experience on the novel techniques, by using either the transcystic approach or by formal CBD exploration during surgery. [30, 31]

Intestinal Obstruction

Husain et al. referred that the incidence of bowel obstruction was found to be 4·4 per cent, with a mean period of presentation of 313 days after RYGB. [32] Increased risk of intestinal obstruction is correlated the surgical approach, which will affect the degree of adhesions as well as the position of the Roux limb, in close association with the limb position, retrocolic or antecolic. [32] The most frequent causes of bowel obstruction consist in internal hernias (53 per cent), Roux limb compression due to scarring (20 per cent) and adhesions (14 per cent). [33] Stricture at the gastrojejunal anastomosis, incisional hernia, intestinal intussusception and kinking of the alimentary limbcan also considered possible causes of obstruction. The clinical symptoms of these patients are central colicky abdominal pain (82 per cent), nausea and vomiting (46–48 per cent), abdominal distension and absolute constipation. [32] It is crucial to enquire about the volume and character of the emesis in patients with RYGB as this may provide a clue about the site of the obstruction. Furthermore, the type of the vomit will differ in relation to the site of obstruction. Copious amounts of bilious vomiting are indications of obstruction at the common channel (CC) distal to the jejunojejunal anastomosis. Dilatation of the CC proximal to the obstruction, of the biliopancreatic limb, the gastric remnant and the Roux limb are signs that can be evident with CT. Smaller quantity of non-bilious vomit is suggestive of obstruction at the Roux limb or above the jejunojejunal anastomosis. CT, at this type of obstruction, will make evident a dilated Roux limb and a collapsed CC and biliopancreatic limb. Absence or little amount of vomit, combined with abdominal distension are generally signs of obstruction at biliopancreatic limb. In addiction, symptoms include postprandial left upper abdominal quadrant pain. Dilatation of the biliopancreatic limb and at the remnant of the stomach, combined with normal CC and Roux limb caliber can also be evident with CT. Patients with a RYGB can present a number of mesenteric defects through which even a small bowel loop is in position to pass and provoke obstruction or in the worst case strangulation. Paroz et al. showed that the most frequent sites for internal herniation are localized at the mesojejunal mesenteric window (56 per cent), the Peterson's window (27 per cent) and the mesocolic window (17 per cent). [33] The incidence of symptomatic internal herniation variates from 1·6 to 4·1 per cent. [33,34] Failure to close the mesenteric defects, the closure technique in combination with the type of suture used, and the variations of these defects as patients lose weight are some of the factors that can assist to the development of internal hernias. [12] Almost one-third of all patients can present with symptoms and signs of acute intestinal obstruction. [33] The onset of symptoms is generally insidious and presents with intermittent abdominal discomfort, mainly after eating. [34, 35]

Even if laparotomy is often indicated for the diagnosis, laparoscopy is the first option from the invasive techniques. [34, 35] Moreover, it is important for the surgeon to identify all limbs and great attention should be given to mesenteric defects as these should be closed with non-absorbable sutures. The presence of ulceration at the gastrojejunal anastomosis, which may contribute to the formation of anastomotic strictures in 27 per cent of patients, can often be revealed by endoscopy. [36, 37]

Endoscopic balloon dilatations up to 12–15 mm can resolve gastrojejunal strictures, even if there is a risk of perforation (2·1 per cent). [38] 8–10 per cent of patients may present incisional hernias following open bariatric operations. [39] The utilization of laparoscopic surgical approach can low the incidence of port-site incisional hernias, estimated to be up to 0·5 per cent. [40]

Most of the times, in obese patients, port-site hernias can be difficult to detect clinically and ultrasonography could be useful as diagnostic method. Intestinal intussusception, a rare cause of abdominal pain, after open or laparoscopic RYGB, is most often located at the CC of the gastrojejunal anastomosis, due either to alterated motility or the staple line of the anastomosis which acte as a lead point. The utilization of contrast-enhanced CT with is extremely valuable in establishing of diagnosis while the surgical management includes the reduction of the affected limb and resection if there is any evidence of intestinal ischaemia.

Gastrointestinal Bleeding

Gastrointestinal bleeding after RYGB is uncommon outside the postoperative period and generally takes origin by marginal or stomal ulceration. [41] The adequate resuscitation, the assessment of the severity of the bleeding and the close monitoring should be the first steps in managing these patients. [42] Patients with RYGB may be chronically anaemic and thus it is perfectly reasonable to accept lower haemoglobin levels and to withhold blood transfusion and emergency endoscopy, provided the patient is haemodynamically stable. [43]

Endoscopy should constantly be performed immediately in patients with severe bleeding. [44] In cases where the source of the bleeding cannot be identified, the endoscopist should carefully examine the Roux limb, biliopancreatic limb, jejunojejunal anastomosis as well as the gastric remnant.

The endoscopist can The utilization of a push enteroscope or paediatric colonoscope is useful way in order to realize this. [45] An innovative technique such as double-balloon enteroscopy is in position to facilitate the access to the biliopancreatic limb and gastric remnant while permits therapeutic interventions. [46, 47] In cases of endoscopical failure to control bleeding, radiological embolization of the bleeding vessel can be an indication for surgical intervention. [12] Last but not least, if haemostasis cannot be achieved, procedures such as excision and reconstruction of the jejunojejunal or gastrojejunal anastomoses, excision of bleeding gastric ulcer or even resection of the gastric remnant may be considered as alternative options.

Functional Complications

Even though the patients who submit to bariatric surgery experience improvement in functional gastrointestinal disorders, some possibly will develop exacerbations of symptoms. [48] The basic understanding of the origin of these symptoms by the emergency surgeon is critical. 49 per cent of bariatric patients before surgery are affected by eating disorders, such as binge-eating. [49, 50] The first element to the diagnosis is an increase in the patient's weight. Malabsorption can cause diarrhoea, bile salts or dumping syndrome. [51] Dumping syndrome habitually manifests itself as facial flushing and postprandial diarrhoea after the consumption of carbohydrate-rich meals. [52] Moreover, these symptoms tend to improve with time and less than 5 to10 per cent of patients continue to have chronic problems. Other causes of diarrhoea may possibly be irritable bowel syndrome or food intolerance or bacterial overgrowth. In these situations, the treatment of diarrhoea normally includes reduction the amount of carbohydrate consumed, avoiding foods that usually cause intolerance, while the use of probiotics and antibiotics is indicated where bacterial overgrowth is suspected. Many studies report an improvement in patients' reflux symptoms after bariatric surgery. [53, 54] The explanation of this fact is based on the distal diversion of bile, the reduction at the volume of parietal cells in the gastric pouch and weight loss. [55] However, some patients may present with new or exacerbation of the reflux symptoms. [56] In cases where the initial investigations are normal, other clinical hypotheses that should be considered are gastroparesis and oesophageal dysmotility. [57]

Nutritional Complications

Every surgical operation that alters in drastic way the anatomic pathways of nutrient intake may inevitably affect the intake of specific nutrients. Gastric restrictive procedures can induce nutrient deficiencies as a result of inadequate intake as a consequence of frequent vomiting and not due to malabsorption. Consequently, the reduction of the numerous episodes of vomit as well as the replacement of vitamin and mineral requirements are in position to prevent micronutrient deficiencies in these patients. [5, 58] Significantly, greater risk for micronutrient deficiency is present in malabsorptive procedures, in which the not proper micronutrient absorption may occur. In the digestion as well as the absorption of vitamin B12, iron, and calcium, it is important the anatomic integrity of stomach, duodenum, and of the proximal jejunum. In patients who have undergone gastric bypass, the deficiency of vitamin B12 has not presented as a long-term clinical issue. The postoperative recommendation to vitamin B12 supplement, the persistence of intrinsic factor, as the body of the stomach is usually preserved, and the presence of a functioning terminal ileum where vitamin B12 is absorbed, is probably the main reasons for the absence of B12 deficit in gastric bypass. Likewise, the lack of reports on an increased incidence of pathologic fractures demonstrates that the homeostasis of calcium, following this procedure, is preserved. [59] Moreover, the relative young age of patients who have undergone gastric bypass, increased estrogen production present at these patients, the stimulation of enhanced bone mass due to obesity and the usual recommendation to calcium and vitamin D supplementation may represent factors that also prevent pathologic fractures. On the other hand, procedures, such as the biliopancreatic diversion with duodenal switch (BPD/DS), which provoke a greater degree of malabsorption may possibly cause long-term demineralization of bones. Studies that report an increased concentration of parathormone in circulation, despite of a careful replacement protocol of calcium following BPD/DS, seems that at least in short term, serious bone pathology is avoided. [60, 61]

In the early months following bariatric surgery may be presented a reduced dietary protein intake. [5] Deficient of protein intake is considered more complicated to prevent than are micronutrients as its replacement necessitates ingestion of actual protein in order to reach nutritional equilibrium, while the consumption following in general the bariatric procedures can be limited so as protein intake drops below the recommended daily standard of 0. 8 gr/kgr (according to the ideal body weight). The early finding of deficient protein intake is alopecia, therefore should be paid attention on the dietary protein intake during the early months following bariatric operation.

Iron deficiency is considered the most frequent micronutrient deficiency subsequent to gastric bypass. A degree of iron deficiency may be present preoperatively and may be exacerbated by factors, such as the operative blood loss, the postoperative gastrointestinal pathology, the reduced intake of iron and a degree of iron malabsorption as a result of bypass of the stomach and duodenum, can have a great impact on iron homeostasis. As a consequence, the supplementation of iron following bariatric surgery as well as the vigorous monitoring of iron concentration is recommended in order to prevent grave anemia.

Conclusion

The knowledge of normal anatomy and the surgical technique is fundamental for correct interpretation of imaging studies in patients who have undergone bariatric surgery. [62] The type, the pathophysiology and the timing of each complication is predictable and there are precise signs that can assist in their identification. Over the last decade, perioperative morbidity and mortality of bariatric surgery have decreased significantly that is almost equivalent with many well-accepted procedures such as cholecystectomy. [63] In effect, the mortality risk of bariatric surgery is one-tenth that of coronary artery bypass surgery with considerably greater improvement in long-term mortality. Technical advances in laparoscopic surgery and the establishment of surgical centers of excellence have contributed at the improvement in perioperative morbidity and mortality. [64] Consequently, extensive evidence on safety and efficacy has imposed bariatric surgery as the standard for treatment of morbid obesity.

References

[1] Flum DR, Belle SH, King WC, et al. Perioperative safety in the longitudinal assessment of bariatric surgery. *N. Engl. J. Med.* 2009;361:445-54.

[2] Morino M, Toppino M, Forestieri P, Angrisani L, Allaix ME, Scopinaro N. Mortality after bariatric surgery: analysis of 13,871 morbidly obese patients from a national registry. *Ann. Surg.* 2007;246:1002-7; discussion 7-9.

[3] Poulose BK, Griffin MR, Zhu Y, et al. National analysis of adverse patient safety for events in bariatric surgery. *Am. Surg.* 2005;71:406-13.

[4] Cotter SA, Cantrell W, Fisher B, Shopnick R. Efficacy of venous thromboembolism prophylaxis in morbidly obese patients undergoing gastric bypass surgery. *Obes. Surg.* 2005;15:1316-20.

[5] Elder KA, Wolfe BM. Bariatric surgery: a review of procedures and outcomes. *Gastroenterology*, 2007;132:2253-71.

[6] Brethauer SA, Hammel JP, Schauer PR. Systematic review of sleeve gastrectomy as staging and primary bariatric procedure. *Surg. Obes. Relat. Dis.* 2009;5:469-75.

[7] Podnos YD, Jimenez JC, Wilson SE, Stevens CM, Nguyen NT. Complications after laparoscopic gastric bypass: a review of 3464 cases. *Arch. Surg.* 2003;138:957-61.

[8] Tice JA, Karliner L, Walsh J, Petersen AJ, Feldman MD. Gastric banding or bypass? A systematic review comparing the two most popular bariatric procedures. *Am. J. Med.* 2008;121:885-93.

[9] Mehran A, Szomstein S, Zundel N, Rosenthal R. Management of acute bleeding after laparoscopic Roux-en-Y gastric bypass. *Obes. Surg.* 2003;13:842-7.

[10] Nguyen NT, Longoria M, Chalifoux S, Wilson SE. Gastrointestinal hemorrhage after laparoscopic gastric bypass. *Obes. Surg.* 2004;14:1308-12.

[11] Nguyen NT, Rivers R, Wolfe BM. Early gastrointestinal hemorrhage after laparoscopic gastric bypass. *Obes. Surg.* 2003;13:62-5.

[12] Hamdan K, Somers S, Chand M. Management of late postoperative complications of bariatric surgery. *Br. J. Surg.* 2011;98:1345-55.

[13] Lancaster RT, Hutter MM. Bands and bypasses: 30-day morbidity and mortality of bariatric surgical procedures as assessed by prospective, multi-center, risk-adjusted ACS-NSQIP data. *Surg. Endosc.* 2008;22:2554-63.

[14] Galvani C, Gorodner M, Moser F, et al. Laparoscopic adjustable gastric band versus laparoscopic Roux-en-Y gastric bypass: ends justify the means? *Surg. Endosc.* 2006;20:934-41.

[15] Jan JC, Hong D, Pereira N, Patterson EJ. Laparoscopic adjustable gastric banding versus laparoscopic gastric bypass for morbid obesity: a single-institution comparison study of early results. *J. Gastrointest. Surg.* 2005;9:30-9; discussion 40-1.

[16] Mehanna MJ, Birjawi G, Moukaddam HA, Khoury G, Hussein M, Al-Kutoubi A. Complications of adjustable gastric banding, a radiological pictorial review. *AJR Am. J. Roentgenol.* 2006;186:522-34.

[17] Spivak H, Rubin M. Laparoscopic management of lap-band slippage. *Obes. Surg.* 2003;13:116-20.

[18] Chevallier JM, Zinzindohoue F, Douard R, et al. Complications after laparoscopic adjustable gastric banding for morbid obesity: experience with 1,000 patients over 7 years. *Obes. Surg.* 2004;14:407-14.

[19] Tran D, Rhoden DH, Cacchione RN, Baldwin L, Allen JW. Techniques for repair of gastric prolapse after laparoscopic gastric banding. *J. Laparoendosc. Adv. Surg. Tech. A.* 2004;14:117-20.

[20] Hainaux B, Agneessens E, Rubesova E, et al. Intragastric band erosion after laparoscopic adjustable gastric banding for morbid obesity: imaging characteristics of an underreported complication. *AJR Am. J. Roentgenol.* 2005;184:109-12.

[21] Silecchia G, Restuccia A, Elmore U, et al. Laparoscopic adjustable silicone gastric banding: prospective evaluation of intragastric migration of the lap-band. *Surg. Laparosc. Endosc. Percutan. Tech.* 2001;11:229-34.
[22] Fobi M, Lee H, Igwe D, et al. Band erosion: incidence, etiology, management and outcome after banded vertical gastric bypass. *Obes. Surg.* 2001;11:699-707.
[23] Kiewiet RM, Durian MF, van Leersum M, Hesp FL, van Vliet AC. Gallstone formation after weight loss following gastric banding in morbidly obese Dutch patients. *Obes. Surg.* 2006;16:592-6.
[24] Arias IE, Radulescu M, Stiegeler R, et al. Diagnosis and treatment of megaesophagus after adjustable gastric banding for morbid obesity. *Surg. Obes. Relat. Dis.* 2009;5:156-9.
[25] Lalor PF, Tucker ON, Szomstein S, Rosenthal RJ. Complications after laparoscopic sleeve gastrectomy. *Surg. Obes. Relat. Dis.* 2008;4:33-8.
[26] Shiffman ML, Sugerman HJ, Kellum JM, Brewer WH, Moore EW. Gallstone formation after rapid weight loss: a prospective study in patients undergoing gastric bypass surgery for treatment of morbid obesity. *Am. J. Gastroenterol.* 1991;86:1000-5.
[27] Villegas L, Schneider B, Provost D, et al. Is routine cholecystectomy required during laparoscopic gastric bypass? *Obes. Surg.* 2004;14:206-11.
[28] Caruana JA, McCabe MN, Smith AD, Camara DS, Mercer MA, Gillespie JA. Incidence of symptomatic gallstones after gastric bypass: is prophylactic treatment really necessary? *Surg. Obes. Relat. Dis.* 2005;1:564-7; discussion 7-8.
[29] Ukleja A, Stone RL. Medical and gastroenterologic management of the post-bariatric surgery patient. *J. Clin. Gastroenterol.* 2004;38:312-21.
[30] Phillips EH, Toouli J, Pitt HA, Soper NJ. Treatment of common bile duct stones discovered during cholecystectomy. *J. Gastrointest. Surg.* 2008;12:624-8.
[31] Lyass S, Phillips EH. Laparoscopic transcystic duct common bile duct exploration. *Surg. Endosc.* 2006;20 Suppl 2:S441-5.
[32] Husain S, Ahmed AR, Johnson J, Boss T, O'Malley W. Small-bowel obstruction after laparoscopic Roux-en-Y gastric bypass: etiology, diagnosis, and management. *Arch. Surg.* 2007;142:988-93.
[33] Paroz A, Calmes JM, Giusti V, Suter M. Internal hernia after laparoscopic Roux-en-Y gastric bypass for morbid obesity: a continuous challenge in bariatric surgery. *Obes. Surg.* 2006;16:1482-7.
[34] Parakh S, Soto E, Merola S. Diagnosis and management of internal hernias after laparoscopic gastric bypass. *Obes. Surg.* 2007;17:1498-502.
[35] Iannelli A, Buratti MS, Novellas S, et al. Internal hernia as a complication of laparoscopic Roux-en-Y gastric bypass. *Obes. Surg.* 2007;17:1283-6.
[36] Carrodeguas L, Szomstein S, Zundel N, Lo Menzo E, Rosenthal R. Gastrojejunal anastomotic strictures following laparoscopic Roux-en-Y gastric bypass surgery: analysis of 1291 patients. *Surg. Obes. Relat. Dis.* 2006;2:92-7.
[37] Matthews BD, Sing RF, DeLegge MH, Ponsky JL, Heniford BT. Initial results with a stapled gastrojejunostomy for the laparoscopic isolated roux-en-Y gastric bypass. *Am. J. Surg.* 2000;179:476-81.
[38] Ukleja A, Afonso BB, Pimentel R, Szomstein S, Rosenthal R. Outcome of endoscopic balloon dilation of strictures after laparoscopic gastric bypass. *Surg. Endosc.* 2008;22:1746-50.

[39] Nguyen NT, Goldman C, Rosenquist CJ, et al. Laparoscopic versus open gastric bypass: a randomized study of outcomes, quality of life, and costs. *Ann. Surg.* 2001;234:279-89; discussion 89-91.
[40] Schauer PR, Ikramuddin S. Laparoscopic surgery for morbid obesity. *Surg. Clin. North Am.* 2001;81:1145-79.
[41] Braley SC, Nguyen NT, Wolfe BM. Late gastrointestinal hemorrhage after gastric bypass. *Obes. Surg.* 2002;12:404-7.
[42] Rockall TA, Logan RF, Devlin HB, Northfield TC. Risk assessment after acute upper gastrointestinal haemorrhage. *Gut,* 1996;38:316-21.
[43] Hebert PC, Wells G, Martin C, et al. Variation in red cell transfusion practice in the intensive care unit: a multicentre cohort study. *Crit. Care,* 1999;3:57-63.
[44] Non-variceal upper gastrointestinal haemorrhage: guidelines. *Gut*, 2002;51 Suppl 4:iv1-6.
[45] Flickinger EG, Sinar DR, Pories WJ, Sloss RR, Park HK, Gibson JH. The bypassed stomach. *Am. J. Surg.* 1985;149:151-6.
[46] Kuno A, Yamamoto H, Kita H, et al. Double-balloon enteroscopy through a Roux-en-Y anastomosis for EMR of an early carcinoma in the afferent duodenal limb. *Gastrointest. Endosc.* 2004;60:1032-4.
[47] Yamamoto H, Sekine Y, Sato Y, et al. Total enteroscopy with a nonsurgical steerable double-balloon method. *Gastrointest. Endosc.* 2001;53:216-20.
[48] Clements RH, Gonzalez QH, Foster A, et al. Gastrointestinal symptoms are more intense in morbidly obese patients and are improved with laparoscopic Roux-en-Y gastric bypass. *Obes. Surg.* 2003;13:610-4.
[49] Crowell MD, Cheskin LJ, Musial F. Prevalence of gastrointestinal symptoms in obese and normal weight binge eaters. *Am. J. Gastroenterol.* 1994;89:387-91.
[50] Mitchell JE, Lancaster KL, Burgard MA, et al. Long-term follow-up of patients' status after gastric bypass. *Obes. Surg.* 2001;11:464-8.
[51] Kaplan LM. Gastrointestinal management of the bariatric surgery patient. *Gastroenterol. Clin. North. Am.* 2005;34:105-25.
[52] Abell TL, Minocha A. Gastrointestinal complications of bariatric surgery: diagnosis and therapy. *Am. J. Med. Sci.* 2006;331:214-8.
[53] Frezza EE, Ikramuddin S, Gourash W, et al. Symptomatic improvement in gastroesophageal reflux disease (GERD) following laparoscopic Roux-en-Y gastric bypass. *Surg. Endosc.* 2002;16:1027-31.
[54] Tolonen P, Victorzon M, Niemi R, Makela J. Does gastric banding for morbid obesity reduce or increase gastroesophageal reflux? *Obes. Surg.* 2006;16:1469-74.
[55] Mason EE, Munns JR, Kealey GP, et al. Effect of gastric bypass on gastric secretion. *Am. J. Surg.* 1976;131:162-8.
[56] Mejia-Rivas MA, Herrera-Lopez A, Hernandez-Calleros J, Herrera MF, Valdovinos MA. Gastroesophageal reflux disease in morbid obesity: the effect of Roux-en-Y gastric bypass. *Obes. Surg.* 2008;18:1217-24.
[57] Salameh JR, Schmieg RE, Jr., Runnels JM, Abell TL. Refractory gastroparesis after Roux-en-Y gastric bypass: surgical treatment with implantable pacemaker. *J. Gastrointest. Surg.* 2007;11:1669-72.
[58] Chaves LC, Faintuch J, Kahwage S, Alencar Fde A. A cluster of polyneuropathy and Wernicke-Korsakoff syndrome in a bariatric unit. *Obes. Surg.* 2002;12:328-34.

[59] Riedt CS, Brolin RE, Sherrell RM, Field MP, Shapses SA. True fractional calcium absorption is decreased after Roux-en-Y gastric bypass surgery. *Obesity* (Silver Spring) 2006;14:1940-8.

[60] Marceau P, Biron S, Lebel S, et al. Does bone change after biliopancreatic diversion? *J. Gastrointest. Surg.* 2002;6:690-8.

[61] Slater GH, Ren CJ, Siegel N, et al. Serum fat-soluble vitamin deficiency and abnormal calcium metabolism after malabsorptive bariatric surgery. *J. Gastrointest. Surg.* 2004;8:48-55; discussion 4-5.

[62] Quigley S, Colledge J, Mukherjee S, Patel K. Bariatric surgery: a review of normal postoperative anatomy and complications. *Clin. Radiol.* 2011;66:903-14.

[63] Eldar S, Heneghan HM, Brethauer SA, Schauer PR. Bariatric surgery for treatment of obesity. *Int. J. Obes.* (Lond) 2011;35 Suppl 3:S16-21.

[64] DeMaria EJ, Pate V, Warthen M, Winegar DA. Baseline data from American Society for Metabolic and Bariatric Surgery-designated Bariatric Surgery Centers of Excellence using the Bariatric Outcomes Longitudinal Database. *Surg. Obes. Relat. Dis.* 2010;6:347-55.

In: Bariatric Surgery
Editor: Christos R. Iavazzo

ISBN: 978-1-62618-995-9

Chapter VI

Hepatobiliary Complications of Bariatric Surgery

Omar Khan[1], K. M. Reddy[1] and Khaled Hamdan
[1]Department of Upper GI Surgery, St George's Healthcare NHS Trust, London, UK
[2]Brighton and Sussex University Hospitals, Brighton, England, UK

Abstract

Bariatric surgery has a number of systemic metabolic and physiological consequences which can directly and indirectly affect the hepatobiliary system. The most common hepatobiliary complication following bariatric surgery is the formation of gallstones which occurs as a consequence of a number of factors including rapid weight loss; reduced food intake leading to gallbladder stasis; changes in food preference and malabsorption. Gallstone formation can potentially be prevented by medical treatment with post-operative ursodeoxycholic acid or prophylactic cholecystectomy. However, because only a small number of patients who develop gallstones become symptomatic, the majority of surgeons currently do not perform laparoscopic cholecystectomy at the time of bariatric surgery. Laparoscopic cholecystectomy for gallstones can be done in the normal fashion but management of patients with choledocholithiasis or gallstone pancreatitis can be challenging. This is particularly true of patients following gastric bypass and duodenal switch surgery. These patients cannot undergo conventional endoscopic retrograde cholangiopancreatography (ERCP) and as a result require hybrid endoscopic techniques such as laparoscopic-assisted trans-gastric ERCP to allow cannulation of the common bile duct.

Introduction

Although a plethora of bariatric operations have been described and performed, all of these procedures are designed to restrict dietary intake and/or absorption of food. By definition, these processes lead to alterations in both weight and nutritional uptake and these in turn can have consequences on the functional status of the hepatobiliary system. The purpose of this chapter is to discuss in detail the hepatobiliary complications associated with bariatric surgery and the potential strategies to prevent and manage these complications.

Biliary Complications

Gallstone Disease

Of all of the hepatobiliary complications following bariatric surgery, gallstone formation and its subsequent sequalae are by far the most common and merit detailed discussion. The details of bile salt formation and cholesterol handling by the body are well described and are outside the scope of this chapter. In brief, bile acids (chenodeoxycholic acid and cholic acid) are formed from cholesterol in hepatocytes. The bile acids are then conjugated with glycine or taurine to form bile salts which results in the conversion of the acids into their ionised forms thus increasing the hydrophilicity. [1] Bile salts in combination with lecithin then act as emulsifying agents to allow the cholesterol to form stable vesicles and these vesicles are what is conventionally referred to as bile. [2] Bile is stored in the gallbladder and secreted into the intestine where it emulsifies luminal fat and hence aids lipid digestion and absorption. Following this process the bile salts are reabsorbed predominantly at the terminal ileum and recycled by means of the hepatic portal system.

Composition of Gallstones

Gallstones may be classified as cholesterol stones, mixed stones or pigmented stones depending on their predominant component. The formation of cholesterol and mixed gallstones is a multi-factorial process that has both environmental and genetic components. The causes of lithogenesis can be categorised as follows:

1. Super-saturation of Cholesterol

This can occur as a consequence of either excess cholesterol or decreased levels of bile acids. With reference to excess cholesterol, the bile is forced into a state of super-saturation, as the cholesterol can no longer be incorporated into the vesicles. This causes the formation of cholesterol-supersaturated agglomerations and the deposition of cholesterol microcrystals. Over time there is layering on one or two core stones that go on to form compact gallstones.

2. Gallbladder Dysfunction

The contraction of the gall bladder has been shown to agitate and excrete cholesterol crystals helping to prevent lithogenesis. A large gallbladder volume is associated with poor motility which in turn results in impaired filling and emptying; potentially resulting in cholestasis. [3] Ineffective or non-frequent contraction also leads to increase stasis which provides a perfect lactogenic environment. One naturally occurring cause for the dysfunction is age. It has been speculated that a decline in receptor sensitivity, primarily those involved in motor activity stimulation, i.e. cholecystokinin (CCK) and motile can cause decreased gall bladder contractility. [4]

3. Enter hepatic Circulation

Bile acids are recycled when they are absorbed in the terminal ileum and returned to the hepatocytes via the hepatic portal system. Therefore any condition that causes malabsorption leading to a compromise and potentially decreased bile acid absorption results in dysphonia. For example patients with active terminal ileal Crohn's disease have been shown to have a 25% incidence of gallstones. [5]

Bariatric Surgical Patients and Gallstones

As a population group, bariatric patients have a high risk of developing gallstones both before and after weight-loss surgery. The reasons for the high incidence of gallstones pre-operatively may be attributable to:

1. Obesity

Patients with morbid obesity have been shown to have an increased dietary consumption of cholesterol. [6] Previous studies have demonstrated that morbidly obese patients prior to bariatric surgery have elevated amounts of super-saturated bile in both the gall bladder and hepatic duct. [7] This in turn increases the risk of developing gallstones due to the mechanisms previously described. In addition, the relationship between gallstone formation and increased body mass index (BMI) is particularly strong in young females and this demographic makes up the majority of patients undergoing bariatric surgery. One explanation for the association between young obese females and gallstone formation may lie in their genetics. For example a number of studies have focused on the role of the beta (3) - adrenergic receptor (*ADRB 3*). This protein is excessively expressed in adipose tissue and there is an increase in prevalence of polymorphisms of ADRB 3 in both the obese and patients with gallstones. [8,9]

2. Low Calorie Diets and Weight Fluctuations

Weight cycling and large weight fluctuations (independent of BMI) are risk factors for lithogenesis in both men and women. [12,13] This is due to several different pathogenic mechanisms - at times of weight gain, there is an increase in weight and abdominal fat accumulation resulting in super-saturation of the bile due to the increased calorie intake. [14] In times of weight loss with very low calorie diets, there is normally a low fat content and consequently a net reduction in gall bladder stimulated contraction leading to gall bladder stasis. Therefore with weight cycling involving rapid weight loss and weight gain, the rate of weight loss causes an increase in the risk of lithogenesis. [12] This is particularly relevant to bariatric surgical patients as the majority have a history of yo-yo dieting prior to surgery. In addition, patients undergoing bariatric surgery typically consumea pre-operative low calorie liver shrinking diet that may lead to gallbladder stasis. These factors may be responsible for the high rate of asymptomatic gallstone in pre-operative bariatric patients-26% of all these patients exhibit evidence of gallbladder disease with either cholelithiasis on preoperative trans-abdominal ultrasound or a history of cholecystectomy. [15]

Post Bariatric Surgery

In terms of discussing the factors for gallstone formation followingbariatric surgery, it should be noted at the outset that many patients remain obese following surgery which as previously discussed is a risk factor for lithogenesis. However bariatric surgery itself has been identified to carry a five-fold increase in developing symptomatic gallstones, with each form of bariatric surgery carrying its own risk profile as shown below. [16]

Surgery	Risk of post-operative symptomatic gallstone disease
Gastric banding	7% [10]
Sleeve gastrectomy	4% [13]
Roux-en-Y bypass	7% - 16% [11]

The potential mechanisms underlying these associations are not entirely clear but are likely to include:

1. Weight Loss

By definition, the purpose of bariatric surgery is to promote weight loss. However as discussed rapid weight loss is associated with the formation of gallstones. Moreover it has been shown that increasing rates of weight loss results in an exponential rise in the incidence of gallstones. [17] Hence any procedure which results in rapid weight loss, such as a duodenal switch or a gastric bypass are most likely to result in the formation of new gallstones.

2. Food Restriction

A number of bariatric procedures have a restrictive component designed to reduce overall dietary intake. With respect to purely restrictive procedures, adjustable gastric bands have been shown to reduce intake which in turn leads to a decrease in gallbladder emptying and a fall in gallbladder refilling thus encouraging stasis in the gall bladder, both of which increase the risk of developing gallstones. [18] However, following gastric banding it is still possible to consume foods with a high fat density, which although detrimental from a weight-loss perspective, may paradoxically lower risk of developing gallstones by promoting gallbladder emptying.

3. Food Preferences Changes

It has been suggested that both sleeve gastrectomy and Roux-en-Y bypass lead to changes in food preferences. Animal models using rats have shown that following sleeve gastrectomy and gastric bypass, there is a marked decrease in dietary fat intake. This effect has been attributed to alterations in the rat's food preferences towards foods with a lower calorie intake as well as the restrictive effects of the surgery. This change in food preference has been replicated in Roux-en-Y bypass patients. Studies have demonstrated that this surgery has led to both a decrease in the patients' preoccupation with food and an increased satisfaction with smaller portion sizes. The net consequence of these changes in food preferences and overall decreased intake leads to highly lithogenic environment. [19]

4. Malabsorption

As discussed previously bile salts are reabsorbed in the terminal ileum. Hence any bariatric operations that have a malabsorbative element may alter recycling of bile salts.

A) Gastric Bypass

For patient undergoing the Roux-en-Y bypass, particularly in the super obese patients who may have a tailored long Roux limb, there is some exclusion of the proximal ileum. This causes a net reduction in ileal absorption which may impact on the reabsorption of bile salts. It should however be noted that the majority of the absorption of bile salts occurs in the terminal as opposed to proximal ileum.

B) Duodenal Switch

This operation involves the exclusion of a significant portion of the terminal ileum and hence significantly disrupts the enterohepatic circulation, consequently causing bile acid loss and lithogenesis. [20]

Prevention of Gallstone Disease

Given the preceding discussion, it is clear that bariatric surgical patients have a high incidence of gallstones. Decreasing the formation of gallstones and its associated complications following surgery is therefore a clearly an important therapeutic strategy. This may be achieved by:

Medical Prophylaxis

Ursodeoxycholic acid is a bile acid that facilitates gallstone dissolution by reducing biliary cholesterol secretion in turn leading to lower bile cholesterol saturation. [21] Moreover even among those patients on urosedeoxycholic acid who do develop gallstones, this medication reduced the risk of symptomatic stone disease and hence the requirement for cholecystectomy. [22] The main shortfall of this medical management is however patient's poor compliance. [21] A number of studies have examined the role of this medication following bariatric surgery:

A) Restrictive Procedures

Miller et al. conducted a single centered, randomized, double-blind placebo controlled trial on patients who had undergone either a vertical banded gastroplasty or adjustable gastric banding who were given either a daily dose of 500 mg of ursodeoxycholic acid or placebo for

6 months. The formation of gallstones in the treatment group was significantly less than with placebo at both 12 months (3% vs. 22%) and 24 months (8% vs. 30%). In addition the requirement for cholecystectomy was reduced in the treatment group (4. 7% vs. 12%). [23]

B) Roux-en-Y Gastric Bypass

A multi-centered, double blinded, randomised prospective trial concluded that a daily dose of 600 mg of ursodeoxycholic acid is an effective prophylaxis treatment option for gallstone formation following a gastric bypass. The incidence of gallstones was markedly raised in the placebo group (32%) in comparison to the 600 mg treatment group (2%). A dose dependent response was seen with 600 mg being most effective in lowering the incidence of gallstones. [21] A recent meta-analysis including 5 randomised control trials with a total of 512 patients concluded that 8. 8% of the treatment group (on ursodeoxycholic acid) developed gallstones in comparison to 27. 7% of placebo group. [24]

C) Duodenal Switch

Although there is no high quality prospective data in this group of patients, a retrospective study of 219 duodenal switch patients looked at those taking 600 mg ursodeoxycholic acid for 6 months post-operatively noted a very low incidence of post-operative symptomatic gallstones. [25]

Surgical Prophylaxis

The role of prophlyactic cholecystectomy during baraitric surgery is controversial. [26] Proponents of this procedure argue that given the high risk of developing gallstones following baraitric surgery and the potential technical difficulties of mobilising the gallbladder due to adhesions following surgery, the gallbladder should be routinely removed. However others argue that cholecystectomy is a time consuming and potentially hazardous procedure with serious complications in up to 3% of cases. [21] Moreover the technical challenge of performing concomitant cholecystectomy is greater in the era of laparoscopic as opposed to open surgery as port positions are optimised for the primary bariatric procedure.

The role of prophylactic cholecystectomy for particular bariatric procedures is summarised below:

A) Gastric Banding

Although prophylactic cholecystectomy is technically feasible in patients undergoing insertion of a gastric band, there are concerns that inadvertent bile spillage during cholecystectomy may lead to infection of the implant. In addition, given the relatively low incidence of symptomatic gallstone disease following banding, most authors do not advocate prophylactic cholecystectomy. [27]

B) Roux-en-Y Gastric Bypass

As previously discussed, Roux-en-Y gastric bypass is associated with a high rate of post-operative symptomatic gallstone disease, and as such, there have been a number of studies on the subject of prophylactic cholecystectomy. The largest cohort comparison study on this subject involving 274 patients demonstrated that 18. 6% of the patients who did not have a prophylactic cholecystectomy went on to require a cholecystectomy. Of the 134 patients that underwent a simultaneous prophylactic cholecystectomy there was no increase in the rate for conversion to open, operative time, hospital stay or post-operative morbidity. [28]

C) Duodenal Switch

Unlike gastric bypass, there is a smaller evidence base for the use of prophylactic cholecystectomy in patients undergoing a duodenal switch. Michielson et al. reported that out of 33 patients who underwent a duodenal switch without prophylactic cholecystectomy, 2 (6%) went on to develop acute cholecystitis. [29] Similarly Ren et al. reported a series of 40 consecutive patients undergoing laparoscopic biliopancreatic diversion without cholecystectomy, of whom only 1 subsequently required cholecystectomy. [30]

On reviewing all of this data, it does appear that a selective approach to prophylactic cholecystectomy is indicated. For example a strategy of pre-operative ultrasound screening and prophylactic cholecystectomy in those cases where gallstones are detected has been shown to lower the probability of gallbladder-related morbidity and the need for future surgical intervention. [31]

Gallstone Disease in the Emergency Setting

For bariatric patients who do not undergo prophylactic cholecystectomy, a significant proportion will end up as emergency admissions to hospital with complications related to gallstones. The majority of these patients will present with either biliary colic or acute cholecystitis and require acholecystectomy. Although there have been debates in the past as to the benefits of urgent vs. delayed surgery, a number of groups have demonstrated the feasibility and desirability of surgery during the patients' index admission. Although this principle also applies to patients who have undergone bariatric surgery, these patients do pose additional challenges. For a start these patients may well be morbidly obese despite their bariatric surgery. In addition there may be adhesions in the upper abdomen restricting access to the gallbladder.

As a consequence of this, although there is good evidence to support the concept that urgent laparoscopic cholecystectomy in bariatric patients is feasible; it should only be performed by specialist Upper GI surgeons. In cases where the patient is too unwell to undergo laparoscopy, radiologically-guided percutaneous cholecystostomy may be useful either as a temporising measure to decompress the gallbladder and control sepsis prior to medical optimisation and cholecystectomy or in some cases as a definitive treatment.

For patients who do undergo urgent cholecystectomy, we advocate the routine use of intra-operative cholangiogram, particularly in those patients with a history of jaundice, deranged liver function test or ultrasound findings of a dilated biliary tree. Stones discovered at the time of on table cholangiogram may be flushed with normal saline following the administration of IV glucagon. Should persistant filling defects remain following flushing, a number of techniques such as trans-cystic insertion of a Fogarty catheter and sphincterototomy may be used. The gold standard for removal of stones is trans-cystic exploration of the common bile duct. This should be undertaken using a flexible choledochoscope and has been shown to have a 70-80% success rate in expert hands.

Pancreatitis

Bariatric patients with gallstone pancreatitis can pose a particular therapeutic challenge. Those with mild pancreatitis can be managed with laparoscopic cholecystectomy and on table cholangiogram during the index admission; and if common bile duct stones are detected intra-operatively they should be dealt with as outlined above. The main issues relate to patients with severe pancreatitis. A number of randomised controlled trials have demonstrated clinical benefit from ERCP within 48 hours of the onset of symptoms, particularly if there is concomitant obstruction of the biliary tree. Although laparoscopic gastric banding and sleeve gastrectomy should not preclude the performance of ERCP, for patients who have previously undergone a gastric bypass standard ERCP is not possible. Novel hybrid endoscopic techniques such as the laparoscopic-assisted trans-gastric insertion of an endoscope through the defunctioned stomach in order to access the biliary tree have been reported. This hybrid approach is not however suitable for patients who have undergone duodenal switch and hence in these patients the only techniques which can be used for instrumenting the biliary tree are radiologically-guided percutaneous trans-hepatic approach or surgical common bile duct exploration.

Hepatic Complications Following Bariatric Surgery

Fatty changes in the liver have been well described in the morbidly obese. This phenomenon mimics the spectrum of alcoholic liver disease and hence has been given the name non-alcoholic fatty liver disease (NAFLD). This umbrella term encompasses simple steatosis, non-alcoholic steatohepatitis (characterised by hepatocyte ballooning and inflammatory changes) and frank cirrhosis. Bariatric surgery has been shown to improve the histological features of NAFLD through a number of mechanisms including weight loss and resolution of the metabolic syndrome. [32] However, there have been reports of bariatric surgery leading to severe hepatic complications. The vast majority of these relate to jejunoileal bypass procedures. Although a number of varaitions of this operation have been described, all essentially involved connecting the jejunum with the ileum and forming a long bypassed small bowel loop. This resulted in massive weight loss but a number of serious complications including kidney stones, diarrhoea, electrolyte disturbances and vitamin deficiencies. With respect to the hepatic complications, long term follow-up of these patients showed hepatic structural abnormalities in 29% of patients and cirrhosis in 7%. [32] Experimental studies on rats seem to suggest that these hepatic complications were attributable to the presence of the excluded limb, possibly through changes in the bacterial flora. In terms of clinical studies, reversal of the bypass was shown to reduce hepatic inflammation, fibrosis and cirrhosis. Although this operation was abandoned for precisely this reason, there remains a cohort of unrevised patients who may develop hepatic complications in the future.

In terms of the common currently performed bariatric procedures, gastric banding, sleeve gastrectomy and gastric bypass have not been associated with hepatic complications. With respect to the duodenal switch procedure, there have been some reports of liver failure following surgery but the incidence is very rare. The few reported cases of this have been arrested by total parenteral nutrition and amino acid infusion or reversing the duodenal switch. Although it is possible that in the future there may be some long-term deleterious effect of bariatric surgery on liver function, the literature at present seems to suggest that gastric bypass in particular has a beneficial long-term effect on liver function over and above that seen due to weight loss.

Conclusion

Bariatric surgery has a number of effects on hepatic function and the biliary system. Although many of these changes are beneficial, some do have the potential to result in serious medical and surgical complications. Of these by far the most common is the formation of gallstones and its subsequent sequelae. Although general surgeons can deal with the majority of these complications, successful management requires a broad understanding of the anatomical and physiological changes following surgery and there should be a low threshold for involving an appropriately experienced bariatric unit.

References

[1] Marschall H. Einarsson C. Gallstone disease. *J Intern Med.* 2007; 261 (6): 529-542.

[2] Reshetnyak V. Concept of the pathogenesis and treatment of cholelithiasis. *World J Hepatol.* 2012;4(2):18–34.

[3] Olokoba AB. et al. The relationship between gallstone disease and gall bladder volume. *Niger J ClinPract.* 2008;11(2):89-93.

[4] Srivastava A. et al. Cholecystokinin receptor A gene polymorphism in gallstone disease and gallbladder cancer. *J Gastroenterol Hepatol.* 2008;23(6):970-975.

[5] Dowling RH. Pathogenesis of gallstones. *Aliment PharmacolTher.* 2000;2:39-47.

[6] Völzke H. et al. Independent risk factors for gallstone formation in a region with high cholelithiasis prevalence. *Digestion.* 2005;71(2):97-105.

[7] Freeman J. et al. Analysis of gallbladder bile in morbid obesity. *Am J Surg.* 1975; 129(2): 163-166.

[8] Klass M. et al. Arg64 variant of the beta3-adrenergic receptor is associated with gallstone formation. *Am J Gastroenterol.* 2007;102(11):2482-2487.

[9] Yamakita M. Ando D. Tang S. Yamagata Z. The Trp64Arg polymorphism of the beta3-adrenergic receptor gene is associated with weight changes in obese Japanese men: a 4-year follow-up study. *J Physiol Anthropol.* 2010;29(4):133-139.

[10] Kiewiet RM. et al. Gallstone formation after weight loss following gastric banding in morbidly obese Dutch patients. *Obes Surg.* 2006;16(5):592–596.

[11] Li VK. et al. Predictors of gallstone formation after bariatric surgery: a multivariate analysis of risk factors comparing gastric bypass, gastric banding, and sleeve gastrectomy. *Surg Endosc.* 2009;23(7):1640-1644.

[12] Syngal S. et al. Long-term weight patterns and risk for cholecystectomy in women. *Ann Intern Med.* 1999;130(6):471-477.

[13] Tsai J. Leitzmann F. Willett C. Giovannucci L. Weightcycling and risk of gallstone disease in men. *Arch Intern Med.* 2006;166(21):2369-2374.

[14] Cereda E. et al. Weightcycling is associated with body weight excess and abdominal fat accumulation: a cross-sectional study. *Clin Nutr.* 2011;30(6):718-723.

[15] Li VK. et al. Symptomatic gallstones after sleeve gastrectomy. *Surg. Endosc.* 2009;23(11):2488-2492.

[16] Jonas E. et al. Incidence of postoperative gallstone disease after antiobesity surgery: population-based study from Sweden. *Surg Obes Relat Dis.* 2010;6(1):54-58.

[17] Weinsier L. Wilson J. Lee J. Medically safe rate of weight loss for the treatment of obesity: a guideline based on risk of gallstone formation. *Am J Med.* 1995;98(2):115-7.

[18] Al-Jiffry BO. et al. Changes in gallbladder motility and gallstone formation following laparoscopic gastric banding for morbid obesity. *Can J Gastroenterol.* 2003;17(3):169-174.

[19] Shin AC. Berthoud HR. Food reward functions as affected by obesity and bariatric surgery. *Int J Obes(Lond).* 2011;35(3):40-4.

[20] Scopinaro N. et al. Two years of clinical experience with biliopancreatic bypass for obesity. *Am J ClinNutr.* 1980;33:506-14.

[21] Sugerman HJ. Brewer WH. Shiffman ML. et al. A multicenter, placebo-controlled, randomized, double-blinded, prospective trial of prophylactic ursodiol for the prevention of gall stone formation following gastric-bypass induced rapid weight loss. *Am J Surgery.* 1995;169:91-97.

[22] Quesada B. et al. Management of gallstones and gallbladder disease in patients undergoing gastric bypass. *World J Gastroenterol.* 2010;16(17):2075–2079.

[23] Miller K. Hell E. Lang B. Lengauer E. Gallstone formation prophylaxis after gastric restrictive procedures for weight loss: a randomized double-blind placebo-controlled trial. *Ann Surg.* 2003;238(5):697-702.

[24] Uy MC. et al. Ursodeoxycholic acid in the prevention of gallstone formation after bariatric surgery: a meta-analysis. *Obes Surg.* 2008;18(12):1532-1538.

[25] Bardaro SJ. et al. Routine cholecystectomy during laparoscopic biliopancreatic diversion with duodenal switch is not necessary. *Surg Obes Relat Dis.* 2007;3(5):549-553.

[26] Mason EE. Renquist KE. Gallbladder management in obesity surgery. *Obes Surg.* 2002;12:222–229.

[27] Sakcak I. Avsar FM. Cosgun E. Yildiz BD. Management of concurrent cholelithiasis in gastric banding for morbid obesity. *Eur J Gastroenterol Hepatol.* 2011;23(9):766-769.

[28] Tarantino I. et al. Is routine cholecystectomy justified in severely obese patients undergoing a laparoscopic Roux-en-Y gastric bypass procedure? A comparative cohort study. *Obes Surg.* 2011;21(12):1870-1878.

[29] Michielson D. Van Hee R. Hendrickx L. Complications of Biliopancreatic Diversion Surgery as Proposed by Scopinaro in the Treatment of Morbid Obesity. *Obes Surg.* 1996;6(5):416-420.

[30] Ren C. Patterson E. Gagner M. Early results of laparoscopic biliopancreatic diversion with duodenal switch: a case series of 40 consecutive patients. *Obes Surg.* 2000;10:514-523.

[31] Tucker ON. Fajnwaks P. Szomstein S. Rosenthal RJ. Is concomitant cholecystectomy necessary in obese patients undergoing laparoscopic gastric bypass surgery? *Surg Endosc*. 2008;22(11):2450-2454.
[32] Liu X et al. Resolution of non-alcoholic steatohepatits after gastric bypass surgery. *Obes Surg*. 2007;17(4):486-492.

In: Bariatric Surgery
Editor: Christos R. Iavazzo
ISBN: 978-1-62618-995-9

Chapter VII

Intestinal Obstruction after Bariatric Surgery

Khaled Hamdan[1] and Manish Chand[2]
[1]Brighton and Sussex University Hospitals, Brighton, England, UK
[2]The Royal Marsden Hospital, London, UK

Abstract

Intestinal obstruction is a recognised complication of abdominal surgery which includes bariatric procedures. The symptoms and signs when related to bariatric surgery can be subtle and knowledge of the type of surgery aids in diagnosis. Details of the surgery will help in understanding the anatomy and the potential causes of the obstruction. Internal hernia, adhesions, stricture and kinking of the Roux limb are all potential causes which produce a characteristic but subtle pattern of presentation. Technical factors such as surgical approach (laparoscopic versus open) and positioning of the Roux limb may influence the risk of obstruction. It may be appropriate to seek specialist advice from the local bariatric unit, however immediate treatment and initial investigations must not be delayed or risk perforation. This chapter describes the causes, presentation and treatment of intestinal obstruction in patients who have previously undergone bariatric surgery.

1. Introduction

The past decade has witnessed an exponential increase in the number of bariatric operations and as a result an increasing number of patients will present with complications that may be directly or indirectly related to their original bariatric procedure. Many of these patients travel long distances to have their surgery in specialized units and may not be local to a bariatric surgical unit if complications arise. This means that regular follow-up of these patients may not be possible and the original surgeon may not be immediately contactable. As such, patients with complications will invariably present to primary care physicians and surgeons who may not necessarily be familiar with bariatric surgery or have the knowledge and experience to deal with potential complications. Therefore, it is imperative that all those who are involved in the care of these patients should be familiar with the potential complications that may develop after bariatric surgery.

Small bowel obstruction (SBO) is one such complication which may occur any time after bariatric surgery and in particular after Roux-en-Y gastric bypass (RYGB). SBO is a major cause of morbidity and mortality and can be one of the most challenging complications to deal with. Failure to recognize and treat SBO in a timely fashion can in itself lead to serious consequences such as short gut syndrome and in some cases, death.

This chapter provides an overview of the causes, clinical presentation, investigations and treatment of postoperative intestinal obstruction after bariatric procedures with a particular emphasis on Roux-en-Y gastric bypass (RYGB).

2. Presentation and Investigation – General Considerations

The importance of obtaining a detailed history in patients with SBO cannot be overemphasized as specific features within the history may direct the surgeon as to the underlying cause and the most appropriate investigations. This includes the onset of symptoms and whether the obstruction is intermittent and incomplete or acute in nature. Furthermore, ascertaining the details of the actual procedure a patient has undergone will not only help the surgeon in deciding the most appropriate management but also aid the radiologist in interpreting any subsequent complex imaging. Such details include whether the procedure was laparoscopic or open, whether the procedure was restrictive or absorptive and whether there were any immediate post-operative concerns.

2.1. Presentation

Patients with intestinal obstruction may present at any time after surgery. This is best illustrated by the findings of a large study in which patients developed SBO from as early as 3 days after surgery to 1215 days [1].

In the acute setting the general features of bowel obstruction after bariatric surgery are no different to those of other general surgical procedures. The key features include colicky abdominal pain, vomiting, abdominal distension and absolute constipation. However, it is important to appreciate that in the bariatric population presentation may be less than typical with symptoms that are far less specific. For example, a significant proportion of patients with SBO secondary to internal hernia present with intermittent, undulating symptoms rather than acute unremitting ones. In addition, symptoms of SBO such as pain and vomiting may be wrongly attributed to non-surgical conditions that are common in bariatric patients. These include overeating, side effects of medications, vitamin B1 or zinc deficiency and gallstones which should all be considered in the assessment of patients presenting with vomiting after bariatric surgery.

It is also important to appreciate that obese patients may not develop many of the clinical signs and symptoms traditionally associated with SBO and a high index of suspicion is required in order to prevent potentially fatal complications caused by delayed diagnosis. For example, the clinician should be aware of the fact that signs such as abdominal tenderness and distention may be difficult to elicit in the morbidly obese patients with SBO. Another pitfall is the assumption that abdominal pain is a common complaint in bariatric patients and that it most often results from functional GI disturbances as a direct consequence of the surgery. It is true that abdominal pain in these patients may be attributed to a long list of non-surgical causes, but one must always exclude potentially serious and life threatening conditions in particular intestinal obstruction.

The site or level of the SBO after RYGB can produce specific symptoms which can aid diagnosis. *A full description of the anatomy of RYGB can be found in another chapter of this book* and only the salient features will be discussed here. RYGB involves the formation of three limbs of small bowel anastomosed in a particular fashion as part of the surgery. These are the Roux limb, the bilio-pancreatic limb (BP) and the common channel (CC). The Roux limb is anastomosed to the stomach while the BP limb is anastomosed to the Roux limb and the common channel continues as the conduit to the terminal ileum.

Patients with obstruction of the common channel distal to the jejuno-jejunal (JJ) anastomosis present with abdominal pain and, if not obscured by the patient's habitus, prominent distention. Except in closed loop obstruction, obstruction at this site causes copious amounts of bilious vomiting mainly because bile from the BP limb drains into the common channel proximal to the site of obstruction. In patients in whom obstruction involves the Roux limb proximal to the JJ anastomosis, vomiting is non-bilious as bile drains into the non-obstructed common channel distal to the site of obstruction. Vomiting is usually induced by eating and there may be little or no abdominal distention. Obstruction of the BP limb causes a specific set of symptoms. The main complaint is that of abdominal pain and nausea with little or no vomiting. Abdominal distension and absolute constipation are rarely present which may lead to the diagnosis of intestinal obstruction being fatally missed.

2.2. Investigations

As mentioned previously, patients with SBO after RYGB may not always present with characteristic history and physical signs of obstruction rendering the clinical diagnosis difficult. In addition, routine investigations including blood tests and plain radiographs may not always show any abnormalities in these patients. In one study white blood-cell count (WBC) was normal in up to three quarters of patients with SBO and up to two-thirds of these patients had "non-specific" findings on plain radiographs [2]. In these scenarios, radiological studies including upper gastrointestinal (UGI) contrast studies and computed tomography (CT) are essential in establishing the diagnosis and guiding treatment. However, the radiological evaluation of patients with SBO after RYGB may be hampered by certain technical challenges such as table weight limit, available scanner space and exceeding the radiological field resulting in artifacts [3].

Generally, CT is considered to be a more accurate diagnostic tool with significantly more cases of partial SBO being identified compared to UGI contrast studies [4]. However, in selected cases UGI contrast studies are useful in evaluating patients with SBO particularly in the first few months after surgery [5].

Although CT scan are highly accurate in establishing the diagnosis of acute SBO [6], the radiological findings in patients with incomplete and intermittent SBO are subtle and therefore can be missed by those not intimately familiar with post gastric bypass anatomy. The diagnosis of SBO may be missed in up to 20 % of patients even in the hands of experienced radiologists [7]. This is particularly the case in patients with internal hernias (IH) in whom the typical radiological features of SBO are not always present at the time of presentation [8]. For example, a study has shown that although the most common intraoperative finding in patients with SBO was IH (35% of all causes) it was also the most frequently missed cause of SBO on preoperative CT scans [9].

3. Causes

3.1. Incidence

The incidence of SBO after bariatric surgery ranges from 0. 5% -15%. In a large study with a long follow up period, the incidence of SBO was reported to be as low as 1. 27% [10]. Another study reported that up to 15% of patients who were admitted with SBO had previous bariatric surgery [11]. This wide variation in the reported incidence of SBO after bariatric surgery may be explained by the different follow up periods reported in published studies. For example studies with follow up periods of less than 1 year have shown low incidence of SBO mainly due to the under reporting of IHs which tend to develop months or years after surgery [12]. In addition, there is evidence that the incidence of SBO is greater in patients who achieve greater than 50% excess weight loss [13]which is usually achieved after the first year of the surgery. This is mainly because of the reopening of the mesenteric defects associated with weight loss which in turn leads to an increase in the risk of internal herniation. These factors mean that studies with short follow up periods do not represent the true incidence of SBO after bariatric surgery. Other factors which contribute to this wide variation between studies include variations in the surgical techniques used and the anatomical alterations that follow surgery and these will be discussed in a later section [14, 15].

3.2. Causes: General Overview

The most frequently encountered causes of SBO after RYGB are adhesions, internal hernias, anastomotic strictures and incisional hernias and these will be discussed in some details. In a cohort of 835 patients the incidence of SBO was 5% and the most common cause was IH (35%), followed by adhesions (25%), incisional hernias (17%) and JJ stricture (9%) [9]. In the early post-operative period SBO most frequently results from technical problems occurring at the time of the original surgery such as anastomotic stricture, whereas late SBO tends to result from adhesions or internal hernias.

Other less frequent causes of SBO include kinking of the small bowel, volvulus, intussusception, and food bolus or bezoar. Obstruction in patients who previously had laparoscopic adjustable gastric banding (LAGB) and sleeve gastrectomy can also occur and this will also be discussed.

It is important to emphasize that although the attending surgeon should be familiar with procedure-specific causes and that the etiology of obstruction in bariatric patients may be related to previous bariatric surgery, intestinal obstruction may be due to a completely unrelated pathology. As more bariatric procedures are performed the size of the elderly population who previously had weight loss surgery will increase. Consequently conditions that commonly lead to intestinal obstruction in the elderly population must also be considered. These include colorectal cancer, complicated diverticular disease, colonic volvulus and pseudo-obstruction. It is therefore important not to get fixated on the previous bariatric surgery as a cause but be aware of the long-term complication the procedures may entail. In addition, it is important for the general surgeon to realize that although bariatric and non-bariatric patients share the same etiologies of SBO there are differences in the frequency of these causes in each group. In one study abdominal wall and internal hernias accounted for 23% of all causes of SBO in bariatric patients compared to only 8% in the non-bariatric patients [11].

3.3. Predisposing Factors

As mentioned previously, the risk of SBO after RYGB may be influenced by the surgical technique used and the changes in anatomy that result after surgery. The most important factors that have been shown to increase the risk of SBO after RYGB include using the ante colic route, laparoscopic surgery and failure to close the mesenteric defects [7, 15].

The choice of operative approach (open or laparoscopic) has been shown to influence the risk of developing small bowel obstruction after RYGB. In fact, the type and frequency of complications after open Roux-en-Y gastric bypass (GBP) have changed dramatically with the development of laparoscopic technique.

It is postulated that the introduction of laparoscopy to bariatric surgery has contributed to the marked increase in the number of bariatric operations performed worldwide [12]. This is mainly attributed to the well proven advantages of laparoscopic surgery which include shorter hospital stay, quicker recovery, lower incidence of wound infection, and fewer incisional hernias. With regards to SBO, factors that may be expected to lower the incidence of this complication after laparoscopic bariatric procedures include the well demonstrated reduction in adhesion formation and the decrease in the risk of incisional hernias which are the two main cases of SBO after open surgery [2, 16].

Despite these advantages several studies have shown that laparoscopic RYGB is associated with an equal or greater incidence of SBO [14, 16-19]. Some studies have reported the incidence of SBO after laparoscopic and open surgery to be the same [17]while the preponderance of the evidence indicates that laparoscopic surgery is associated with a significantly higher incidence (<15%) [14]. In a study that compared a large cohort of 25,000 patients who underwent open RYGB with patients who underwent laparoscopic surgery the incidence of SBO was found to be significantly lower in the open group [11]. Another study demonstrated a large difference between the two approaches with an incidence of 9. 7% in the laparoscopic group compared to 0% in the open group [20]. Nelson et al. found a 50% increase in the incidence of SBO in the laparoscopic group with adhesions accounting for half of all cases of obstruction in the open group [21]. It is postulated that the increase in the incidence of SBO after laparoscopic RYGB is related to the reduction in adhesion formation [20]. This paradox can be explained by the fact that adhesions serve to fix small bowel loops thereby reducing their mobility and the risk of internal herniation. This explains the observation that the most common cause of SBO after laparoscopic bariatric surgery in most published studies is internal hernias [14]. Open surgery, on the other hand, is known to produce diffuse adhesions which in the case of RYGB may serve to reduce the risk internal herniation. However, this increases the risk of adhesion obstruction which has been shown to be the most common cause of intestinal obstruction after open RYGB [22]. The position of the Roux limb also appears to influence the incidence of small bowel obstruction after RYGB. Although the placement of the Roux limb in the retrocolic position may be necessary and technically more feasible in some patients [23] this route seems to be associated with a higher risk of SBO compared to the antecolic route [13, 24]. This is attributed to fact that the antecolic route eliminates one of the most common sites for intestinal obstruction, the mesocolic defect. The mesocolic defect has been sown to be the site of SBO in over 20% of the cases either due to the development of internal herniation through the mesocolic defect or external compression as the Roux limb traverses the mesocolic window [25]. Other studies have identified the use of the retrocolic technique as a risk factor for intestinal obstruction with 9. 3% of patients developing SBO mainly due to internal hernias compared to only 1. 8% in the antecolic group [26]. It has also been clearly demonstrated that switching the placement of the Roux limb from the retrocolic route into the antecolic route resulted in a 4-10 fold decrease in the overall incidence of small bowel obstruction [23, 26-28].

3.4. Cause of SBO after RYGB

Tucker et al. devised a simple classification system for the causes of SBO after RYGB, a modified form of which is presented in table [3, 29].

Table 1. The ABC classification system of the causes of SBO after RYGB

	Acute	Chronic
Roux limb	Anastomotic stricture Internal hernia Intussusception Intraluminal blood clot Mesocolic window stricture	Internal hernia Mesocolic window stricture
BP limb	JJ stricture Intussusception Intraluminal blood clot Mesocolic window stricture Volvulus	Internal Hernia Anastomotic stricture
Common channel	Internal hernia Volvulus Intraluminal clot	Internal hernia Adhesions

This classification system, which is referred to as the ABC system, is based on the site of SBOalimentary limb (A), biliopancreatic limb (B), or common channel (C)), the time of presentation after surgery (acute if less than 30 days and late or chronic if more than 30 days), and also according to the etiology of the obstruction.

Internal Hernias

Patients with a RYGB have several mesenteric defects that can potentially allow the passage of small bowel loops from one abdominal compartment to another *(see anatomy chapter).* As mentioned previously, herniation through these mesenteric defects is the most common cause of SBO after laparoscopic RYGB with an incidence ranging from 1·6 and 4·1 per cent [30, 31]. Gandhi e et al. reported an overall incidence of SBO of 3. 8% after laparoscopic RYGB with internal hernias accounting for more than half of all causes [12]. Factors that contribute to the development of internal herniation and subsequent SBO include failure to close the mesenteric defects, closure of these defects with absorbable rather than non-absorbable suture material, significant weight loss and laparoscopic surgery.

There is accumulating evidence to suggest that closure of the mesenteric defects significantly reduces the incidence of IHs and SBO after RYGB [8, 22]. In one study the risk of internal herniation was completely eliminated after the authors changed their practice to fully closing the mesenteric defects [11]. It has also been shown that patients in whom the mesenteric windows were routinely closed using non-absorbable sutures had significantly fewer hernias (1. 3%) compared to those in whom the defects were not closed or closure was done using absorbable sutures (5. 6%) [22].

As previously mentioned, abdominal adhesions form less commonly after laparoscopic RYGB and as such small bowel loops move more freely which increases the chances of a loop becoming trapped in one of the aforementioned mesenteric defects. The incidence of SBO secondary to IHs is also higher in patients who are most successful in losing weight [1]. This is thought to be due to the suggestion that with weight loss there is "melting of the mesenteric fat " which leads to reopening of the mesenteric defects and elongation of the bowel mesentery which in turn increase the risk of internal herniation [11].

The reported incidence of internal hernias at each of the known mesenteric defects varies widely and, as previously mentioned, largely depends on the surgical approach (open or laparoscopic) and whether the antecolic or the retrocolic route was used. The most frequent site of internal herniation in patients who previously had retrocolic RYGB has been shown to be the mesocolic defect (65%), followed by mesojejunal defect (22%) and Peterson defect (8%) [12, 26]. In patients who previously had antecolic RYGB IHs were found to account for more than half of all causes of SBO and all of these IHs were found to occur at the meso-jejunal mesenteric defect [11]. This has been confirmed in two other studies which reported that the most common location of IHs was the meso-jejunal mesenteric defect (56-95%)followed by Petersen's window (5-27%) [8, 31, 32].

Patients with IHs usually present months or years after surgery with a mean time to presentation of about 20 months [12]. This is in contrast to SBO secondary to other causes such as anastomotic stricture and intussusception where presentation is more likely to be earlier [17].

It is estimated that only a quarter to a third of patients with internal hernias present with the classic features of acute intestinal obstruction. The diagnosis of IHs in these patients is usually easily established and the radiological features on CT scan which include dilated small bowel loops and swirled appearance of the mesenteric fat and blood vessels at the site of obstruction are obvious [33]. More frequently however patients with internal hernias present with signs of incomplete bowel obstruction and recurrent vague symptoms rather than a single acute episode. These patients report symptoms such as intermittent abdominal pain, bloating and nausea before they present acutely. The symptoms in these patients develop when a loop of small bowel becomes temporarily trapped in one of the mesenteric defects. Abdominal pain may occur shortly after eating and is occasionally relieved by vomitingor lying on the right side, a manoeuvre that possibly allows the dislodgment of the trapped bowel from the mesenteric defect [12]. Patients may also recall similar episodes in the past that had spontaneously resolved. It has been shown that the development of acute SBO secondary to IHs is nearly always preceded by at least one episode of intermittent abdominal problems which highlights the importance of taking a thorough history from these patients [12].

Establishing the correct diagnosis of IH is challenging and CT scans are often difficult to interpret. Features on CT that are common to all types of internal hernias include the presence of small bowel dilatation, volvulus and the presence of a cluster of small bowel loops [9, 31]. In addition, mesenteric swirl is considered a very helpful CT sign of internal hernia, with high sensitivity and specificity [33]. Other CT features such as the position of cluster small bowel loops and a shift in the position of the SMV may give a clue to the type hernia [34].

Most surgeons advocate immediate surgical exploration of the abdomen as the only reliable means of establishing the correct diagnosis and preventing serious complications [13, 24, 35]. Furthermore, elective laparoscopic exploration in patients who presented with intermittent abdominal pain following RYGB is likely to reveal the presence of IH in a significant proportion of these patients. This has been highlighted in a study which interestingly showed that patients with early symptoms who turned down early elective intervention later presented with acute SBO and required emergency surgery [12].

Incisional and Port Site Hernias

Morbid obesity is a risk factor for wound dehiscence and the development of incisional hernia after abdominal surgery. Incisional hernia is one of the most common complications after open RYGB occurring in up to 26% of patients [36]. In a study which included a large cohort of over 25000 patients the incidence of incisional hernia after open RYGB was 6. 4% for the standard midline incision and 0. 3% for the left subcostal incision [15].

Incisional hernias can potentially lead to incarceration and or strangulation of the bowel. Although surgical repair will be required in most patients it is often advisable to postpone this until significant weight loss has been achieved as this makes the surgery technically easier and improves outcome. Of course earlier repair is required if there is significant pain or the patient develops bowel obstruction.

The development of minimally invasive surgical techniques have dramatically decrease but not eliminated the risk of abdominal wall hernias as trocar-wound hernias still occur in laparoscopic weight loss surgery with an incidence of less than 1% [37]. The presence of a thick pre-peritoneal adipose tissue in obese patients means that trocar defects may still exist even after fascial closure [38]. This predisposes to the development of Richter hernia in which part of the circumference of the bowel herniates through the defect. Although this type of hernia is uncommon it has a high risk of strangulation and the diagnosis may easily be overlooked. It is therefore mandatory to close all trocar sites particularly if they are 10mm or larger. However, closure of the fascial layer of trocar wounds may be technically difficult and alternative techniques including closure under direct vision and the placement of a surgical plug into the muscle layer have been suggested as means to reduce the incidence of port site hernias [37].

Anastomotic Stricture

Anastomotic stricture at the gastro-jejunal (GJ) or JJ anastomoses is a recognizable cause of obstruction in patients undergoing RYGB. The most common site of anastomotic stricture after RYGB is the GJ anastomosis with a reported incidence of 6-10% [26]. Factors that increase the likelihood of post-operative anastomotic stricture at the GJ anastomosis include technical problems at the time of surgery such as poor blood supply and ischemia at the anastomosis, post-operative anastomotic leak and the use of small diameter anvil [26, 39]. Marginal ulcers around the GJ anastomosis also predisposes to anastomotic strictures. They occur in up to 15% of patients mainly as a result of tension or poor tissue perfusion at the anstomotic site, smoking and NSAIDs. A rare but important predisposing factor is the presence gastro-gastric fistula which leads to the presence of excessive amounts of acid in the stomach pouch thereby increasing the risk of stomal ulceration and stricture formation.

Patients with anastomotic stricture may present in the first few days after surgery as result of inflammatory changes and edema or later as a result of ischemia, fibrosis or chronic ulceration. Patients with GJ anastomotic stricture present with progressive nausea, regurgitation and reflux. They may have upper abdominal discomfort but sever pain and abdominal distension are not usually present. A previous history of marginal ulceration or anastomotic leak at the time of original surgery may give a clue to the diagnosis.

The incidence of obstruction at the JJ anastomosis appears to be higher after laparoscopic RYGB compared to open surgery [20]. SBO secondary to JJ stricture tends to develop early in the post-operative period with an incidence of about 1. 2% [39]. In one study of 1400 patients who underwent laparoscopic antecolic RYGB, stricture at the JJ anastomosis was found to be the most common cause of SBO [4]. One of the predisposing factors to JJ stricture is misalignment of the bowel edges during stapled closure of the enterotomy. This leads to narrowing of the lumen of the BP limb which leads to dilatation of the BP limb, duodenum and the excluded stomach. This problem can be minimized by using suture rather than stapled closure of the enterotomy [40].

Patients with JJ stricture present in a manner that is indistinguishable from other causes of SBO with nausea, vomiting and abdominal pain. Anastomotic stricture at the JJ anastomosis that leads obstruction of the Roux limb produces non-bilious vomiting which distinguishes it from more distal obstruction. An uncommon but serious complication of obstruction of the BP limb secondary to stricture at the site of JJ is acute dilatation of the gastric remnant which if not treated promptly can potentially result in gastric necrosis and blow out, pancreatitis and biliary sepsis [41].

UGI contrast study and endoscopy are the investigations of choice for diagnosing a suspected GJ stricture. Fluoroscopy shows narrowing at the GJ anastomosis, distended gastric pouch, and delayed emptying of the gastric pouch. Endoscopy may reveal an underlying cause such as marginal ulceration and may also be used for therapeutic balloon dilatation. Balloon dilatation must be undertaken by an experienced endoscopist as the risk of perforation can be up to 2% [42, 43]. In the case of JJ stricture the radiological features include a dilated Roux limb, narrowing at the site of the anastomosis and possibly retrograde flow of contrast medium into the BP limb [44].

Treatment of patients with JJ stricture depends on the timing and severity of the symptoms. The majority of patients can be successfully treated conservatively but those who are acutely unwell or if conservative treatment fails operative intervention is indicated [39]

Obstruction at the Mesocolic Window

In addition to internal herniation through the mesocolic window SBO in patients with retrocolic Roux limb can be caused by extrinsic compression of the Roux limb as it traverses mesocolic window. This is usually caused by the formation of thickened cicatrix which results from excessive or continuous suturing during closure of the defect or hematoma at this site [45]. Post-operative inflammatory changes and edema at this site can also cause early post-operative obstruction but this tends to be transient and self-limiting. In one series 0. 9% of patients developed SBO at the mesocolic window and, unlike IH, presentation tended to be early after surgery [46]. The diagnosis is readily established using UGI contrast study or CT scan. Imaging findings include dilatation of the Roux limb above the constriction point which can be seen at the level of the mesocolon [44]. Endoscopic dilatation may be helpful but patients often require division of the constricting fibrotic scar around the Roux limb [45].

Bowel Kink and Twists

SBO can also result from kinking of the small bowel at the JJ anastomosis or a twist of the Roux limb which leads to narrowing of the bowel lumen and intermittent SBO [20]. Techniques which have been employed to reduce the risk of obstruction from kinking of the bowel at the JJ anastomosis include suture closure of the enterotomy and placement of the so called anti-obstruction or anti kink stich [40]. The anti- obstruction stich is placed between the common channel and the stapled end of the BP limb immediately distal to the JJ anastomosis limb thereby fixing the position of the staple line and preventing the common channel from folding. This suture can be continued distally to the root of the mesentery to close the JJ mesenteric defect.

The diagnosis of SBO caused by a kink or a twist of the small bowel is extremely difficult to establish or distinguish from true JJ stricture and it is best to avoid these problems by careful inspection of the JJ anastomosis and the orientation of the bowel limbs at the time of surgery.

Intussusception

Small bowel intussusception is an uncommon cause of intestinal obstruction after RYGB [47]. The reported overall incidence of intussusceptions after Roux-en-Y gastric bypass is 0. 1% which is higher after open surgery [48, 49]. Contributing factors include abnormal motility of the bowel limbs and the presence of lead points at the site of suture or staple lines [50, 51]. The condition is characterized by retrograde intussusception or internal prolapse of a segment of small bowel proximally which occurs most commonly at the site of the JJ anastomosis [52, 53]. The rarity of this condition coupled with the fact that presentation may be nonspecific makes the diagnosis difficult to establish. It is therefore important to be aware of this entity and have a high index of suspicion in order to avoid the catastrophic complication of intestinal necrosis and perforation. A clue to the diagnosis is the presence on

CT of the classic target sign in which one bowel segment (intussusceptum) is seen to telescope into the lumen of the receiving bowel segment (intussuscipient) [54]. Early recognition with the aid of CT scan or immediate laparoscopy may allow the diagnosis to be made in a timely manner. At surgery the affected segment may be simply reduced but, off course, bowel resection of the affected segment will be required if there are signs of necrosis [52].

Intraluminal Obstruction

Intraluminal causes of SBO include bezoars and blood clots. Bezoars are an unusual but well documented underlying cause of SBO after bariatric surgery. Predisposing factors include the composition of food, previous gastric surgery and gastric dysmotility [55, 56]. Bezoars can form at any site of the GIT including the gastric pouch and the small bowel [57-60]. CT scan findings that suggest the presence of bezoar include an ovoid mass of a mottled appearance at the site of obstruction [61] Intraluminal clots can cause obstruction at the GJ or JJ anastomoses and the symptoms are often indistinguishable from anastomotic stricture [50]. Treatment depends on the site of bezoar or blood clot and includes endoscopic or surgical removal.

3.5. Obstruction after Other Bariatric Procedures

Sleeve gastrectomy and LAGB involve little or no manipulation of the small bowel and therefore are not expected to expose the patient to the risk of SBO. Although SBO after these procedures is rare [62] several studies have reported this complication.

Although vomiting after LAGB may be the result of behavioral and eating disorders such as overeating and bulimia, band slippage and erosion are two causes that should be considered in this setting. Band slippage occurs when the anterior or anterolateral wall of the fundus of the stomach prolapses upward underneath the band resulting in an enlarged pouch above the band and a tight stoma. Patients with this condition often present with vomiting shortly after meals with pain and discomfort in the epigastrium and left upper quadrant. Patients with band erosion may present with signs of sepsis and occasionally infection around the band port which results from infection tracking up the band tube.

In the case of sleeve gastrectomy stenosis or stricture formation along the staple line can lead to abdominal discomfort and vomiting which are often triggered by eating. This condition results from the formation of excessively narrow tube at the time of surgery or from post-operative staple line leak and sepsis. The investigation of choice in patients presenting with obstructive symptoms after gastric banding and sleeve gastrectomy is endoscopy and barium contrast study. In the case of band slippage contrast study shows a dilated stomach pouch above a horizontally lying band with little or no contrast passing through it.

The management of band slippage includes immediate deflation of the band which relieves symptoms in the majority of the cases. If symptoms do not improve with simple band deflation immediate intervention becomes mandatory. In the presence of an experienced surgeon one option would be to re-site the band which can be done laparoscopically. However, in the presence of significant edema and inflammation or if an experienced surgeon is not available immediate re-siting of the band is not advisable. Instead, the locking mechanism of the band can be unbuckled and the band is left in situ for later repositioning. Alternatively, the band can be removed particularly in the presence of band erosion or sepsis.

The management of patients with obstruction after sleeve gastrectomy should be in a specialist bariatric center. Endoscopic dilatation or stenting may be attempted but some patients may require re-operative intervention which may include conversion to RYGB.

Complete or partial band erosion is a well-recognized complication of gastric banding. Occasionally complete internalization and migration of the band can occur and obstruction at the level of the duodenum or even further distally by the impacted band has been described [63-65]. The diagnosis may be difficult to establish and the condition can lead to serious and potentially fatal consequences secondary to bowel wall erosion and perforation [66]. Treatment involves dividing the band tube followed by removal of the band either endoscopically or via an enterotomy [67].

There has been several reports of intestinal obstruction secondary to bowel constriction caused by the connection tubing of the gastric band [68-70]. SBO results when a bowel loop becomes incarcerated between and around the silicon tube and the anterior abdominal wall [71]. Patients present with signs and symptoms of intestinal obstruction which may be preceded by pain at the port site as a result of traction on the connection tube by affected bowel.

4. Management

4.1. General Considerations

As the number of bariatric procedures is increasing worldwide the number of patients who will be at risk of short and long term complication including SBO will also increase. This is best highlighted by the findings of a study which showed that over a period of two years 15% of all patients who were admitted by general surgeons with SBO actually had a history of bariatric surgery [11]. Therefore, surgeons including those not performing bariatric surgery, will be treating more patients with bowel obstruction following RYGB in the future.

SBO is arguably one of the most challenging complications to manage after bariatric surgery. The consequences of SBO in this patient population can be catastrophic and as such early recognition of this complication and timely operative intervention is of paramount importance if adverse outcomes are to be minimised. Prompt diagnosis and treatment of SBO is of paramount importance in order to prevent catastrophic and potentially fatal complications, such as bowel infarction, peritonitis, short gut syndrome and death. Thus the general surgeon must have an appreciation of the effect of previous bariatric surgery on the presentation, evaluation, management and outcomes of common surgical emergencies encountered in bariatric patients [11].

One of the concerns leveled at the management of patients who have previously undergone bariatric surgery is the complicated underlying anatomy and that they should be immediately treated in a specialist unit. Whilst it may be sensible to transfer a patient to a specialist bariatric unit when stable and in need of specialist treatment, most cases of intestinal obstruction regardless of the cause should be managed using the same basic principles. This may also include surgical management which should not be delayed in the attempt to seek specialist advice. Once the immediate danger has subsided and the patient is stable, specialist bariatric advice should be sought. Most patients will be able to be entirely managed in the local hospital with advice only needed. However, in rare cases it may be necessary to transfer the patient for complex investigations or treatment to a specialist bariatric unit.

4.2. Conservative Management

General surgical patients who present with SBO are managed in a manner that largely depends on the underlying pathology and patient factors [72]. A trial of conservative management is a widely accepted practice as an initial treatment option in carefully selected general surgical patients [73]. This involves immediate resuscitation with intravenous fluids and placement of a naso-gastric tube particularly if the patient is vomiting. Bladder catheterization will aid in the accurate charting of fluid balance and therefore allows for appropriate fluid prescription. The patient should remain "nil by mouth" and anti-emetic and analgesic medication should be prescribed for symptom relief. Whilst these measures are being carried out, routine investigations including blood tests and radiological imaging may be ordered. After initial assessment and resuscitation the most important decision to make is whether an urgent operative intervention is required which is indicated in patients with suspected bowel ischemia, perforation or systemic illness. This approach has been shown to be successful in up to three-quarters of patients in whom operative intervention was avoided [74].

In certain circumstances conservative treatment may have a place in the management of patients with SBO after RYGB. This is particularly the case in patients who are not acutely unwell, and those with no radiological evidence of complete obstruction. However, lengthy periods of conservative management may not be appropriate and the management algorithms often used in general surgical patients may not be suitable in bariatric patients. In one study non-operative management of SBO was successful in 72% of general non-bariatric patients while 62 % of bariatric patients with SBO required surgical intervention [11]. In another study all patients who presented with SBO after laparoscopic RGBY required surgical intervention and none were successfully treated with simple NGT decompression and fluid resuscitation [12]. Most non-bariatric patients with SBO can be successfully decompressed by the insertion of NGT which is an essential step in treating these patients. However, internal hernias and obstruction of the BP limb and sometimes the common channel distal the JJ anastomosis results in closed loop obstruction which cannot be effectively decompressed by the mere insertion of NGT. If the underlying anatomy is not fully understood and the possibility of closed loop obstruction is not entertained prolonged and futile attempts at managing SBO will result in catastrophic and fatal consequences [75, 76].

4.3. Timing of Intervention

Another factor that contributes to the concerns raised about bariatric patients presenting with possible SBO is the difficulty in establishing the diagnosis particularly when the cause is related to internal herniation or small incisional and port site hernias that are often difficult to clinically detect in obese patients [11]. As mentioned previously, the presentation of patients with internal hernias is often atypical and symptoms may be insidious and intermittent which may be mistaken for non-surgical GI disturbances. In addition, even if the diagnosis is considered, imaging techniques including CT scans frequently fail to demonstrate the presence of internal hernias in a significant proportion of patients [9, 77].

These considerations have led to the increased acceptance of the notion that bariatric patients require earlier surgical exploration compared to non-bariatric patients [12, 78]. This is highlighted in a large study in which the majority of bariatric patients suspected of having SBO underwent surgical intervention within the first 24 hours of admission while non-bariatric patients underwent intervention at a later stage (> 3 days) [11]. In another study, elective laparoscopy revealed the presence of IH in all patients presenting with abdominal pain and that up to one-third of these patients turned out to have small bowel volvulus emphasizing the importance of early intervention in these patients [10]. It was therefore concluded that a high index of suspicion, based mainly on the clinical history of recurrent colicky abdominal pain, and early surgical exploration are the only means to reduce the number of acute complications [8].

It has been shown that morbidity in patients who present acutely with SBO can be as high as 30% compared to no morbidity in patients undergoing elective laparoscopic exploration for suspected IHs [12]. Similarly, lower complication rates have been reported in bariatric patients who underwent early surgical intervention compared to non-bariatric patients who were treated conservatively [11]. It was therefore concluded that early surgical intervention in bariatric patients with SBO may be a safer approach than watchful waiting [11]. The reduction in in post-operative morbidity is attributed to early intervention, the use of laparoscopic approach and the reduced need for major bowel resection [11]. An element of delay in establishing the diagnosis and proceeding with surgical exploration is usually present in virtually all the patients who subsequently developed complications after surgery for SBO [12]. In these patients the need for bowel resection, length of ITU stay and mortality are significantly increased.

SBO may occur within the first few days after surgery or months or years later. Making a distinction between these different patterns of presentation is useful as the etiologies and the management options may be different. For example early SBO that results from inflammatory changes and edema at the site of the anastomoses is usually self-limiting and a period of conservative treatment may be tried to allow edema to subside. Nelson et al. reported that conservative treatment is likely to be more successful in patients presenting in the early postoperative period [21]. The majority of these patients gradually improve in which case operative intervention will not be required. Early SBO may also be secondary to early internal hernias or technical problems at the time of surgery such as anastomotic stricture or bowel kinking. In these patients conservative treatment is unlikely to be successful and operative intervention is almost always required. Up to 80% of these patients will require surgical intervention and bowel resection indicating that conservative treatment in the early postoperative period can be a dangerous policy [79]. Similarly, SBO occurring months or years after RYGB as a result of adhesions or abdominal wall or internal hernias almost always requires surgical intervention [79].

Operative Management

Laparoscopy is considered to be a reasonable and acceptable option for the treatment of patients with SBO provided an experienced laparoscopist is available [80]. Although laparoscopy was once considered an absolute contraindication in patients with SBO with increasing experience it is now developing into a valuable diagnostic and therapeutic tool particularly in patients with chronic intermittent abdominal pain [81]. The utilization of laparoscopy in the diagnosis and treatment of patients with SBO has been reported in a number of studies. Generally, bariatric patients with SBO are more likely to be treated laparoscopically. This was highlighted in a study that reported that bariatric patients were 5 times more likely to undergo laparoscopic intervention for SBO compared to non-bariatric patients (3. 3 vs. 0. 7% p>0. 001) [11]. In another study, laparoscopy identified the cause of SBO in almost all patients (250/253 patients) and over two thirds of these patients (169/253 of patients) were managed totally laparoscopically [82]. Other studies reported that 70-85% of patients with SBO secondary to internal hernias were successfully managed laparoscopically with a conversion rate of around 10% [12, 20, 32].

The main challenge of using laparoscopy in patients with SBO is establishing pneumoperitoneum safely and the ability to adequately inspect the abdominal cavity in the presence of multiple dilated loops of bowel. This is not necessarily an issue related to laparoscopy in the post-bariatric patient but specific to laparoscopy in the presence of acute intestinal obstruction. If there are any safety concerns, a formal open laparotomy should be performed without unnecessary delay.

Regardless of the approach, abdominal inspection should be done in a systematic manner and a sound understanding of the surgical anatomy of bariatric procedure is essential for the correct identification of the source of the problem. The three limbs of the RYGB must be accurately identified. An approach to this is to start at the terminal ileum and proximally to the JJ anastomosis, the Roux and BP limbs and the GJ anastomosis and ligament of Trietz. One must be careful when handling the bowel whether this is with laparoscopic instruments or manually as the distended loops of bowel may become vulnerable to trauma. If the cause can be readily identified then this must be treated. All sites of mesenteric defects must be carefully inspected and the presence of herniating bowel loops should be considered. If the mesenteric defects are found to be enlarged they should be closed with non-absorbable suture even in the absence of internal herniation.

If on surgical exploration the obstructed bowel is found to be viable the surgeon must aim to deal with the causes of the obstruction which may involve division of adhesions or reduction of the herniated bowel and closure of the mesenteric defect. Management is more complicated in cases where the affected bowel is found be irreversibly ischemic with no signs of viability. In this situation a great deal of judgment and experience will be required as the anatomy can be confusing and the patient is often very sick.

If a significant proportion of the alimentary limb is to be resected intestinal continuity is obviously interrupted and oral intake postoperatively is not possible. In this situation it is advisable not to attempt any form of immediate reconstruction. Instead the affected segment is resected and either a feeding gastrostomy through the gastric remnant or a feeding jejunostomy distal to the ligament of Trietz should be inserted and a wide bore NGT is inserted to decompress the gastric pouch. Definitive reconstruction, which in this situation requires specialist input, can be attempted at a later stage when the patient's general condition and nutritional state improve. An alternative would be to attempt immediate restoration of intestinal continuity by creating an anastomosis between the gastric pouch and the gastric remnant. Although this is an attractive option it is technically challenging and in the acute situation there is a significant risk of anastomotic leakage.

If the alimentary limb is affected and a portion of it has to be resected several options are available depending on the length of the remaining bowel. If primary anastomosis is considered to be unsafe an end ileostomy should be created. Reversal or reconstruction can be attempted at a later stage. If, however, a significant portion of the common channel has to be resected the patient may be left a short common channel which predisposes to short gut syndrome. In this case a feeding gastrostomy or jejunostomy should be inserted to provide the patient with adequate nutrition post operatively. Again reconstruction can be attempted at a later stage. One has to remember that it is the surgeon's responsibility to perform the kind of surgery that will save the patient's life and temporize the situation until the patient recovers from the acute episode.

References

[1] Husain S, Ahmed AR, Johnson J, Boss T, O'Malley W: Small-bowel obstruction after laparoscopic Roux-en-Y gastric bypass: etiology, diagnosis, and management. *Archives of surgery,* 2007, 142(10):988-993.

[2] Srikanth MS, Keskey T, Fox SR, Oh KH, Fox ER, Fox KM: Computed tomography patterns in small bowel obstruction after open distal gastric bypass. *Obesity surgery,* 2004, 14(6):811-822.

[3] Sunnapwar A, Sandrasegaran K, Menias CO, Lockhart M, Chintapalli KN, Prasad SR: Taxonomy and imaging spectrum of small bowel obstruction after Roux-en-Y gastric bypass surgery. *AJR American journal of roentgenology,* 2010, 194(1):120-128.

[4] Cho M, Carrodeguas L, Pinto D, Lascano C, Soto F, Whipple O, Gordon R, Simpfendorfer C, Gonzalvo JP, Szomstein S *et al.*: Diagnosis and management of partial small bowel obstruction after laparoscopic antecolic antegastric Roux-en-Y gastric bypass for morbid obesity. *Journal of the American College of Surgeons,* 2006, 202(2):262-268.

[5] Merkle EM, Hallowell PT, Crouse C, Nakamoto DA, Stellato TA: Roux-en-Y gastric bypass for clinically severe obesity: normal appearance and spectrum of complications at imaging. *Radiology,* 2005, 234(3):674-683.

[6] Esmailzadeh H, Powell W, Lourie D: Use of computed tomography in diagnosis of major postoperative gastrointestinal complications of laparoscopic Roux-en-Y gastric bypass surgery. *The American surgeon,* 2004, 70(11):964-966.

[7] Higa KD, Ho T, Boone KB: Internal hernias after laparoscopic Roux-en-Y gastric bypass: incidence, treatment and prevention. *Obesity surgery,* 2003, 13(3):350-354.

[8] Paroz A, Calmes JM, Giusti V, Suter M: Internal hernia after laparoscopic Roux-en-Y gastric bypass for morbid obesity: a continuous challenge in bariatric surgery. *Obesity surgery,* 2006, 16(11):1482-1487.

[9] Gunabushanam G, Shankar S, Czerniach DR, Kelly JJ, Perugini RA: Small-bowel obstruction after laparoscopic Roux-en-Y gastric bypass surgery. *Journal of computer assisted tomography,* 2009, 33(3):369-375.

[10] Rogula T, Yenumula PR, Schauer PR: A complication of Roux-en-Y gastric bypass: intestinal obstruction. *Surgical endoscopy,* 2007, 21(11):1914-1918.

[11] Martin MJ, Beekley AC, Sebesta JA: Bowel obstruction in bariatric and nonbariatric patients: major differences in management strategies and outcome. Surgery for obesity and related diseases : *official journal of the American Society for Bariatric Surgery,* 2011, 7(3):263-269.

[12] Gandhi AD, Patel RA, Brolin RE: Elective laparoscopy for herald symptoms of mesenteric/internal hernia after laparoscopic Roux-en-Y gastric bypass. Surgery for obesity and related diseases : *official journal of the American Society for Bariatric Surgery,* 2009, 5(2):144-149; discussion 149.

[13] Ahmed AR, Rickards G, Husain S, Johnson J, Boss T, O'Malley W: Trends in internal hernia incidence after laparoscopic Roux-en-Y gastric bypass. *Obesity surgery,* 2007, 17(12):1563-1566.

[14] Rodriguez A, Mosti M, Sierra M, Perez-Johnson R, Flores S, Dominguez G, Sanchez H, Zarco A, Romay K, Herrera MF: Small bowel obstruction after antecolic and antegastric laparoscopic Roux-en-Y gastric bypass: could the incidence be reduced?*Obesity surgery,* 2010, 20(10):1380-1384.

[15] Jones KB, Jr., Afram JD, Benotti PN, Capella RF, Cooper CG, Flanagan L, Hendrick S, Howell LM, Jaroch MT, Kole K et al.: Open versus laparoscopic Roux-en-Y gastric bypass: a comparative study of over 25,000 open cases and the major laparoscopic bariatric reported series. *Obesity surgery,* 2006, 16(6):721-727.

[16] Smith SC, Edwards CB, Goodman GN, Halversen RC, Simper SC: Open vs laparoscopic Roux-en-Y gastric bypass: comparison of operative morbidity and mortality. *Obesity surgery,* 2004, 14(1):73-76.

[17] Dresel A, Kuhn JA, McCarty TM: Laparoscopic Roux-en-Y gastric bypass in morbidly obese and super morbidly obese patients. *American journal of surgery,* 2004, 187(2):230-232; discussion 232.

[18] Marema RT, Perez M, Buffington CK: Comparison of the benefits and complications between laparoscopic and open Roux-en-Y gastric bypass surgeries. *Surgical endoscopy,* 2005, 19(4):525-530.

[19] Podnos YD, Jimenez JC, Wilson SE, Stevens CM, Nguyen NT: Complications after laparoscopic gastric bypass: a review of 3464 cases. *Archives of surgery,* 2003, 138(9):957-961.

[20] Capella RF, Iannace VA, Capella JF: Bowel obstruction after open and laparoscopic gastric bypass surgery for morbid obesity. *Journal of the American College of Surgeons,* 2006, 203(3):328-335.

[21] Nelson LG, Gonzalez R, Haines K, Gallagher SF, Murr MM: Spectrum and treatment of small bowel obstruction after Roux-en-Y gastric bypass. Surgery for obesity and related diseases : *official journal of the American Society for Bariatric Surgery*, 2006, 2(3):377-383, discussion 383.

[22] Brolin RE, Kenler HA, Gorman JH, Cody RP: Long-limb gastric bypass in the superobese. A prospective randomized study. *Annals of surgery,* 1992, 215(4):387-395.

[23] Taylor JD, Leitman IM, Hon P, Horowitz M, Panagopoulos G: Outcome and complications of gastric bypass in super-super obesity versus morbid obesity. *Obesity surgery,* 2006, 16(1):16-18.

[24] Carmody B, DeMaria EJ, Jamal M, Johnson J, Carbonell A, Kellum J, Maher J: Internal hernia after laparoscopic Roux-en-Y gastric bypass. Surgery for obesity and related diseases : *official journal of the American Society for Bariatric Surgery,* 2005, 1(6):543-548.

[25] Swartz DE, Felix EL: Acute mesenteric venous thrombosis following laparoscopic Roux-en-Y gastric bypass. JSLS : *Journal of the Society of Laparoendoscopic Surgeons / Society of Laparoendoscopic Surgeons,* 2004, 8(2):165-169.

[26] Escalona A, Devaud N, Perez G, Crovari F, Boza C, Viviani P, Ibanez L, Guzman S: Antecolic versus retrocolic alimentary limb in laparoscopic Roux-en-Y gastric bypass: a comparative study. Surgery for obesity and related diseases : *official journal of the American Society for Bariatric Surgery,* 2007, 3(4):423-427.

[27] Felsher J, Brodsky J, Brody F: Small bowel obstruction after laparoscopic Roux-en-Y gastric bypass. *Surgery,* 2003, 134(3):501-505.

[28] Champion JK, Williams M: Small bowel obstruction and internal hernias after laparoscopic Roux-en-Y gastric bypass. *Obesity surgery,* 2003, 13(4):596-600.

[29] Tucker ON, Escalante-Tattersfield T, Szomstein S, Rosenthal RJ: The ABC System: a simplified classification system for small bowel obstruction after laparoscopic Roux-en-Y gastric bypass. *Obesity surgery,* 2007, 17(12):1549-1554.

[30] Hope WW, Sing RF, Chen AY, Lincourt AE, Gersin KS, Kuwada TS, Heniford BT: Failure of mesenteric defect closure after Roux-en-Y gastric bypass. JSLS : *Journal of the Society of Laparoendoscopic Surgeons / Society of Laparoendoscopic Surgeons,* 2010, 14(2):213-216.

[31] Garza E, Jr., Kuhn J, Arnold D, Nicholson W, Reddy S, McCarty T: Internal hernias after laparoscopic Roux-en-Y gastric bypass. *American journal of surgery,* 2004, 188(6):796-800.

[32] Eckhauser A, Torquati A, Youssef Y, Kaiser JL, Richards WO: Internal hernia: postoperative complication of roux-en-Y gastric bypass surgery. *The American surgeon,* 2006, 72(7):581-584; discussion 584-585.

[33] Lockhart ME, Tessler FN, Canon CL, Smith JK, Larrison MC, Fineberg NS, Roy BP, Clements RH: Internal hernia after gastric bypass: sensitivity and specificity of seven CT signs with surgical correlation and controls. *AJR American journal of roent genology,* 2007, 188(3):745-750.

[34] Kawkabani Marchini A, Denys A, Paroz A, Romy S, Suter M, Desmartines N, Meuli R, Schmidt S: The four different types of internal hernia occurring after laparascopic Roux-en-Y gastric bypass performed for morbid obesity: are there any multidetector computed tomography (MDCT) features permitting their distinction? *Obesity surgery,* 2011, 21(4):506-516.

[35] Cho M, Pinto D, Carrodeguas L, Lascano C, Soto F, Whipple O, Simpfendorfer C, Gonzalvo JP, Zundel N, Szomstein Set al.: Frequency and management of internal hernias after laparoscopic antecolic antegastric Roux-en-Y gastric bypass without division of the small bowel mesentery or closure of mesenteric defects: review of 1400 consecutive cases. Surgery for obesity and related diseases : official *journal of the American Society for Bariatric Surgery,* 2006, 2(2):87-91.

[36] Reddy RM, Riker A, Marra D, Thomas R, Brems JJ: Open Roux-en-Y gastric bypass for the morbidly obese in the era of laparoscopy. *American journal of surgery* 2002, 184(6):611-615; discussion 615-616.

[37] Chiu CC, Lee WJ, Wang W, Wei PL, Huang MT: Prevention of trocar-wound hernia in laparoscopic bariatric operations. *Obesity surgery,* 2006, 16(7):913-918.

[38] Cottam DR, Gorecki PJ, Curvelo M, Weltman D, Angus LD, Shaftan G: Preperitoneal herniation into a laparoscopic port site without a fascial defect. *Obesity surgery,* 2002, 12(1):121-123.

[39] Lewis CE, Jensen C, Tejirian T, Dutson E, Mehran A: Early jejunojejunostomy obstruction after laparoscopic gastric bypass: case series and treatment algorithm. Surgery for obesity and related diseases *: official journal of the American Society for Bariatric Surgery,* 2009, 5(2):203-207.

[40] Brolin RE: The antiobstruction stitch in stapled Roux-en-Y enteroenterostomy. *American journal of surgery,* 1995, 169(3):355-357.

[41] Torrens AS, Born PW, Naver L: [Gastric blow-out: complication after obesity surgery]. *Ugeskrift for laeger,* 2009, 171(49):3624-3625.

[42] Gill RS, Whitlock KA, Mohamed R, Sarkhosh K, Birch DW, Karmali S: The role of upper gastrointestinal endoscopy in treating postoperative complications in bariatric surgery. *Journal of interventional gastroenterology,* 2012, 2(1):37-41.

[43] Ukleja A, Afonso BB, Pimentel R, Szomstein S, Rosenthal R: Outcome of endoscopic balloon dilation of strictures after laparoscopic gastric bypass. *Surgical endoscopy,* 2008, 22(8):1746-1750.

[44] Chandler RC, Srinivas G, Chintapalli KN, Schwesinger WH, Prasad SR: Imaging in bariatric surgery: a guide to postsurgical anatomy and common complications. *AJR American journal of roentgenology,* 2008, 190(1):122-135.

[45] Ahmed AR, Rickards G, Johnson J, Boss T, O'Malley W: Radiological findings in symptomatic internal hernias after laparoscopic gastric bypass. *Obesity surgery,* 2009, 19(11):1530-1535.

[46] Ahmed AR, Rickards G, Messing S, Husain S, Johnson J, Boss T, O'Malley W: Roux limb obstruction secondary to constriction at transverse mesocolon rent after laparoscopic Roux-en-Y gastric bypass. Surgery for obesity and related diseases : *official journal of the American Society for Bariatric Surgery,* 2009, 5(2):194-198.

[47] Simper SC, Erzinger JM, McKinlay RD, Smith SC: Laparoscopic reversal of gastric bypass with sleeve gastrectomy for treatment of recurrent retrograde intussusception and Roux stasis syndrome. Surgery for obesity and related diseases : *official journal of the American Society for Bariatric Surgery,* 2010, 6(6):684-688.

[48] Sandrasegaran K, Maglinte DD, Lappas JC, Howard TJ: Small-bowel complications of major gastrointestinal tract surgery. *AJR American journal of roentgenology,* 2005, 185(3):671-681.

[49] Shaw D, Huddleston S, Beilman G: Anterograde intussusception following laparoscopic Roux-en-Y gastric bypass: a case report and review of the literature. *Obesity surgery,* 2010, 20(8):1191-1194.

[50] Hocking MP, McCoy DM, Vogel SB, Kaude JV, Sninsky CA: Antiperistaltic and isoperistaltic intussusception associated with abnormal motility after Roux-en-Y gastric bypass: a case report. *Surgery,* 1991, 110(1):109-112.

[51] Daellenbach L, Suter M: Jejunojejunal intussusception after Roux-en-Y gastric bypass: a review. *Obesity surgery,* 2011, 21(2):253-263.

[52] Simper SC, Erzinger JM, McKinlay RD, Smith SC: Retrograde (reverse) jejunal intussusception might not be such a rare problem: a single group's experience of 23 cases. Surgery for obesity and related diseases: *official journal of the American Society for Bariatric Surgery,* 2008, 4(2):77-83.
[53] McAllister MS, Donoway T, Lucktong TA: Synchronous intussusceptions following Roux-en-Y Gastric Bypass: case report and review of the literature. *Obesity surgery,* 2009, 19(12):1719-1723.
[54] Ver Steeg K: Retrograde intussusception following Roux-en-Y gastric bypass. *Obesity surgery,* 2006, 16(8):1101-1103.
[55] Parameswaran R, Ferrando J, Sigurdsson A: Gastric bezoar complicating laparoscopic adjustable gastric banding with band slippage. *Obesity surgery,* 2006, 16(12):1683-1684.
[56] Robles R, Parrilla P, Escamilla C, Lujan JA, Torralba JA, Liron R, Moreno A: Gastrointestinal bezoars. *The British journal of surgery,* 1994, 81(7):1000-1001.
[57] Pinto D, Carrodeguas L, Soto F, Lascano C, Cho M, Szomstein S, Rosenthal R: Gastric bezoar after laparoscopic Roux-en-Y gastric bypass. *Obesity surgery,* 2006, 16(3):365-368.
[58] Ionescu AM, Rogers AM, Pauli EM, Shope TR: An unusual suspect: coconut bezoar after laparoscopic Roux-en-Y gastric bypass. *Obesity surgery,* 2008, 18(6):756-758.
[59] Pratt JS, Van Noord M, Christison-Lagay E: The tethered bezoar as a delayed complication of laparoscopic Roux-en-Y gastric bypass: a case report. *Journal of gastrointestinal surgery : official journal of the Society for Surgery of the Alimentary Tract,* 2007, 11(5):690-692.
[60] Koulas SG, Zikos N, Charalampous C, Christodoulou K, Sakkas L, Katsamakis N: Management of gastrointestinal bezoars: an analysis of 23 cases. *International surgery,* 2008, 93(2):95-98.
[61] Zissin R, Osadchy A, Gutman V, Rathaus V, Shapiro-Feinberg M, Gayer G: CT findings in patients with small bowel obstruction due to phytobezoar. *Emergency radiology,* 2004, 10(4):197-200.
[62] Himpens J, Dapri G, Cadiere GB: Laparoscopic conversion of the gastric bypass into a normal anatomy. *Obesity surgery,* 2006, 16(7):908-912.
[63] Shah KG, Molmenti EP, Nicastro J: Gastric band erosion and intraluminal migration leading to biliary and small bowel obstruction: case report and discussion. Surgery for obesity and related diseases : *official journal of the American Society for Bariatric Surgery,* 2011, 7(1):117-118.
[64] Offodile AC, 2nd, Okafor P, Shaikh SN, Lautz D, Thompson CC: Duodenal obstruction due to erosion and migration of an adjustable gastric band: a novel endoscopic approach to management. Surgery for obesity and related diseases : *official journal of the American Society for Bariatric Surgery,* 2010, 6(2):206-208.
[65] Lantsberg L, Kirshtein B, Leytzin A, Makarov V: Jejunal obstruction caused by migrated gastric band. *Obesity surgery,* 2008, 18(2):225-227.
[66] Egbeare DM, Myers AF, Lawrance RJ: Small bowel obstruction secondary to intragastric erosion and migration of a gastric band. *Journal of gastrointestinal surgery : official journal of the Society for Surgery of the Alimentary Tract,* 2008, 12(5):983-984.

[67] Bueter M, Thalheimer A, Meyer D, Fein M: Band erosion and passage, causing small bowel obstruction. *Obesity surgery,* 2006, 16(12):1679-1682.

[68] Strobos E, Antanavicius G, Josloff R: Unusual complication: small bowel obstruction caused by tubing of gastric band. Surgery for obesity and related diseases : *official journal of the American Society for Bariatric Surgery,* 2009, 5(5):637-640.

[69] Fass G, Simoens C, da Costa PM: Diffuse abdominal and port site pain caused by the connecting tube in gastric banding. *Obesity surgery* 2010, 20(8):1183-1185.

[70] Egberts K, Brown WA, O'Brien PE: Systematic review of erosion after laparoscopic adjustable gastric banding. *Obesity surgery,* 2011, 21(8):1272-1279.

[71] Shipkov CD, Uchikov AP, Uchikova EH: Small bowel obstruction by the silicone tube of the gastric band. *Obesity surgery,* 2004, 14(9):1280-1282.

[72] Zerey M, Sechrist CW, Kercher KW, Sing RF, Matthews BD, Heniford BT: Laparoscopic management of adhesive small bowel obstruction. *The American surgeon,* 2007, 73(8):773-778; discussion 778-779.

[73] Trevino C: Small bowel obstruction: the art of management. *AACN advanced critical care,* 2010, 21(2):187-194.

[74] Williams SB, Greenspon J, Young HA, Orkin BA: Small bowel obstruction: conservative vs. surgical management. *Diseases of the colon and rectum,* 2005, 48(6):1140-1146.

[75] Abell TL, Minocha A: Gastrointestinal complications of bariatric surgery: diagnosis and therapy. *The American journal of the medical sciences,* 2006, 331(4):214-218.

[76] Macgregor AM: Small Bowel Obstruction Following Gastric Bypass. *Obesity surgery,* 1992, 2(4):333-339.

[77] Parakh S, Soto E, Merola S: Diagnosis and management of internal hernias after laparoscopic gastric bypass. *Obesity surgery,* 2007, 17(11):1498-1502.

[78] Frezza EE, Wachtel MS: Laparoscopic re-exploration in mechanical bowel obstruction after laparoscopic gastric bypass for morbid obesita. *Minerva chirurgica,* 2006, 61(3):193-197.

[79] Hwang RF, Swartz DE, Felix EL: Causes of small bowel obstruction after laparoscopic gastric bypass. *Surgical endoscopy,* 2004, 18(11):1631-1635.

[80] Lauter DM: Treatment of nonadhesive bowel obstruction following gastric bypass. *American journal of surgery,* 2005, 189(5):532-535; discussion 535.

[81] Chousleb E, Shuchleib S, Chousleb A: Laparoscopic management of intestinal obstruction. *Surgical laparoscopy, endoscopy and percutaneous techniques,* 2010, 20(5):348-350.

[82] Chowbey PK, Panse R, Sharma A, Khullar R, Soni V, Baijal M: Elective laparoscopy in diagnosis and treatment of recurrent small bowel obstruction. *Surgical laparoscopy, endoscopy and percutaneous techniques,* 2006, 16(6):416-422.

In: Bariatric Surgery
Editor: Christos R. Iavazzo
ISBN: 978-1-62618-995-9

Chapter VIII

Bariatric Surgery and Infectious Diseases

Fotinie Ntziora
A' Academic Department of Medicine, Laiko General Hospital
Medical School, University of Athens, Athens, Greece

Abstract

Obese patients do not appear to have a greater risk of perioperative death. However, the risk of postoperative infection clearly is higher, in particular, their risk of SSI, as shown in multiple studies of diverse populations of patients. As obesity is more often considered a serious medical condition, studies with similar conclusions likely will proliferate. Stratification of infection risk for obese surgical patients with different and specific tools (e. g., scores for obese patients) may be necessary. From the existing data, it is clear that there are at least four strategies that should be considered in order to decrease the risk of SSI when operating on obese patients. First, tight perioperative glucose control is key to minimizing episodes of hyperglycemia that are associated with a higher rate of SSI. Second, optimizing tissue oxygen tension through increased perioperative FIO_2 and appropriate resuscitation improves the perfusion of tissues and oxygen radical-mediated defense mechanisms against infection. Third, larger doses of prophylactic antibiotics maximize serum and tissue concentrations, providing a real (and expected) decrease in SSI. Fourth, performing laparoscopic operations whenever feasible certainly decreases the area at risk and has a demonstrated ability to reduce SSI. Infectobesity is a relatively novel, yet extremely significant concept. Obesity management strategies mainly target behavioural components of the disorder, but are only marginally effective. If infections contribute to human obesity, then entirely different prevention and treatment strategies and public health policies could be needed to address this subtype of the disorder. While inflammation is a shared and key characteristic of both chronic inflammatory diseases and infections, infectious diseases have long been associated directly with obesity [i. e., Canine distemper virus (CDV), Rous-associated virus-7 (RAV-7), Borna disease virus (BDV), Scrapie agent and adenoviruses SMAM-1 and 36] as well as the consequences of obesity such as metabolic syndrome, diabetes and atherosclerosis [i. e. *Helicobacter pylori* (*H. pylori*), *Chlamydia pneumoniae* (*C. pneumoniae*), *Porphyromonas gingivalis* (*P. gingivalis*), hepatitis B virus (HBV), hepatitis C virus (HCV) and human immunodeficiency virus (HIV)]. Obesity and exposure to infectious agents overlap in large population segments and therefore may mutually influence each other.

Introduction

In recent years it has been developed a new surgical assay in order to treat morbid obesity. Novel surgical techniques have been applied to reduce the size of the gastrointestinal tract and consequently to reduce the absorbing area for the food intake. Various infectious diseases have been associated with bariatric surgery both as part of the surgical site infection and as causal agents.

The increasing use of bariatric procedures in the treatment of morbidly obese patients means that aesthetic plastic surgeons can expect to care for more and more patients who have undergone bariatric surgery. It is important for surgeons to understand the procedures, outcomes, and possible complications to recognize the signs and symptoms of any potential problems. Candidates for bariatric surgery must have a body mass index (BMI) of at least 40 kg/m^2 or a BMI of 35 kg/m^2 with at least one comorbidity, plus demonstrated failure of nonsurgical means of weight control to control weight and no significant psychiatric disorders. Surgical procedures can be categorized as restrictive or malabsorptive and include adjustable gastric band, Roux-en-Y gastric bypass, and biliopancreatic diversion with or without duodenal switch. There are no definitive criteria for choosing any single procedure, although in general restrictive procedures may be more appropriate for those patients with lower BMIs and malabsorptive procedures for those with higher BMIs. Results of bariatric surgery are impressive and include not only significant and sustained weight loss but also improvement or resolution of major comorbid conditions. Significant complications include anastomotic leak, marginal ulceration, and internal herniation, as well as wound infection, incisional hernia, hemorrhage, deep venous thrombosis, and pulmonary embolus.

Innovative procedures now under study include gastrointestinal neuromodulation, sleeve gastrectomy, intragastric balloons, intraluminal sleeves, and other endoscopic procedures [1].

Mechanisms that Predispose Obese Patients to Infection

Obesity increases morbidity and mortality through its multiple effects on nearly every human system. Obesity has a clear but not yet precisely defined effect on the immune response through a variety of immune mediators, which leads to susceptibility to infections. Data on the incidence and outcome of specific infections, especially community-acquired infections, in obese people are limited.

The available data suggest that obese people are more likely than people of normal weight to develop infections of various types including postoperative infections and other nosocomial infections, as well to develop serious complications of common infection [49].

Possible mechanisms have been suggested in the recent bibliography and molecul interactions seem to play crucial role in pathogenesis.

The hormonal connection between immunity and nutrition becomes equally evident in nutritional dysregulatory eating disorders such as obesity, which is becoming alarmingly common in high income countries and is also spreading to transitional societies at an unexpectedly high speed. Obesity in humans is correlated with high concentrations of leptin, often associated with leptin resistance. Patients with obesity present with increased tumor necrosis factor (TNF) α production, altered T cell subset ratios, repressed T cell responses, and higher incidence of infectious diseases, all of which can be reversed by weight loss. Diet-induced or inherite obesity in rodents causes natural killer (NK) and T cell suppression and increased TNF-α secretion. Leptin-induced production of proinflammatory cytokines by macrophages causes neutrophil activation and T-helper (TH) 1-derived interferon (IFN) γ secretion.

The obese phenotype in leptin-deficient *ob/ob* mice is also associated with diminished circulating T cells, reduced T cell responses, and lymphoid atrophy. Although seemingly in a committed stage, macrophages from *ob/ob* mice have reduced phagocytic activity. Furthermore, the natural ligand of the secretagogue receptor of the pituitary gland, ghrelin, which regulates fat storage and consumption, is directly linked to immune functions by its counteraction of leptin-induced activation of monocytes and T cells [76]. Recently, the cytokine interleukin (IL) 18, which usually drives TH1 responses in synergy with IL-12, has been linked to obesity. IL-18 knockout mice became obese through overeating and resistant to insulin through increased gluconeogenesis in the liver. Consequently, intracerebrally administered IL-18 inhibited food intake. Another study demonstrated that a differential gut flora with distinct metabolic requirements was found in obese versus lean humans as well as mice. Even more intriguingly, when transferred to germ-free mice, the “obese” but not the “lean” gut flora caused an increase of total body fat. These reports add two more components to the already complex relationship of nutrition, inflammation, immunity, and infection: cytokine patterns and gut flora compositions.

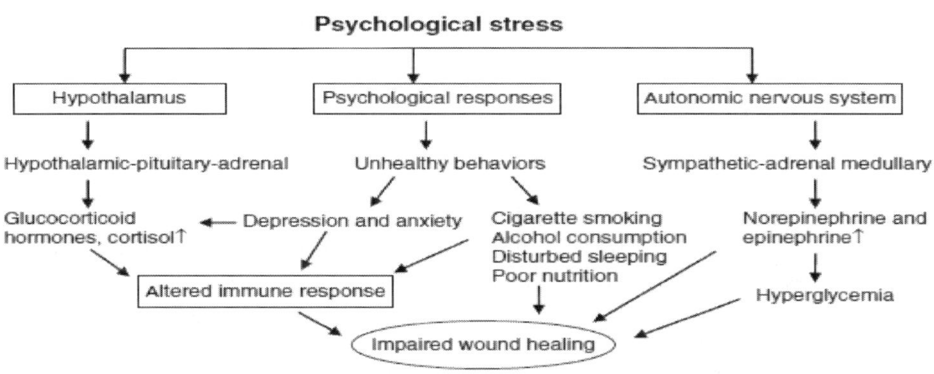

Figure 1. Stress-impaired wound healing is mediated primarily through the hypothalamic-pituitary-adrenal, sympathetic-adrenal medullary axes, and psychological-response-induced unhealthy behaviors (adapted from Guo et al.,2010).

Thus, regulation of food uptake and storage is closely intermingled with immune functions. However, a higher nutrient uptake may also be beneficial for the host response, likely due to higher energy requirements, as illustrated by a recent study showing that a cholesterol-rich diet accelerates clearance of bacilli during the treatment of tuberculosis. Diabetes mellitus is a hormonally regulated metabolic disease which affects immunity to infection. Neutrophils and macrophages from patients with diabetes have suppressed functions, including phagocytosis, chemotaxis, and extravasation. T cell activation is also affected, as evidenced by reduced delayed-type hypersensitivity reactions. Patients with diabetes are more prone to diseases caused by *Staphylococcus aureus* and *Mycobacterium tuberculosis*, and show higher mortality and morbidity from infections with *Streptococcus. pneumoniae* and influenza virus.

In patients with diabetes, diseases due to urogenital tract and opportunistic infections by *Enterococcus*, *Mucor mucedo,* and *Candida albicans* are common. *Pseudomonas aeruginosa* is a frequent cause of abscesses in patients with diabetes, as are polybacterial infections causing skin ulcers (diabetic foot), and severe osteomyelitis. There is clear evidence that proper control of hyperglycemia improves immune functions and resistance to infection [118] [66]. Chronic inflammation present in obesity may predispose the obese to cancer through Fas-receptor over-expression and L-selectin under-expression in leukocytes, and elevated Fas-ligand secretion in tumors affecting the morbidly obese. In one study leukocytes from 25 patients having gastric bypass surgery were compared to 15 normal controls preoperatively and at 1, 3, 6, and 12 months postoperatively using flow cytometry to measure CD3, CD4, CD8, CD56, CD62 (L-selectin), CD69, and CD95 (Fas antigen) expression on T lymphocytes, B lymphocytes, NK cells, and neutrophils. The percentage of CD95 + T cells was significantly elevated from controls and this difference persisted through 1 month postoperatively. Furthermore, expression of CD95 per cell, was significantly greater in these patients than that of the controls preoperatively, and this continued to 1 month. The reduced expression of L-selectin combined with the elevated levels of CD95 suggested that morbid obesity predisposes patients to sites of immune privilege. This could be the mechanism for increased rates of cancer and wound infections seen in obesity [34].

Obesity and Clinical Infections

Nosocomial Infections

The association between obesity and postoperative infections has been the focus of recent studies. In a retrospective review by Choban *et al.* the effect of obesity on nosocomial infections in 849 surgical patients was studied. Age, American Society of Anesthesiologists (ASA) score [83], and mortality were similar for the obese and non-obese groups. Despite a relatively small number of patients with nosocomial infections, obese patients had a significantly higher rate of these complications, including surgical site infections (SSI), *Clostridium difficile* diarrhea, pneumonia, and bacteremia [29]. Other studies also confirmed these finding; Garibaldi *et al.* [59] and, more recently, Canturk *et al.* [22] showed a trend toward a higher risk of pneumonia and nosocomial infections in the obese population. A more recent larger study by Pessaux *et al.*, in which they evaluated the risk factors for nosocomial infections in patients undergoing non-colorectal abdominal operations, found that obesity, among other variables (age, underweight, cirrhosis, vertical abdominal incision, gastrointestinal anastomosis, and prolonged operative time), was an independent predictor of postoperative infection by multivariate analysis. However, obesity did not predict risk of SSI specifically [108, 5].

Respiratory Infections

An intact and functioning immune response is critical for protection against infectious disease. Impairment of the immune response of the obese host would be expected to have an impact on the response to infectious diseases.

Indeed, genetically obese animals have been shown to exhibit decreased resistance to bacterial and viral infections including Mycobacterium abscessus, *Klebsiella pneumoniae, Streptococcus pneumoniae and Mycobacterium tuberculosis* [94].

However, a separate group [146] found no differences in bacterial growth in ob/ob mice challenged with the *K. pneumoniae* and *S. pneumoniae strains*. Db/db mice have been shown to have increased usceptibility to *Staphylococcus aureus* and *H. pylori*. Both ob/ob and db/db mice have been shown to have increased susceptibility to *Listeria monocytogenes*. Obese Zucker rats (fa/fa) have been shown to have increased susceptibility to *Candida albicans* [110].

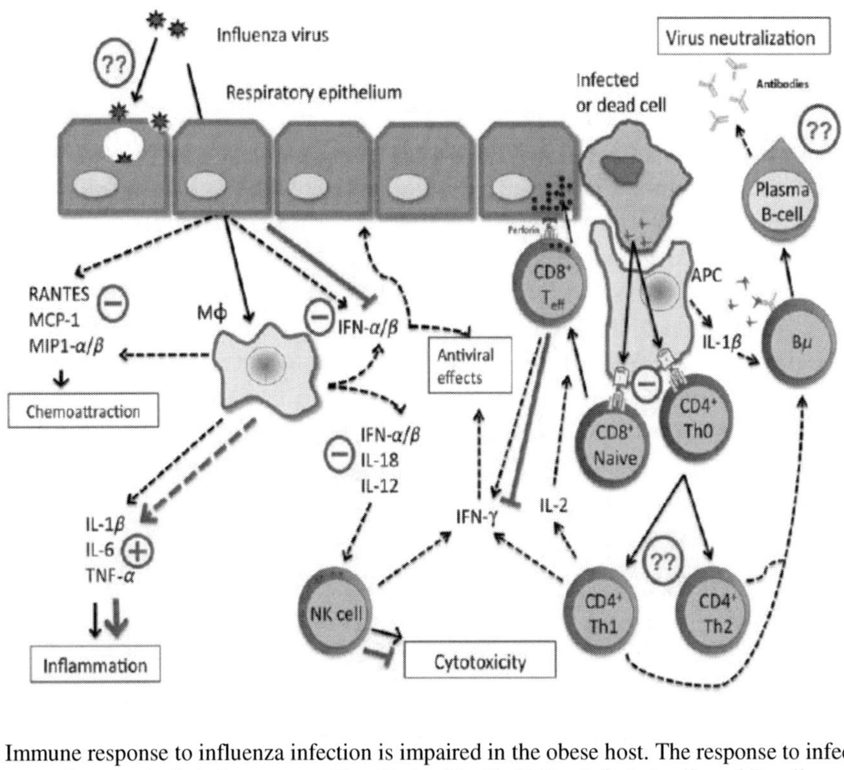

Figure 2. Immune response to influenza infection is impaired in the obese host. The response to infection with influenza virus results in influenza-specific effector T-cells killing infected cells and B-cells producing neutralizing antibody to protect against further infection. Altered responses known to be a result of the obesigenic state are shown in red. IL, interleukin; MCP, monocyte chemoattractant protein; TNF-a, tumor necrosis factor alpha; IFN-g, interferon; NK, natural killer cell (Adopted from Karlsson et al., 2012).

In regards to viral infection, ob/ob mice have been found to have increased susceptibility to viral myocarditis induced by coxsackie virus B468 as well as encephalomyocarditis virus [81]. Similar to genetically obese models, diet-induced obese mice are more susceptible to bacterial infection, including infection with *Porphyromonas gingivalis and Staphylococcus aureus*-induced sepsis (Nilsson 2009). Influenza-infected, diet-induced obese mice had seven times greater mortality, and increased lung pathology compared with infected lean controls. In the lungs of influenza-infected, diet-induced obese mice, a significant decrease in the expression of mRNA for IFN-a/-b and an increase and delay in the expression of proinflammatory cytokines and chemokines was noted [125].

In addition, dendritic cells (DCs) from obese mice failed to efficiently present influenza antigen to T-cells (Figure 2). Overall, it appears that diet-induced obesity can increase susceptibility to bacterial and viral infections [82]. In a meta-analysis aiming to assess the association between obesity and the risk of intensive care unit (ICU) admission and death among patients hospitalized for influenza A (H1N1) viral infection a total of 3059 subjects from six cross-sectional studies were included in this. The study concluded that severely obese H1N1 patients (body mass index ≥ 40 kg/m^2) were as twice as likely to be admitted to ICU or die compared to H1N1 patients who were not severely obese [136].

Gastrointestinal, Liver, and Biliary Infections

Obesity and its metabolic complications are major health problems worldwide, and increasing evidence implicates the microbiota in these important health issues. Indeed, it appears that the microbiota function much like a metabolic "organ," influencing nutrient acquisition, energy homeostasis, and, ultimately, the control of body weight. Moreover, alterations in gut microbiota, increased intestinal permeability, and metabolic endotoxemia likely play a role in the development of a chronic low-grade inflammatory state in the host that contributes to the development of obesity and associated chronic metabolic diseases such as nonalcoholic fatty liver disease (NAFLD). Supporting these concepts are the observations that increased gut permeability, low-grade endotoxemia, and fatty liver are observed in animal models of obesity caused by either high-fat or high-fructose feeding. Consistent with these observations, germ-free mice are protected from obesity and many forms of liver injury. Many agents that affect gut flora/permeability, such as probiotics/prebiotics, also appear to affect obesity and certain forms of liver injury in animal model systems [55].

Infections Following Procedures for the Management of Obesity

Types of Bariatric Surgical Procedures

Historically, the three most common types of bariatric surgical procedures include an open and laparoscopic Roux-en-Y gastric bypass (RYGB) and laparoscopic adjustable gastric banding (LAGB). The laparoscopic sleeve gastrectomy has become a popular procedure in the past 4–5 years but the number of procedures that have been performed for this type of surgery and the number of published reports have been small in comparison with the other bariatric surgical procedures. A recent multicenter prospective study of 4776 bariatric procedures showed that the combined end point of 30-day mortality, major thrombotic complication, re-intervention and prolonged hospitalization was 1. 0% for LAGB, 4. 8% for laparoscopic RYGB and 7. 8% for open RYGB, with overall mortality 0. 3% (52). The major risk factors for increased complication rates in this study were obstructive sleep apnea, poor functional status or a history of prior thrombotic events. The introduction of laparoscopic RYGB has been associated with a significant reduction in perioperative mortality and complications. The complication rate associated with LAGB is even lower than that seen with laparoscopic RYGB [87].

Surgical Site Infections, Skin Infections and Wound Healing

Although risk factors for SSIs have been well described for various types of surgical procedures, scant data exist describing risk factors for SSIs following bariatric surgery [5]. In a retrospective review addressing the incidence of and risk factors for SSI in patients undergoing open bariatric surgery the use of epidural analgesia and delay in the appropriate timing of prophylactic antibiotics was associated with a higher risk of SSI [32]. The SSI among RYGBs performed were categorized as superficial, deep incisional and organ/space according to a study performed in order to determine the risk factors for SSI following open RYGB surgical procedures [30]. Bivariate predictors of SSIs included morbid obesity (defined by the authors as BMI ≥50), asthma, smoking, sleep apnea, increased duration of surgery, and presence of urinary incontinence in the preoperative setting and needing assistance with ambulation in the preoperative setting. In multivariate analysis, Type 2 diabetes, morbid obesity (BMI ≥50), preoperative urinary incontinence and sleep apnea were each associated with an approximate twofold increase in SSI risk [143]. SSI following RYGB was associated with an increased risk for emergency department visits for all causes, hospital re-admissions, outpatient procedures and 30-day mortality [30]. Important patient-related factors for SSI include existing infection, low serum albumin concentration, older age, obesity, smoking, diabetes mellitus, and ischemia secondary to vascular disease or irradiation. Surgical risk factors include prolonged procedures and inadequacies in either the surgical scrub or the antiseptic preparation of the skin. Physiological states that increase the risk of SSI include trauma, shock, blood transfusion, hypothermia, hypoxia, and hyperglycemia. Parameters that may be associated independently with an increased risk of SSI, and that may predict infection, include abdominal surgery, a contaminated or dirty operation, and more than three diagnoses at the time of discharge.

The rise of bariatric surgery has led to an increasing number of reoperations for failed bariatric procedures. Examples of secondary bariatric operations include vertical banded gastroplasties, mini-gastric bypasses, non-divided bypasses, RYGBP and sleeve gastrectomies converted to RYGBP. Other patients with jejunoileal bypasses and bilio-pancreatic diversions had to undergo sleeve gastrectomies, re-anastomotic rings had to be removed due to erosion, pouch trimmings, redo gastrojejunostomies, redo jejunojejuno-stomies, remnant gastrectomies and gastrogastric fistula takedowns had to be performed for pouch enlargements, strictures, and gastrogastric fistulas, as well as combinations of these procedures. In a case of gastroesophageal junction leak after gastric bypass with serious sepsis and hemodynamic instability minimally invasive treatment was performed without the need for open surgery (Martin-Malagon 2010). Based on previous meta-analyses, most of the more frequently seen complications from bariatric surgery are gastrointestinal: dumping, vitamin/mineral deficiencies, vomiting (and nausea), staple line failure, infection, stenosis (and bowel obstruction), ulceration, bleeding, splenic injury, and perioperative death. Other gastrointestinal complications of bariatric surgery are indirect consequences of the surgery: bacterial overgrowth and diarrhea [2, 141]. Serious subnutrition, associated to intestinal bacterial overgrowth, in patients submitted to bariatric surgery has also been reported. The patients reported asthenia, hair fallout, and edema, and one also reported diarrhea, but none was feverish. Bacterial overgrowth is an important complication that can compromise clinical evolution of patients submitted to intestinal surgery like gastroplasty with Y-Roux anastomosis [92, 12]. Complications includ wound infection, intra-abdominal abscess formation, trocar site hernias, salmonella infection associated with vomiting, and postoperative pneumonia associated with coughing [57, 107]. Compared with open surgery, laparoscopic surgery is associated with lower risk of wound infection and incisional hernia [114]. However, there is no significant difference in the 30-day reoperation rate, 30-day mortality and 30-day readmission rate between the open and laparoscopic groups [122].

Surgical site infection is one of the most common complications of bariatric surgery. The relatively low rates of SSI published in large series of both open and laparoscopic gastric bypass procedures underestimate the magnitude of the problem. Large series of open gastric bypass operations have described SSI rates between 15% and 25% [95], and a pooled analysis of outcomes in open and laparoscopic bypasses showed a rate of SSI of only 6. 6% in open procedures [111]. Christou *et al.* did a retrospective review of their prospectively collected database specifically addressing the incidence of and risk factors for SSI in patients undergoing open bariatric surgery. The authors correlated the administration of epidural analgesia and delay in appropriate timing of prophylactic antibiotics with a higher risk of SSI. A high correlation between SSI and incisional hernia, another common complication after surgery was also seen in obese patients [32]. Incisional hernia was described by Sugerman *et al.* to be more common after gastric bypass in morbidly obese patients than in patients receiving chronic corticosteroids and undergoing colectomy for inflammatory bowel disease [127]. Laparoscopic procedures, particularly in high-volume centers, have reduced the high risk of SSI in patients undergoing bariatric operations [103]. Schauer *et al.* [119] have published the results with their first few hundred laparoscopic bariatric operations, and reported incidences of SSI of 5% and 1. 5%, respectively. Other series have had incidences of SSI of 1% and 9%, and the pooled analysis published by Podnos *et al.* showed an SSI rate of 2. 98%, all considerably lower than those described for open procedures [148, 72, 124].

The major sources of infection are microorganisms on the patient's skin and, less often, the alimentary tract or female genital tract [27]. The most common source of pathogens causing SSIs post-gastrointestinal surgeries is endogenous patient flora (including staphylococcal and streptococcal species) and flora of the gastrointestinal tract (including aerobic and anaerobic Gram-negative bacilli). As similar with other gastrointestinal surgeries, SSI following bariatric surgery can be polymicrobial. The most common organisms causing SSI following bariatric surgery include staphylococcal species such as *Staphylococcus aureus* and coagulase-negative staphylococci. The most commonly isolated bacteria are streptococci, Enterococcus spp., coagulase-negative staphylococci, Enterobacteriaceae, *S. aureus* and Eikenella spp. The most common anaerobes isolated are *Prevotella*, followed by

Peptostreptococcus, *Bacteroides* and *Veillonella* [30]. Peritoneal contamination during laparoscopic gastric bypass has also been reporte. Culture results were positive for streptococcus species, anaerobes, staphylococcus species, and enterobacter. Prophylactic intravenous antibiotics and antibiotic irrigation may reduce the risk of clinically significant infections in this small as shown in uncontrolled series [147]. Risk factors for the development of SSIs following bariatric surgery have to be recognized in order to improve risk stratification for SSIs. Novel scoring systems, such as the BULCS score, have been suggested as predictosr and risk adjusters for SSI following bariatric surgery. SSI following bariatric surgery has been associated with receipt of antibiotic prophylaxis other than cefazolin and comorbid conditions including sleep apnea and bipolar disorder [31]. Morbidly obese individuals should be offered bariatric surgery before major co-morbid conditions develop as a strategy to decrease the operative risk [75].

Obese patients are at higher risk than nonobese patients for surgical site infections and other complications such as dehiscence, pressure ulcers, deep tissue injury, and rhabdomyolysis [13]. Cellulitis is one of the most common infections encountered by physicians in outpatient settings and is usually treated with oral antibiotics. The increase in methicillin resistance among these organisms worldwide has made the treatment more complicated and challenging. Whether empiric antibiotic therapy needs to be active against methicillin resistant *Staphylococcus aureus* (MRSA) is difficult to determine but evaluation of risk factors can help. Patients with MRSA cellulitis were significantly more obese, present with abscesses and have lesions that involved the head and neck compared with those who had other bacteria. The presence of abscesses may represent a manifestation of virulence factors such as Panton-Valentine Leukocidin (PVL) or unique characteristics associated with the new CA-MRSA strains [85]. Necrotizing fasciitis associated with bariatric surgery is another important issue. Necrotizing fasciitis is a progressive soft tissue infection (skin, subcutaneous tissue and fascia) caused in the main by *Streptococcus pyogenes,* which gains entry into the organism through any type of wound and even through intact skin. Diagnosis is essentially clinical, being the sum of non-specific, insidious skin lesions, associated with intense pain and multiorgan failure. Treatment is radical surgical excision of the affected tissues, combined antibiotic therapy and supportive care. However, mortality rates are still very high. Several cases have been reported in the current literature; one case reported by Heinz *et al.* occurred as a complication of liposuction surgery, and the second presented after minor trauma [69].

Other cases initially presented with toxic shock-like syndrome with necrotising fasciitis and myositis, caused by Lancefield-group-A beta-haemolytic streptococci. Radical debridement of the skin, subcutis, fasciae and part of the pectoral muscle, plus antibiotics and sequencially transplantation of autologous skin were necessary for the patient to survive; however, serious difiguration remained [63, 101, 135].

Cases of patients experiencing post surgical infection with a specific pathogen have been reported in the current litterature and some of them are presented here in summary. Two patients who underwent abdominal body-contouring surgery in a specifc surgical center later experienced a severe deep infection and a methicillin-resistant *Staphylococcus aureus* (MRSA) superinfection resulting to a massive retractile and painful scar despite appropriate antibiotic treatment applied [8, 7]. A rare case of group A streptococcal fasciitis complicating tumescent liposuction was also reported highlighting the importance of early diagnosis and treatment of this condition as by using early aggressive medical and surgical treatments, the disease was prevented to progress to necrotizing fasciitis [14]. Laparoscopic adjustable gastric banding represents a safe and effective bariatric surgical method. Nevertheless, complications such as band infection due to colon microperforation during endoscopic polypectomy or peritonitis by *Streptococcus milleri, Streptococcus viridans* or other streptococcal species may occur [126, 33, 28]. A case of *Pseudomonas aeruginosa* infection of the abdominoplasty flap that complicated the wound closure and jeopardized the aesthetic outcome has also been reported [9].

In case series, it was reported a high prevalence of Mycobacterial infections in patients who traveled in specific to undergo cosmetic surgery for fat removal, a practice referred to as "lipotourism". *Mycobacterium abscessus* can cause postsurgical wound infection and painful, erythematous, draining subcutaneous abdominal nodules [58, 102]. In other case series, microorganisms isolated from the purulent drainage obtained from wounds or fistulas following laparoscopic gastric banding procedures were identified as *Mycobacterium fortuitum* in patients exhibited signs of inflammation, microabscesses, and purulent wound drainage within 24 months of abdominal and/or thigh liposuction or homologous fat tissue injection [113, 99, 15, 25]. Cases of *Mycobacterium chelonae* infection in the buttock after combined liposuction and lipo injection have also been reported [40, 61, 96]. These organisms are most often known to cause skin, bone, and soft tissue infections associated with local trauma, surgical procedures, and in patients with immunodeficiency [21]. Another patient who underwent a gastric bypass for morbid obesity developed 1 year after the surgery as severe vomiting that was attributed to a severe stenosis of the gastrojejunal anastomosis by radiological studies.

The patient underwent resection of the stenotic anastomosis and histology showed an intact mucosa and beneath it an abscess filled with numerous filamentous microorganisms leading to the diagnosis of gastric actinomycosis [50].

Table 1. Factors affecting wound healing

Local Factors	Systemic Factors
Oxygenation	Age and gender
Infection	Sex hormones
Foreign body	Stress
Venous sufficiency	Ischemia
	Diseases: diabetes, keloids, fibrosis, hereditary healing disorders, jaundice, uremia
	Obesity
	Medications: glucocorticoid steroids, non-steroidal anti-inflammatory drugs, chemotherapy
	Alcoholism and smoking
	Immunocompromised conditions: cancer, radiation therapy, AIDS
	Nutrition

In adult humans, optimal wound healing involves the following the events: [1] rapid hemostasis; [2] appropriate inflammation; [3] mesenchymal cell differentiation, proliferation, and migration to the wound site; [4] suitable angiogenesis; [5] prompt re-epithelialization (re-growth of epithelial tissue over the wound surface); and [6] proper synthesis, cross-linking, and alignment of collagen to provide strength to the healing tissue. Multiple factors can lead to impaired wound healing.

In general terms, the factors that influence repair can be categorized into local and systemic. Local factors are those that directly influence the characteristics of the wound itself, while systemic factors are the overall health or disease state of the individual that affect his or her ability to heal (Table 1).

Many of these factors are related, and the systemic factors act through the local effects affecting wound healing [67]. Risk factors for wound infection included history of coronary artery diseases, diabetes, chronic respiratory illness and malignant disease [133]. Another important factor for SSI is inadequate dosing of antibiotic prophylaxis as supported in a large prospective cohort study on obese patients who underwent bariatric surgery (BS) at nine community hospitals in the USA between 2007 and 2008. Patients who received vancomycin prophylaxis as a single agent at a dose less than 2 g were more likely to develop SSI than patients who received other antibiotic regimens. It was thus suggested that if an antibiotic is to be used for prophylaxis, then the appropriate dose should be calculated using actual bodyweight rather than lean bodyweight in accordance with Infectious Disease Society of America recommendations [56].

Obesity and Infections in Specific Populations

Children

The intestinal microbiota has been implicated in adult diseases ranging from obesity to cancer, but there have been relatively few investigations of bacteria in surgical diseases of infancy and childhood. Recent studies have pointed out the clinical significance of the unique features of the pediatric microbiota and the contribution of gut microbes to common diseases for the pediatric surgeons: necrotizing enterocolitis, obesity, and inflammatory bowel disease [23]. A meta-analysis in obese pediatric population with average age of 16. 8 years (range, 9-21) concluded that bariatric surgery results in sustained and clinically significant weight loss, but also has the potential for serious complications. For laparoscopic adjustable gastric banding (LAGB), band slippage and micronutrient deficiency were the most frequently reported complications, with sporadic cases of band erosion, port/tube dysfunction, hiatal hernia, wound infection, and pouch dilation. For Roux-en-Y gastric bypass (RYGB), more severe complications have been documented, such as pulmonary embolism, shock, intestinal obstruction, postoperative bleeding, staple line leak, and severe malnutrition [134]. Those patients with sleep apnea have had resolution of their sleep apnea [19]. Little is known, however, about the relationship between obesity and otitis media with effusion (OME). Obesity may result in altered cytokine expression, gastroesophageal reflux disease, or fat accumulation, all of which may contribute to OME. Conversely, OME may induce taste changes through middle ear cavity inflammation, thus contributing to obesity. A similar pattern of taste change has been shown in patients with gustatory nerve anesthesia [88].

Pregnancy

Obesity is a global health problem that is increasing in prevalence. The World Health Organization characterizes obesity as a pandemic issue, with a higher prevalence in females than males. Many pregnant patients are seen with high body mass index (BMI). Obesity during pregnancy is considered a high-risk state because it is associated with many complications. Compared with normal-weight patients, obese patients have a higher prevalence of infertility. Once they conceive, they have higher rate of early miscarriage and congenital anomalies, including neural tube defects. Besides the coexistence of preexisting diabetes mellitus and chronic hypertension, obese women are more likely to have pregnancy-induced hypertension, gestational diabetes, thromboembolism, macrosomia, and spontaneous intrauterine demises in the latter half of pregnancy. Obese women also require instrument or cesarean section delivery more often than average-weight women. Following cesarean section delivery, obese women have a higher incidence of wound infection and disruption. Irrespective of the delivery mode, children born to obese mothers have a higher incidence of macrosomia and associated shoulder dystocia, which can be highly unpredictable. In addition to being large at birth, children born to obese mothers are also more susceptible to obesity in adolescence and adulthood. Prevention is the best way to prevent this problem. As pregnancy is the worst time to lose weight, women with a high BMI should be encouraged to lose weight prior to conceiving. During preconception counseling, they should be educated about the complications associated with high a BMI. Obese women should also be screened for hypertension and diabetes mellitus. In early pregnancy, besides being watchful about the higher association of miscarriage, obese women should be screened with ultrasound for congenital anomalies around 18 to 22 weeks.

The ultrasound should be repeated close to term to check on the estimated fetal weight to rule out macrosomia. Obese pregnant women are screened for gestational diabetes around 24 to 28 weeks. During the second half of pregnancy, one needs to closely watch for signs and symptoms of pregnancy-induced hypertension. Once in labor, an early anesthesia consultation is highly recommended irrespective of delivery mode. When cesarean section is performed, many obstetricians prefer an incision above the pannus to avoid skin infection.

However, the incision should be decided upon the discretion of the surgeon. Peripartum, special attention is given to avoid thromboembolism by using compression stockings and early ambulation [117].

There are limited data to support the use of prophylactic antibiotic before cesarean delivery, closure of subcutaneous space >2 cm, and maintaining normothermia intraoperatively to help reduce the incidence of postoperative wound complications. Either primary or secondary closure of wounds is preferred to healing by secondary intention. Antibiotics should be administered in the presence of cellulitis or systemic toxicity. Use of vacuum-assisted wound closure devices may be useful in wound management (132). Gastric bypass surgery, by definition, changes the absorption capability of stomach and small intestine. The use of oral medications in patients post gastric bypass may need to be adjusted by medical providers to account for this absorption change. Cases of peritonitis on gastric banding due to *Klebsiella pneumoniae* complicated with fetal death have also been described [60]. In cases of complicated infections in post gastric bypass surgery pregnant patient the route of antibiotics administration should be taken into account [93].

Elderly

More information is needed on the role and the outcome of bariatric surgery in the elderly. Compared with nonelderly patients, elderly patients who underwent bariatric surgery are expected to have more comorbidities, longer lengths of stay, more overall complications, pulmonary complications, hemorrhagic complications and wound complications. In a recent study however it was shown that although the morbidity and mortality were higher in the elderly, bariatric surgery in this specific population was considered as safe as other gastrointestinal procedures because the observed mortality is better than the expected (risk-adjusted) mortality [139]. Older patients had more pre- and post-operative comorbidities and lost less weight than younger patients. Complications included major wound infections, anastomotic leaks, symptomatic marginal ulcers, stomal stenoses, bowel obstructions, incisional hernias (nonlaparoscopic), and pulmonary embolism. However the weight loss and improvement in comorbidities in older patients were clinically significant [128].

Super Obese Patients (BMI>50kg/m^2)

The safety of laparoscopic bariatric procedures in superobese patients is still debatable. Using the American College of Surgeons National Surgical Quality Improvement Program's participant-use file, the patients who had undergone laparoscopic Roux-en-Y gastric bypass and laparoscopic adjustable gastric banding for morbid obesity were identified and data were compared within each procedure after dividing the patients according to the body mass index: <50 kg/m^2 (morbidly obese group and ≥50 kg/m^2 (superobese group) in a recent study by Kakarla *et al.* Overall, compared with the morbidly obese group, the superobese group had a greater incidence of co-morbidities (e. g., hypertension and dyspnea), a significantly increased length of stay, and a greater rate of 30-day. In the gastric bypass group, the superobese group had a significantly greater incidence of postoperative complications, including superficial wound infections, reintubation, pulmonary embolism, myocardial infarction, deep vein thrombosis, septic shock, and 30-day mortality. In the laparoscopic adjustable gastric banding group, the superobese group had a significantly greater incidence of postoperative complications, including superficial and deep wound infections, sepsis, septic shock and 30-day mortality [79]. These results are supported by other syudies concluding that Roux-en-Y gastric bypass can be performed safely, even at the extremes of weight. Postoperative complications were fewand no cases of intra-abdominal sepsis were reported althought the operation in this group may be technically challenging. Need for ICU and hospital LOS was greater. Weight loss was significant and appeared to be sustained in most patients [70].

Critically Ill Patients and Sepsis

In contrast to the common prejudice that obese patients probably have a higher ICU mortality than lean patients, convincing meta-analyses have revealed that this is not the case. Mechanical ventilation may prove to be a big challenge in ICU patients not only because of obesity-related anatomical problems that may complicate intubation, but also due to obstructive sleep apnoea, obesity hypoventilation syndrome and increased intra-abdominal pressure are of major relevance concerning ventilation, weaning and successful extubation. The risk of infections is increased in obese ICU patients. Sepsis is the number one cause of morbidity and mortality in noncoronary artery disease critical care units all over the world and is associated with a high cost of care. An increase in morbidity in obese septic patients compared with lean people is a cause of growing concern. Laboratory evidence suggests that there is exaggeration in the inflammatory and prothrombogenic phenotype assumed by obese compared with lean septic animals [136]. There seem to be interplay of obesity and sepsis; the adipous tissue is not just a passive reservoir of energy but an active endocrine and immunomodulating organ but the exact interactions between adipokines, inflammation and coagulation in sepsis have to be clarified [97].

Infections and Metabolic Disorders

Novel, culture-independent, molecular and metagenomic techniques have provided new insight into the complex interactions between the mammalian host and gut microbial species. It is increasingly evident that gut microbes may shape the host metabolic and immune network activity and ultimately influence the development of obesity and diabetes. Evidence connects gut microflora to obesity and to type 1 and type 2 diabetes. Potential mechanisms underlying this relationship may include increased nutrient absorption from the diet, prolonged intestinal transit time, altered bile acid entero-hepatic cycle, increased cellular uptake of circulating triglycerides, enhanced de novo lipogenesis, reduced free fatty acid oxidation, altered tissue composition of biologically active polyunsaturated fatty acid, chronic low-grade inflammation triggered by the endotoxin toll-like receptor 4 axis, and altered intestinal barrier function [100].

Diabetes mellitus (DM) is a risk factor for SSI, well known complications of gastro-intestinal surgery associated with an increased morbidity, mortality and overall cost. The type of hypoglycemic regimen, immunosuppression, and emergency surgery has not been associated with an increased rate of SSI. On the other hand, higher than normal glucose control at all postoperative time intervals has been associated with SSI [121]. The impact of abdominal fat and insulin resistance on arterial hypertension in non-obese women is also discussed in various studies and main findings are that arterial hypertension is associated with insulin resistance, central fat distribution, and higher leptin levels [115]. The link between diabetes mellitus and tuberculosis has also been recognised for centuries. In recent decades, tuberculosis incidence has declined in high-income countries, but incidence remains high in countries that have high rates of infection with HIV, high prevalence of malnutrition and crowded living conditions, or poor tuberculosis control infrastructure. At the same time, diabetes mellitus prevalence is soaring globally, fuelled by obesity. There is growing evidence that diabetes mellitus is an important risk factor for tuberculosis and might affect disease presentation and treatment response. Furthermore, tuberculosis might induce glucose intolerance and worsen glycaemic control in people with diabetes. Recent studies describe potential mechanisms by which diabetes mellitus can cause tuberculosis, the effects of tuberculosis on diabetic control, and pharmacokinetic issues related to the co-management of diabetes and tuberculosis [45].

Infections and Malignancy

The human gastrointestinal tract harbors a complex and abundant microbial community reaching as high as 10^{13}-10^{14} microorganisms in the colon. This endogenous microbiota forms a symbiotic relationship with their eukaryotic host and homeostasis is maintained by performing essential and non-redundant tasks (e. g. nutrition/energy and, immune system balance, pathogen exclusion). Although this relationship is essential and beneficial to the host, various events (e. g. infection, diet, stress, inflammation) may impact microbial composition, leading to the formation of a dysbiotic microbiota, further impacting on health and disease states. As an example, Crohn's disease and ulcerative colitis, collectively termed inflammatory bowel diseases (IBD), have been associated with the establishment of a dysbiotic microbiota. Extra-intestinal disorders such as obesity and metabolic syndrome have also been associated with the development of a dysbiotic microbiota. Recent studies provide evidence to the emerging relationship between the microbiota and development of colorectal cancer and suggest that microbial manipulation (probiotic, prebiotic) may have an impact in disease development and progression [151]. Obesity has been shown to be an independent risk factor for other malignancies too including breast cancer, endometrial cancer, renal cell carcinoma, esophageal adenocarcinoma, pancreatic ductal adenocarcinoma, and hepatocellular carcinoma.

Although HBV and HCV infections are considered as major hepatocellular carcinoma risk factors worldwide, obesity is likely to be the primary risk factor along with other non-viral factors, such as type 2 diabetes mellitus, alcohol, tobacco, and oral contraceptives. Obesity also represents an independent hepatocellular carcinoma risk factor in patients with alcoholic cirrhosis and cryptogenic cirrhosis. A follow-up study in Taiwan has implicated synergistic effects between metabolic disorders (obesity and diabetes) and viral hepatitis, with hepatocellular carcinoma risk increasing by more than 100-fold in HBV or HCV carriers with obesity and diabetes. Obesity has been implicated in the genesis of metabolic syndromes including insulin resistance and type 2 diabetes, and a spectrum of non-cancerous liver diseases, such as NAFLD and NASH, hepatic fibrosis and cirrhosis. NAFLD is strongly associated with type 2 diabetes mellitus and dyslipidemia. Without proper management, NAFLD may progress to chronic liver inflammation, termed as steatohepatitis (NASH), which is a severe condition of inflamed fatty liver that can further progress to liver fibrosis and cirrhosis causing serious complications, including liver failure and hepatocellular carcinoma [129].

Obesity of Infectious Origin

The aetiology of obesity is multifactorial. An understanding of the contributions of various causal factors is essential for the proper management of obesity. Although it is primarily thought of as a condition brought on by lifestyle choices, recent evidence shows there is a link between obesity and viral infections. Numerous animal models have documented an increased body weight and a number of physiologic changes, including increased insulin sensitivity, increased glucose uptake and decreased leptin secretion that contribute to an increase in body fat and support that infection may be a possible cause of obesity [98]. In the last two decades, more than 10 adipogenic pathogens have been reported, including human and nonhuman viruses, scrapie agents, bacteria, and gut microflora. Some of these pathogens are associated with human obesity, but their causative role in human obesity has not been established. The two most likely mechanisms are either a peripheral effect on fat cell differentiation and storage or a central effect on appetite and energy expenditure. Potential changes in specific areas within the brain involved in appetite control have been suggested. These are not novel concepts nor are they without precedent as encephalitis lethargica which was described by Constantin von Economo after a viral outbreak in the winter of 1916–1917, a condition where the substantia nigra was damaged with severe reduction in dopamine production, while other brain regions such as the cerebral cortex remained unaffected. Thus it is possible for a virus to affect specific neuronal pathways involved with energy balance without other obviously detrimental effects. Viruses should thus be considered as a possible contributing factor to obesity as not to do so would deprive us of a potential new avenue of investigating and treating the everincreasing epidemic of obesity. Moreover the treatment of obese patients infected with the implicated viruses may also change significantly. For the moment, studies to confirm or refute the existing data are required, while further work to unravel the mechanism would persuade more scientists to acknowledge the possibility that certain viruses may cause weight gain [140, 11].

If relevant to humans, "Infectobesity" would be a relatively novel, yet extremely significant concept [106]. Obesity management strategies mainly target behavioural components of the disorder, but are only marginally effective. A comprehensive understanding of the causative factors of obesity might provide more effective management approaches. If infections contribute to human obesity, then entirely different prevention and treatment strategies and public health policies could be needed to address this subtype of the disorder [44].

While inflammation is a shared and key characteristic of both chronic inflammatory diseases and infections, infectious diseases have long been associated directly with obesity [i. e. Canine distemper virus (CDV), Rous-associated virus-7 (RAV-7), Borna disease virus (BDV), Scrapie agent and adenoviruses SMAM-1 and 36] as well as the consequences of obesity such as metabolic syndrome, diabetes and atherosclerosis [i. e. *Helicobacter pylori* (*H. pylori*), *Chlamydia pneumoniae* (*C. pneumoniae*), *Porphyromonas gingivalis* (*P. gingivalis*), hepatitis B virus (HBV), hepatitis C virus (HCV) and human immunodeficiency virus (HIV)]. Obesity and exposure to infectious agents overlap in large population segments and therefore may mutually influence each other.

Canine Distemper Virus

Canine distemper virus (CDV) was the first virus linked to obesity [91]. CDV is a morbillivirus antigenically related to measles, which infects dogs and a wide range of carnivores. Like all morbilliviruses, CDV is highly contagious, and transmission occurs predominantly via aerosols. In susceptible hosts, acute febrile and multisystemic disease is induced; neuroinvasiveness and severe immunosuppression are hallmarks of CDV infection [68]. Lyons *et al.* investigated the pathological consequences of CDV infection on the central nervous system (CNS) of mice [91]. Researchers noticed that an obesity syndrome developed in 26% of the study animals who survived the acute CNS disease. Later studies by Bernard *et al.* revealed that CDV can target hypothalamic nuclei and lead to an obesity syndrome in the late stages of infection [16]. Griffond *et al.* [65] suggested that the CDV-related obesity syndrome more probably results from an array of conditions including individual susceptibility, leptin network alteration, imbalance between hypothalamic matrix degrading proteases and their inhibitors and neuropeptide/neurotransmitter impairments. Currently, no evidence exists to link CDV to human obesity.

Rous-Associated Virus Type 7

Avian leucosis viruses (AVL) are retroviruses that may induce neoplastic growth such as B-cell lymphomas, proliferative disorders such as osteopetrosis and chronic degenerative diseases, such as anaemia and immunosuppresion [24]. Rous associated virus 7 (RAV-7) is an AVL that causes an obesity syndrome in chickens. Carter *et al.* [24] discovered that infection of 10-day chicken embryos with RAV-7 resulted in stunting, obesity and hyperlipidemia within 3 weeks after hatching. Histological examination of the liver of infected chickens revealed diffuse panlobular fatty infiltrates while the thyroid and the pancreas were infiltrated with lymphoblastoid cells. An increase in serum triglycerides and cholesterol was also present. At present there is no report of RAV-7 human infection and whether humans are susceptible to AVL infection is a matter that requires investigation [77].

Borna Disease Virus

Borna disease (BD) was first described more than 200 years ago in Southern Germany as a fatal neurologic disease of horses and sheep. Borna disease virus (BDV) is a neurotropic, enveloped, non-segmented, negative-strand RNA virus distinctive in its nuclear localization of replication and transcription [20]. The infection of the rats with the variant BDV-obese (BDV-ob) caused rapid increase of body weight and minimal or absent neurological signs. In rats infected with the strain BDV-ob, inflammatory lesions in the brain were restricted mainly to the septum, hippocampus, ventromedian hypothalamus and amygdala. These areas have also been implicated in appetite control. Until now there has been no report of evidence linking BDV to human obesity.

Scrapie Agent

Scrapie is a fatal degenerative disease affecting the CNS of sheep and goats. The clinical symptoms of scrapie develop very slowly; the affected animals usually show behavioural changes, tremor, rubbing and locomotor incoordination that progress to recumbence and death. The infectious agent responsible for scrapie is an abnormal form of a physiological constituent of the cell membrane (prion) [78]. Several authors have reported an increase in food consumption followed by a subsequent increase in animal body weight during the pre-clinical phase of the disease. Kim *et al.* [86] suggested that changes in the hypothalamic–pituitary–adrenal axis played an important role in the development of scrapie-related obesity This theory was supported by the following three findings: [1] the scrapie obesity effect was augmented when the scrapie strain was injected into the hypothalamus of mice; [2] the weight of the adrenals was significantly greater (because of cortical enlargement) in scrapie-infected obese mice than that of uninfected controls; [3] low-scrapie infectivity titres were found in the adrenals of the obese mice indicating that the obesity effect was probably not due to direct action of the scrapie agent on the adrenals.

SMAM-1 Virus

SMAM-1 is an avian adenovirus that infects chickens and causes excessive fat accumulation [41]. To assess whether SMAM-1 could be associated with human obesity, Dhurandhar *et al.* [42] screened the serum of 52 obese humans in India, for antibodies against SMAM-1 virus. Ten subjects were tested positive to SMAM-1 antibodies, while 42 subjects did not have antibodies. The SMAM-1 positive group had significantly higher BMI and significantly lower serum cholesterol and triglycerides values compared with the SMAM-1 negative group. These findings suggest that SMAM-1, or a serologically similar human virus may be associated with human obesity.

Human Adenoviruses

Adenoviruses are medium-sized, non-enveloped icosahedral viruses containing double-stranded DNA. There are more than 50 immunologically distinct types (six species: A–F) that can cause human infections [37]. Although epidemiological characteristics of the adenoviruses vary by type, all are transmitted by direct contact, faecal-oral transmission and occasionally water-borne transmission. Adenoviruses most commonly cause respiratory disease but they may cause gastroenteritis, conjunctivitis and cystitis [71]. The last decade six human adenoviruses have been investigated in relation to obesity [43, 137].

Human Adenovirus 36

Of the many viruses screened, Adenovirus 36 (Ad-36) has been found to be a strong candidate virus that is associated with obesity, based on evidence in various model systems as well as clinical data. Oxidative stress could be a possible mechanism of how adenovirus might lead to obesity [144].

The adiposity-promoting effect of Ad-36 was first presented in animal models. Although the adipogenic effects of Ad-36 were demonstrated in chickens and rodents, verification in higher mammals was necessary. For ethical reasons humans could not be infected experimentally with Ad-36 to verify its adipogenic effect directly. In the first study with non-human primates, the presence of spontaneously occurring antibodies to Ad-36 in rhesus monkeys (Macaca mulatta) was observed. Moreover, a significant longitudinal association of positive antibody status with weight gain and plasma cholesterol lowering during the 18 months after viral antibody appearance was discovered. In vitro experiments suggested that Ad-36 downregulates leptin expression and secretion in 3T3-L1 cells, as well as leptin secretion from primary adipocytes.

Moreover, there was some experimental evidence that Ad-36 increased de novo lipogenesis in adipocytes. Studies determining the prevalence of Ad-36 antibodies in obese people have been carried out by Atkinson *et al.* [10]. These studies showed that 30% of obese and 11% of non-obese humans have neutralizing antibodies to Ad-36. Antibody positive subjects were heavier compared with their antibody negative counterparts. As expected from the animal studies, serum cholesterol and triglycerides were lower in Ad-36 antibody-positive *vs.* negative subjects.

On the contrary, in a study by Rogers *et al.* it was suggested that Ad-36 proteins may provide novel therapeutic targets that remodel human adipose tissue to a more metabolically favorable profile. It was shown that Ad-36 increased glucose uptake by adipose tissue explants obtained from nondiabetic and diabetic subjects. Without insulin stimulation, Ad-36 upregulated expressions of several proadipogenic genes, adiponectin, and fatty acid synthase and reduced the expression of inflammatory cytokine macrophage chemoattractant protein-1 in a phosphotidylinositol 3-kinase (PI3K)-dependent manner.

In turn, the activation of PI3K by Ad-36 was independent of insulin receptor signaling but dependent on Ras signaling recruited by Ad-36. Natural Ad-36 infection in nondiabetic and diabetic subjects was associated with significantly lower fasting glucose levels and A1C, respectively [116]. The obesity inducing mechanism, specifically in humans was evaluated by Vangipuram [138], realizing that glycerol-3-phosphate dehydrogenase, an adipocyte differentiation marker, was increased in 3T3-L1 and human cells infected by Ad-36 [39].

Human Adenoviruses Ad-37, Ad-31, Ad-9, Ad-5 and Non-Adipogenic Ad-2

Whigham *et al.* studied three human viruses in vitro and in vivo: Ad-37 (classified as a species D adenovirus like Ad-36), Ad-31 (species A) and Ad-2 (species C) [145].

The average food intake was not different between groups. The study of the serum lipids revealed that the Ad-37 group had a significant increase in serum cholesterol from baseline to death ($P \leq 0.01$). Ad-37 had significantly decreased serum triglyceride levels at the end of the study compared with all the other groups. In the control, Ad-31 and Ad-2 groups there were no changes in serum cholesterol and triglyceride levels. Atkinson et al. tested obese and non-obese volunteers for antibodies against Ad-37, Ad-31 and Ad-2 but no association of antibodies with BMI or serum lipids was found. The prevalence of Ad-37 was very low in the population tested and this may have caused a type II statistical error. The results of the experiments using human adenoviruses demonstrate that more than one human adenovirus is capable of producing obesity in animal models but the adipogenic property is not necessarily shared by all human adenoviruses [140] [11].

Table 2. Human and animal obesity related viruses (adopted from Vangipuram et al. 2007)

Virus	Year of report
Animal	
Canine distemper virus	1982
Rous-associated virus type 7	1983
Borna disease virus	1983
Scrapie agent	1987
SMAM-1 aviary adenovirus	1990
Human	
Adenovirus 36	2000
Adenovirus 37	2002
Adenovirus 5	2005

Hepatitis B Virus (HBV)

The safety and efficacy of bariatric surgery in patients with hepatitis B viral (HBV) infection is not clear. In a study by Lee *et al.* morbidly obese patients with HBV infection did not show difference in the outcome of bariatric surgery; however, continuing monitor of the liver function was indicated. Morbidly obese patients positive for HBV infection were associated with older age and higher diastolic blood pressure. The weight loss curves and resolution of obesity-related comorbidities were similar between patients with and without HBV infection apart from the postoperative aspartate transaminase (AST) and alanine transaminase (ALT) that were significantly higher in HBV positive patients. During follow-up, two patients developed fulminating hepatitis after bariatric surgery and one died [89].

Hepatitis C Virus (HCV)

Chronic HCV infection may result in liver cirrhosis and hepatocellular carcinoma and is associated with multifaceted disease such as porphyria cutanea tarda, membranoproliferative glomerulonephritis and cryoglobulinemia. Hepatitis C, NAFLD characterized by hepatic steatosis, and obesity inflict significant health and economic burdens on the Western world. Insulin resistance is the key player in these disease processes. Complex interplay between these conditions results in the ultimate phenotype of liver disease [112]. While epidemiological studies suggested a linkage between HCV infections and type 2 diabetes, other studies confirmed the direct involvement of HCV infection in the development of insulin resistance in a mouse model using mice with the HCV core gene inserted in their genome. A high level of TNF-α was shown to be the main factor to induce insulin resistance in HCV-transgenic mice and insulin sensitivity was restored by administration of anti-TNF-α antibody [142].

Human Immunodeficiency Virus (HIV)

Insulin resistance is common in HIV-infected people and the prevalence of hyperglycemia and diabetes is significantly higher in people with HIV infection treated with antiretrovirals as compared with the general population. The prevalence of insulin resistance in HIV subjects is around 35% and up to 47% when they received protease inhibitor therapy, while the incidence of insulin resistance is only around 5% in the general population. HIV induces an increased inflammatory state, as evident in elevated levels of adiponectin and free fatty acids in HIV-infected individuals [142, 84]. The successful introduction in 1995 of highly active antiretroviral therapy (HAART), a combination of potent antiretroviral agents, has substantially decreased mortality among HIV-infected patients. HAART is the standard of care to avoid selection of viral mutations, and the regimen is typically chosen based on the patient's comorbidities, efficacy and tolerability in clinical trials, potential drug interactions, adverse drug effects, and potential long-term complications. Furthermore, selection of drugs for treatment-naïve and treatment-experienced patients take into account the benefit/risk ratio and the HIV genotype. However, HAART is associated with a number of metabolic and anthropometric abnormalities, including dyslipidemia and insulin resistance as well as subcutaneous fat loss (lipoatrophy) and abdominal obesity (lipohypertrophy), all of which may contribute to an increased risk of cardiovascular disease (CVD).

Besides the side effects from HIV treatment, there is recognition that HIV infection by itself, or in combination with genetic and/or environmental factors, may cause metabolic abnormalities due to the dynamic relationship between the virus and the host. In view of this, it is noteworthy that increased mortality and morbidity rate from CVD has been reported among HIV-infected patients. As the HIV-positive population ages, the combination of cardiovascular risk factors commonly seen in the general population with the presence of HIV infection and its treatment thus pose significant therapeutic and health care challenges. Soon after PIs introduction, safety concerns for lipodystrophy and associated metabolic complications such as insulin resistance and dyslipidemia were raised, and although several studies have established an association between the use of PI therapy and a wide range of adverse effects [26]. Results from cross-sectional studies have shown that compared to healthy subjects, HIV-positive patients receiving antiretroviral therapy have increased secretion and decreased clearance of VLDL particles, increased synthesis and reduced catabolism of apolipoprotein B, the protein backbone of atherogenic lipoproteins, and diminished lipoprotein lipase activity. Hypertriglyceridemia and increased levels of pro-atherogenic remnant lipoproteins have also been noted in HIV-positive patients on HAART. Changes in body fat distribution, often referred to as HIV/HAART-associated lipodystrophy, are common in HIV-infected individuals and typically start to occur after 6–12 months of PI therapy. Importantly, these body fat changes include both lipoatrophy and lipohypertrophy. Lipoatrophy denotes a decrease in adipose tissue volume and is an HIV-specific change that occurs with HIV/HAART therapy affecting all subcutaneous adipose tissue depots; the least amount of subcutaneous fat loss occurs in the upper trunk, contributing to the characteristic "buffalo hump" in HIV-treated patients. Alternatively, lipohypertrophy denotes an increase in adipose tissue volume, and most commonly occurs in visceral adipose tissue (VAT) and adipose tissue depots in the upper trunk, particularly in the breast and dorsocervical fat pads [6].

Different approaches have been tried for the management of the HAART associated adverse effects. These approaches can be categorized in three groups: those intrinsic to the host, some of them modifiable and some not, those associated with antiretroviral therapy, that are sometimes modifiable as well, and finally those related to HIV-1 infection and its consequences, most often not modifiable. The most commonly used strategies for HALS reversion have included host-dependent factors such as lifestyle and dietary modifications and antiretroviral-dependent factors such as switching or avoiding the use of drugs more prone to promote HALS. Lifestyle modifications and switching thymidine analogues have been associated with moderate success. Pharmacological interventions have included the use of insulin-sensitising agents and hormone therapy with disappointing results, whereas treatment with pravastatin or pioglitazone, and uridine supplementation seem to be associated with fat gain in preliminary studies. The only interventions with almost immediate results that may render a patient's appearance similar to his past one have included filling techniques for facial lipoatrophy and ultrasound-assisted liposuction for cervical fat pad hypertrophy. Among the filling options, semipermanent reabsorbable materials and autologous fat transfer have been associated with acceptable outcomes (38). Gastric bypass surgery may be an option for some patients who have failed diet and therapeutic lifestyle changes, changes in ART or other treatment modalities for HIV/ART-related lipohypertrophy and obesity.

Bariatric surgery may provide an effective treatment modality for obesity and its related comorbidities in the HIV-infected population while not sacrificing virologic suppression [123]. Oral administration through the bypass achieved sufficient serum concentrations of lopinavir, whereas administration through the jejunal tube did not an HIV-infected patient with duodenal malignant lymphoma [80]. Surgical interventions may include a combination of ultrasonic-assisted liposuction (UAL) and suction-assisted lipectomy (SAL) of the anterior neck, posterior neck, and trunk; direct excision of mastoid fat pads; direct excision of thigh lipomata; facelift/necklift; browlift; fat injections; and blepharoplasty. UAL/SAL is particularly beneficial in reducing the cervicodorsal fat pad, whereas facelift and necklift may be necessary to adequately address anterior neck lipohypertrophy [73, 62, 109]. Roux-en-Y gastric bypass (RYGB) can be safely performed in HIV-infected individuals. Initial results appear to be comparable to those in noninfected controls. Well-controlled HIV infection must not be a contraindication to bariatric surgery [51].

Helicobacter Pylori (H. pylori)

There is a high prevalence of *H. pylori* infection in morbidly obese patients [3, 35, 47] [64, 150]. Aydemir *et al.* (Aydemir 2005) provided the first association between chronic *H. pylori* infection and insulin resistance. The homeostasis model assessment of insulin resistance was significantly higher in *H. pylori*-positive subjects than in *H. pylori*-negative ones. Epidemiological evidence also supported the association of *H. pylori* seropositivity with cardiovascular diseases and elevated parameters of metabolic syndrome [142]. Decision analysis models suggest preventing acquisition of *H. pylori*, via vaccination in childhood, could be cost-effective and may reduce incidence of gastric cancer by over 40%. As yet, no country has adopted public health measures to treat infected individuals or prevent infection in populations at risk [53].

The relationship between obesity and *H. pylori* infection is controversial. Some studies support that *H. pylori* can be a 'protective' factor against the development of overweight [90]. The risk of *H. pylori* infection is not increased in overweight young persons. Moreover, *H.*

pylori seropositivity or CagA antibody status are not associated with the BMI or fasting serum leptin levels. On the other hand, the speculations on the protective role of *Helicobacter pylori* against gastroesophageal reflux disease (GERD) originated from epidemiological observations. These studies have shown that the rising trend of GERD is coincident with declining prevalence of *H. pylori* and peptic ulcer disease in Asia. Furthermore, most case-control and population-based studies suggest a negative association between *H. pylori* infection and GERD. It is generally believed that the preponderance of cagA+ and vacA+ virulent strains and proinflammatory interleukin-1 beta polymorphism increase the risk of hypochlohydria and protects against the development of GERD in Asian population. Recovery of gastric acid secretion and emergence of reflux esophagitis has been reported after *H. pylori* eradication in patients with corpus gastritis and atrophic gastritis. Recent studies have also reported that *H. pylori* eradication leads to recovery of ghrelin secreting cells in the gastric corpus and a rise in plasma ghrelin levels, which may contribute to obesity through its appetite-stimulating action and predispose to GERD. Modern lifestyle leads to a generation with high gastric acid and ghrelin secretion rates. These physiological changes may contribute to increased dietary calorie intake, obesity and increased prevalence of GERD [149]. An inverse relationship between morbid obesity and *H. pylori* seropositivity has been shown, leading to the hypothesis that the absence of *H. pylori* infection during childhood may enhance the risk of the development of morbid obesity. In contrast, other studies showed that obesity and/or an elevation of the BMI may be associated with an increased incidence of *H. pylori* colonization, probably as a result of reduced gastric motility. In addition, the incidence of *H. pylori* infection in patients undergoing Roux-en-Y gastric bypass surgery for morbid obesity was higher than that found in all patients undergoing endoscopies and biopsy, even though the incidence of infection was not higher in controls matched for age.

The relationship between obesity and *H pylori* eradication is also controversial. There are data which demonstrate that eradication of *H. pylori* significantly increases the incidence of obesity in patients with peptic ulcer disease, since it increases the level of BMI, and/or enhances the appetite of asymptomatic patients, due to an elevation of plasma ghrelin and a reduction of leptin levels. In fact, *H. pylori* infection caused a marked reduction in plasma levels of ghrelin, as a result of a negative effect of this infection on the density of gastric ghrelin-positive cells and an increase in plasma levels of leptin and gastrin. Since ghrelin exerts orexigenic and adipogenic effects in contrast to leptin which exerts anorexigenic effects, alterations in plasma levels of gastric originated appetite-controlling hormones in children and adults infected by *H. pylori* may contribute to chronic dyspepsia and loss of appetite. Consequently, *H. pylori* can be a "protective" factor against the development of becoming overweight. In contrast, other studies showed that there are no differences in plasma ghrelin levels between *H. pylori*+ve and *H. pylori*-ve patients matched for age and BMI and that successful eradication of *H. pylori* had no effect on plasma ghrelin levels [104]. Mean plasma ghrelin levels fell following eradication therapy and were inversely correlated with body weight gain. Gastric ghrelin expression increased following eradication but did not correlate with BMI, suggesting that plasma ghrelin concentration more strongly influences body weight change than increases in gastric ghrelin, and that increased expression of preproghrelin mRNA in the stomach does not directly influence the total plasma ghrelin level. The discrepancy between gastric ghrelin expression and plasma ghrelin concentration may be reconciled by the presence of ghrelin isoforms which affect growth hormone secretagogue receptors differently. Nevertheless, the regulation of gastric ghrelin secretion and the determinants of plasma ghrelin levels have yet to be elucidated.

Obestatin, a novel hormone, and ghrelin are derived from a common precursor, preproghrelin, yet obestatin exhibits opposite effects to those of ghrelin. Obestatin antagonizes growth hormone secretion and reduces food intake. Its discovery in 2005 brought an additional layer of complexity to the understanding of the function of ghrelin. The ghrelin/obestatin balance may be a key factor determining an individual's response to *H. pylori* infection and weight gain following *H. pylori* eradication [17].

Chlamydia Pneumoniae (C. Pneumoniae)

Epidemiological surveys, experimental studies and clinical trials have provided strong evidence for the association between *C. pneumoniae* infection and metabolic syndrome, insulin resistance and cardiovascular disease. The current concept of the influence of *C. pneumoniae* on atherosclerosis is that *C. pneumoniae*-infected macrophages traffic to secondary organs including arterial endothelium, induce persistent infection and lead to the local upregulation of proinflammatory molecules. Subsequently, infected macrophages and smooth muscle cells transform into foam cells and result in plaque destabilization, thrombus formation and myocardial infarction in arterial endothelium. Ased on this notion, antibiotic treatment would reduce cardiovascular events by eliminating *C. pneumoniae* persistent infection and preventing re-infection. However, clinical trials with antibiotic treatment based on this concept failed. This failure to reduce cardiovascular events by antibiotic treatment requires the reformulation of the current mechanistic understanding of the association between *C. pneumoniae* and metabolic syndrome and cardiovascular disease [142]. Wang et al. examined the influence of *C. pneumoniae* infection on progression of insulin resistance in dependence of host genetic background and dietary fat concentration in an obese mouse model. They concluded that murine *C. pneumoniae* infection enhances insulin resistance and diabetes in a genetically and nutritionally restricted manner *via* circulating inflammatory mediators such as TNF-α and proposed a new mechanism of *C. pneumoniae*-induced exacerbation of insulin resistance developed in this investigation. By quantifying the levels of *C. pneumoniae* and TNF-α transcripts in different organs, they concluded that the dispersal of a small number of *C. pneumoniae* organisms to secondary tissues was irrelevant to progression of insulin resistance and the early onset of type 2 diabetes. In contrast, the bulk infection of the lung caused an increase in circulating cytokines that drove the long-term exacerbation of insulin resistance and accelerated the onset of type 2 diabetes. It was reported that combined pathogen burden and positive serology for both *H. pylori* and *C. pneumoniae* showed the strongest association with insulin resistance. These data suggest that exposure to multiple pathogens may potentiate chronic low-grade inflammation and insulin resistance and that the mechanisms whereby the pathogens affect chronic inflammatory diseases are shared [142].

Porphyromonas Gingivalis (P. Gingivalis)

Approximately 35% of the adults in the USA have periodontitis, an inflammation that involves the periodontal ligament and alveolar bone, while about 75% have gingivitis, an inflammation of the gingival tissues surrounding the teeth. Periodontal diseases are initiated by gram-negative and anaerobic bacteria such as *P. gingivalis* residing in biofilms on gingival tissues and teeth. Periodontal diseases had been thought of as localized conditions of concern only to dental health professionals. Emerging evidence now suggests that periodontal diseases also exacerbate systemic conditions such as metabolic syndrome and diabetes. The oral infection causes elevated circulating IL-1β and TNF-α which lead to hyperlipidemia and development of diabetes [142].

Diagnosis

Infections are usually detected in obese patients. They may be divided into common infections such as fungal infections, pulmonary tuberculosis, pneumonia, bacteraemia, urinary tract infections, and diabetic foot infections and specific infections. The latter occur almost exclusively in diabetes and include rhinocerebral mucormycosis, malignant external otitis, emphysematous pyelonephritis, perirenal abscess, emphysematous cystitis and emphysematous cholecystitis. Radionuclide tests have been suggested for the diagnosis and localisation of foot osteomyelitis, as well as the distinction of osteomyelitis from other conditions, notably Charcot osteoarthropathy. Technetium-99m methylene disphosphonate and labelled leukocyte bone scans are the main imaging techniques employed, while emerging techniques include single-photon emission tomography/computed tomography (CT) and positron emission tomography/CT. Nuclear medicine is also useful in the diagnosis and follow-up of specific infections in obese patients like, malignant external otitis, rhinocerebral mucormycosis, acute pyelonephritis, renal papillary necrosis and cholecystitis [105]. A case of infected gastric band was diagnosed by technetium 99m-hexamethyl propilenamine oxime-labeled leukocyte scintigraphy showing the value of integrated interpretation of anatomical and functional imaging modalities obtained by software fusion techniques [131]. Tissue oxygen tension has also been shown to accurately predict SSIs. In a retrospective analysis on patients who developed an SSI after operation there was a significant difference in tissue oxygen saturation at the surgical site between patients who developed an SSI and those who did not [74]. Different diagnostic imaging modalities are crucial for follow-up of patients who have undergone bariatric procedures and detection of the different postoperative complications.

Management of Infection in Obese Patients

Given the rising incidence of obesity, bariatric surgery has proven life sustaining. Surgical-site infections associated with bariatric surgery can be prevented with appropriate pre-operative measures including appropriate prophylactic antibiotics, adequate control of hyperglycemia and utilization of more laparoscopic methods for surgery. Cefazolin is the preferred agent for surgical prophylaxis in bariatric procedures above or including the duodenum, while cefoxitin or cefazolin in combination with metronidazole should be used for bariatric procedures below the duodenum. For patients with IgE-mediated hypersensitivity to penicillin or cephalosporin, antimicrobial surgical prophylaxis often includes a fluoroquinolone or clindamycin in combination with a fluoroquinolone, an aminoglycoside or aztreonam. Metronidazole is added if anaerobic activity is required for bariatric surgeries involving the ileum. Intravenous is preferred over topical, subcutaneous or mechanical bowel preparation as the route of delivery for bariatric antimicrobial surgical prophylaxis. Standard doses of antimicrobial agents may result in low serum and tissue concentrations in obese patients. Hence, the highest dose of prophylactic antimicrobial agent that can be safely administered should be used for bariatric surgical prophylaxis. For cefazolin and cefoxitin, this translates to a minimal initial dose of 2 g, and for metronidazole the initial dose should be 1 g. All intravenous prophylactic antimicrobial agents should be infused within 30 min to 1 h before incision, with the exception of fluoroquinolones or vancomycin. Antimicrobial prophylaxis should be redosed if the bariatric surgery exceeds two half-lives of the drug from the time the first dose was administered or if the operation exceeds 3 h. The duration of antimicrobial prophylaxis for bariatric surgery should not exceed 24 h after surgery is completed [31].

With an aging and obese population, chronic wounds such as diabetic ulcers, pressure ulcers, and venous leg ulcers are of an increasingly relevant medical concern in the developed world. Identification of bacterial biofilm contamination as a major contributor to non-healing wounds demands biofilm-targeted strategies to treat chronic wounds. While the current standard of care has proven marginally effective, there are components of standard care that should remain part of the wound treatment regime including systemic and topical antibiotics, antiseptics, and physical debridement of biofilm and devitalized tissue. Emerging anti-biofilm strategies include novel, non-invasive means of physical debridement, chemical agent strategies, and biological agent strategies. While aging and obesity will continue to be major burdens to wound care, the emergence of wounds associated with war require investigation and biotechnology development to address biofilm strategies that manage multi-drug resistant bacteria contaminating the chronic wound [4].

Malnutrition and Infection

In response to infection, the immune system first executes innate and then subsequently acquired host defense functions of high diversity. Both processes involve activation and propagation of immune cells and synthesis of an array of molecules requiring DNA replication, RNA expression, and protein synthesis and secretion, and therefore consume additional anabolic energy. Mediators of inflammation further increase the catabolic response [118]. Malnutritiona has commonly been associated with secondary immune deficiency and susceptibility to infection in humans. On the other hand infection itself contributes to malnutrition. Examples of how infections can contribute to malnutrition are: [1] gastrointestinal infection can lead to diarrhea; [2] HIV/AIDS, tuberculosis, and other chronic infections can cause cachexia and anemia; and [3] intestinal parasites can cause anemia and nutrient deprivation. Stimulation of an immune response by infection increases the demand for metabolically derived anabolic energy and associated substrates, leading to a synergistic vicious cycle of adverse nutritional status and increased susceptibility to infection. Moreover, malnutrition affects immunity. Severe protein malnutrition in newborns and small children causes atrophy of the thymus with reduced cell numbers and subsequently illdeveloped peripheral lymphoid organs, i. e., lymph nodes and spleen. This causal chain leads to longlasting immune defects characterized by leucopenia, decreased CD4 to CD8 ratio and increased numbers of CD4/CD8 double-negative T cells, and, therefore, the appearance of immature T cells in the periphery. Malnourished children present with diminished functional T cell counts, increased undifferentiated lymphocyte numbers, and depressed serum complement activity. Reduced antibody responses to polysaccharide antigens of encapsulated bacteria such as *Streptococcus pneumoniae* and *Haemophilus influenzae* exacerbate susceptibility to these pathogens. Moreover, immune defense at the epithelial barrier of the undernourished host is compromised due to altered architecture of the gut mucosa, such as flattened hypotrophic microvilli, reduced lymphocyte counts in Peyer's patches, and reduced immunoglobulin A (IgA) secretion [118].

Discussion and Conclusions

Obesity is undoubtedly a surrogate for other known risk factors for SSI, particularly diabetes mellitus [130]. Gastric bypass patients with elevated fasting blood glucose concentrations had a higher risk of SSI, highlighting the importance not only of diabetes mellitus but also of perioperative hyperglycemia [36]. Obesity also has been associated with longer operations, which is one of the few independent predictors of SSI that is commonly significant in multiple series. The magnitude of blood loss has frequently been reported as a risk factor for SSI. Whereas some reports cite greater blood loss in obese patients, others report a lower incidence of reoperation for bleeding [18]. Obesity as an intrinsic risk factor has also been postulated. In general, it is agreed that obese patients have tissue hypoperfusion (subcutaneous adipose tissue), which may predispose to SSI through a greater risk of ischemia/ necrosis and suboptimal neutrophil oxidative killing mainly attributed to a poor balance between tissue oxygen demand and oxygen supply. Another mechanism may be the tissue concentrations of prophylactic antibiotic achieved in obese patients. The importance of antibiotic concentrations in serum and tissue during an operative procedure in prevention of SSI has clearly been demonstrated [120]. Forse *et al.* observed a high rate of SSI in patients undergoing gastric bypass and recorded low serum concentrations of antibiotic in these patients, whilw when the dose of prophylactic antibiotic was doubled, the rate of SSI decreased [54]. More recently, Edmiston *et al.* measured serum and tissue concentrations of prophylactic antibiotics in obese patients at different intervals from incision time. As the BMI increased, there was a significant decrease in antibiotic concentration at closure in adipose tissue and at incision and closure in deep tissues (omentum) [46]. Obese patients need substantially higher doses of prophylactic antibiotics to achieve therapeutic concentrations and adequate protection against SSI. Recent studies support these data and show that in obese patients, antibiotic dose adjustment depending on patient's actual weight rather than ideal weight should be preferred in order to achieve a relative benefit in patients' outcome [48].

References

[1] Abeles D, Shikora SA. Bariatric surgery: current concepts and future directions. *Aesthet. Surg. J.*, 2008;28(1):79-84.

[2] Abell TL, Minocha A. Gastrointestinal complications of bariatric surgery: diagnosis and therapy. *Am. J. Med. Sci.*, 2006;331(4):214-8.

[3] Al-Akwaa AM. Prevalence of Helicobacter pylori infection in a group of morbidly obese Saudi patients undergoing bariatric surgery: a preliminary report. *Saudi. J. Gastroenterol.,* 2010;16(4):264-7.

[4] Ammons CB. Anti-biofilm strategies and the need for innovations in wound care. *Recent. Pat. Antiinfect. Drug. Discov.,* 2010;5(1):10-17.

[5] Anaya DA, Dellinger EP. The obese surgical patient: a susceptible host for infection. *Surg. Infect. (Larchmt),* 2006;7(5):473–480.

[6] Anuurad E, Bremer A, Berglund L. HIV Protease Inhibitors and Obesity. *Curr. Opin. Endocrinol. Diabetes Obes.,* 2010;17(5): 478–485.

[7] Araco A, Gravante G, Araco F, Grimaldi M, Bottini DJ, Cervelli V. Devastating methicillin resistant Staphylococcus aureus wound infection following abdominoplasty in a prior bariatric surgery patient. *Obes. Surg.,* 2007;17(6):828-31.

[8] Araco A, Zaccheddu R, Araco F, Gravante G. Methicillin-resistant superinfection of the wound after body-contouring abdominal surgery. *Aesthetic Plast. Surg.,* 2008;32 (4):681-3.

[9] Araco A, Araco F, Abdullah P, Overton J, Gravante G. Pseudomonas aeruginosa necrotizing infection of the abdominal flap in a post-bariatric patient undergoing body contouring surgery. *Obes. Surg.,* 2009;19(6):812-6.

[10] Atkinson RL, Dhurandhar NV, Allison DB, Bowen RL, Israel BA, Albu JB et al. Human adenovirus-36 is associated with increased body weight and paradoxical reduction of serum lipids. *Int. J. Obes. (London),* 2005; 29: 281–286.

[11] Atkinson RL. Viruses as an etiology of obesity. *Mayo Clin. Proc.,* 2007;82(10):1192-1198.

[12] Balsiger BM, Murr MM, Mai J, Sarr MG. Gastroesophageal reflux after intact vertical banded gastroplasty: correction by conversion to Roux-en-Y gastric bypass. *J. Gastrointest. Surg.,* 2000;4(3):276-81.

[13] Baugh N, Zuelzer H, Meador J, Blankenship J. Wound wise: wounds in surgical patients who are obese. *Am. J. Nurs.,* 2007;107(6):40-50; quiz 51.

[14] Beeson WH, Slama TG, Beeler RT, Rachel JD, Picerno NA. Group A streptococcal fasciitis after submental tumescent liposuction. *Arch. Facial. Plast. Surg.,* 2001;3(4):277-9.

[15] Behroozan DS, Christian MM, Moy RL. Mycobacterium fortuitum infection following neck liposuction: A case report. *Dermatol. Surg.,* 2000;26(6):588-90.

[16] Bernard A, Fevre-Montange M, Bencsik A, Giraudon P, Wild TF, Confavreux C et al. Brain structures selectively targeted by canine distemper virus in a mouse model infection. *J. Neuropathol. Exp. Neurol.,* 1993; 52: 471–480.

[17] Boltin D, Niv Y. Ghrelin, Helicobacter pylori and body mass: Is There an association? *IMAJ,* 2012; 14: 130–132.

[18] Bowditch MG, Villar RN. Do obese patients bleed more? A prospective study of blood loss at total hip replacement. *Ann. R. Coll Surg. Engl.,* 1999;81:198–200.

[19] Breaux CW. Obesity Surgery in Children. *Obes. Surg.,* 1995;5(3):279-284.

[20] Briese T, de la Torre JC, Lewis A, Ludwig H, Lipkin WI. Borna disease virus, a negative-strand RNA virus, transcribes in the nucleus of infected cells. *Proc. Natl. Acad. Sci. USA,* 1992; 89:11486–11489.

[21] Callen EC, Kessler TL. Mycobacterium fortuitum infections associated with laparoscopic gastric banding. *Obes. Surg.,* 2011;21(3):404-6.

[22] Canturk Z, Canturk NZ, Cetinarslan B, et al. Nosocomial infections and obesity in surgical patients. *Obes. Res.*, 2003;11:769–775.

[23] Carlisle EM, Morowitz MJ. Pediatric surgery and the human microbiome. *J. Pediatr. Surg.*, 2011;46(3):577-84.

[24] Carter JK, Ow CL, Smith RE. Rous-associated virus type 7 induces a syndrome in chickens characterized by stunting and obesity. *Infect. Immun.*, 1983; 39: 410–422.

[25] Centers for Disease Control and Prevention (CDC). Rapidly growing mycobacterial infection following liposuction and liposculpture--Caracas, Venezuela, 1996-1998. *MMWR Morb. Mortal. Wkly. Rep.*, 1998 18;47(49):1065-7.

[26] Chastain MA, Chastain JB, Coleman WP. HIV lipodystrophy: review of the syndrome and report of a case treated with liposuction. *Dermatol. Surg.*, 2001;27(5):497-500.

[27] Cheadle WG. Risk factors for surgical site infection. *Surg. Infect. (Larchmt)*, 2006;7 Suppl 1:S7-11.

[28] Chen CC, Huang MT, Wei PL, Liang HH, Chen SC, Wu CH, Wang W. Severe peritonitis due to Streptococcus viridans following adjustable gastric banding. *Obes. Surg.*, 2010;20(11):1603-5.

[29] Choban PS, Heckler R, Burge JC, Flancbaum L. Increased incidence of nosocomial infections in obese surgical patients. *Am. Surg.*, 1995;61:1001–1005.

[30] Chopra T, Zhao JJ, Alangaden G, Wood MH, Kaye KS. Preventing surgical site infections after bariatric surgery: value of perioperative antibiotic regimens. *Expert. Rev. Pharmacoecon. Outcomes. Res.*, 2010;10(3):317–328.

[31] Chopra T, Marchaim D, Lynch Y, Kosmidis C, Zhao JJ, Dhar S, Gheyara N, Turner D, Gulish D, Wood M, Alangaden G, Kaye KS. Epidemiology and outcomes associated with surgical site infection following bariatric surgery. *Am. J. Infect. Control.*, 2012 Feb 10. [Epub]

[32] Christou NV, Jarand J, Sylvestre JL, McLean AP. Analysis of the incidence and risk factors for wound infections in open bariatric surgery. *Obes. Surg.*, 2004;14(1):16–22.

[33] Cone LA, B Waterbor R, Sofonio MV. Purpura fulminans due to Streptococcus pneumoniae sepsis following gastric bypass. *Obes. Surg.*, 2004;14(5):690-4.

[34] Cottam DR, Schaefer PA, Shaftan GW, Angus LD. Dysfunctional immune-privilege in morbid obesity: implications and effect of gastric bypass surgery. *Obes. Surg.*, 2003;13(1):49-57.

[35] Csendes A. Prevalence of Helicobacter pylori seropositivity among patients undergoing bariatric surgery: a preliminary study. *World J. Surg.*, 2009 Jun;33(6):1335.

[36] Czupryniak L, Strzelczyk J, Pawlowski M, Loba J. Mild elevation of fasting plasma glucose is a strong risk factor for postoperative complications in gastric bypass patients. *Obes. Surg.*, 2004;14:1393–1397.

[37] De Jong JC,Wermenbol AG, Verweij-Uijterwaal MW, Slaterus KW, Wertheim-Van Dillen P, Van Doornum GJ et al. Adenoviruses from human immunodeficiency virus-infected individuals, including two strains that represent new candidate serotypes Ad50 and Ad51 of species B1 and D, respectively. *J. Clin. Microbiol.*, 1999;37: 3940–3945.

[38] Del Mar Gutierrez M, Mateo G, Domingo P. Strategies in the treatment of HIV-1-associated adipose redistribution syndromes. *Expert. Opin. Pharmacother.*, 2007;8 (12):1871-84.

[39] De Lacerda Suplicy H, Bornschein A. Infections as the etiology for obesity. *Arq. Bras. Endocrinol. Metab.*, 2009;53/2:159-164.

[40] Dessy LA, Mazzocchi M, Fioramonti P, Scuderi N. Conservative management of local Mycobacterium chelonae infection after combined liposuction and lipofilling. *Aesthetic. Plast. Surg.*, 2006;30(6):717-22.
[41] Dhurandhar NV, Kulkarni P, Ajinkya SM, Sherikar A. Effect of adenovirus infection on adiposity in chicken. *Vet. Microbiol.*, 1992;31: 101–107.
[42] Dhurandhar NV, Kulkarni PR, Ajinkya SM, Sherikar AA, Atkinson RL. Association of adenovirus infection with human obesity. *Obes. Res.*, 1997; 5: 464–469.
[43] Dhurandhar NV, Whigham LD, Abbott DH, Schultz-Darken NJ, Israel BA, Bradley SM et al. Human adenovirus Ad-36 promotes weight gain in male rhesus and marmoset monkeys. *J. Nutr.*, 2002; 132: 3155–3160.
[44] Dhurandhar NV. A framework for identification of infections that contribute to human obesity. *Lancet Infect. Dis.*, 2011;11(12):963-969.
[45] Dooley KE, Chaisson RE. Tuberculosis and diabetes mellitus: convergence of two epidemics. *Lancet Infect. Dis.*, 2009;9(12):737-746.
[46] Edmiston CE, Krepel C, Kelly H, et al. Perioperative antibiotic prophylaxis in the gastric bypass patient: Do we achieve therapeutic levels? *Surgery*, 2004;136:738–747.
[47] Erim T, Cruz-Correa MR, Szomstein S, Velis E, Rosenthal R. Prevalence of Helicobacter pylori seropositivity among patients undergoing bariatric surgery: a preliminary study. *World J. Surg.*, 2008;32(9):2021-5.
[48] Falagas ME, Karageorgopoulos DE. Adjustment of dosing of antimicrobial agents for bodyweight in adults. Lancet, 2010;375(9710):248-251.
[49] Falagas ME, Kompoti M. Obesity and infection. Lancet Infect. Dis., 2006;6(7):438-446.
[50] Fernández-Aceñero MJ, Silvestre V, Fernández-Roldán R, Cortés L, García-Blanch G. Gastric actinomycosis: a rare complication after gastric bypass for morbid obesity. *Obes. Surg.*, 2004;14(7):1012-5.
[51] Flancbaum L, Drake V, Colarusso T, Belsley S. Initial experience with bariatric surgery in asymptomatic human immunodeficiency virus-infected patients. *Surg. Obes. Relat. Dis.*, 2005;1(2):73-6.
[52] Flum DR, Belle SH, King WC, et al. Perioperative safety in the longitudinal assessment of bariatric surgery. *N. Engl. J. Med.*, 2009;361(5):445–454.
[53] Ford AC, Axon AT. Epidemiology of Helicobacter pylori infection and public health implications. *Helicobacter*, 2010;15 Suppl 1:1-6.
[54] Forse RA, Karam B, MacLean LD, Christou NV. Antibiotic prophylaxis for surgery in morbidly obese patients. *Surgery*, 1989;106:750–756.
[55] Frazier TH, DiBaise JK, McClain CJ. Gut microbiota, intestinal permeability, obesity-induced inflammation, and liver injury. *JPEN J. Parenter. Enteral. Nutr.*, 2011;35(5 Suppl):14S-20S.
[56] Freeman JT, Anderson DJ, Hartwig MG, Sexton DJ. Surgical site infections following bariatric surgery in community hospitals: a weighty concern? *Obes. Surg.*, 2011;21(7):836-40.
[57] Frezza EE, Reddy S, Gee LL, Wachtel MS. Complications after sleeve gastrectomy for morbid obesity. *Obes. Surg.*, 2009;19(6):684-7. Martin-Malagon A, Arteaga-
[58] Furuya EY, Paez A, Srinivasan A, Cooksey R, Augenbraun M, Baron M, Brudney K, Della-Latta P, Estivariz C, Fischer S, Flood M, Kellner P, Roman C, Yakrus M, Weiss D, Granowitz EV. Outbreak of Mycobacterium abscessus wound infections among

"lipotourists" from the United States who underwent abdominoplasty in the Dominican Republic. *Clin. Infect. Dis.*, 2008 15;46(8):1181-8.

[59] Garibaldi RA, Britt MR, Coleman ML, et al. Risk factors for postoperative pneumonia. *Am. J. Med.*, 1981;70:677–680.

[60] Gaudry P, Mognol P, Fortin A, Marmuse JP. Reflection on one case of acute peritonitis due to adjustable gastric banding during pregnancy. *Gynecol. Obstet. Fertil.*, 2006;34(5):407-9.

[61] Giannella M, Pistella E, Perciaccante A, Venditti M. Soft tissue infection caused by Mycobacterium chelonae following a liposculpture and lipofilling procedure. *Ann. Ital. Med. Int.*, 2005;20(4):245-7.

[62] Gold DR, Annino DJ Jr. HIV-associated cervicodorsal lipodystrophy: etiology and management. *Laryngoscope,* 2005;115(5):791-5.

[63] Gonzalez I, Rodriguez-Ballester L, Diaz-Romero F. Gastroesophageal junction leak with serious sepsis after gastric bypass: successful treatment with endoscopy-assisted intraluminal esophageal drainage and self-expandable covered metal stent. *Obes. Surg.*, 2010;20(2):240-3.

[64] Gould J. Prevalence of Helicobacter pylori infection among patients undergoing bariatric surgery: a preliminary study. *World J. Surg.*, 2008;32(9):2026-7.

[65] Griffond B, Verlaeten O, Belin MF, Risold PY, Bernard A. Specific alteration of the expression of selected hypothalamic neuropeptides during acute and late mouse brain infection using a morbillivirus: relevance to the late-onset obesity? *J. Brain. Res.*, 2004; 1022: 173–181.

[66] Grimble RF. Symposium 5 (Joint Nutrition Society and BAPEN Symposium): Too many pies: metabolic competencies in obesity. The true cost of in-patient obesity: impact of obesity on inflammatory stress and morbidity. *Proceedings of the Nutrition Society,* 2010;69:511–517.

[67] Guo S, DiPietro LA. Factors affecting wound healing. *J. Dent. Res.*, 2010;89(3):219-229.

[68] Harder TC, Osterhaus ADME. Canine distemper virus – a morbollivirus in search of new hosts? *Trends Microbiol.*, 1997; 5: 120–124.

[69] Heinze S, Püschel K, Tsokos M. Necrotizing fasciitis with fatal outcome: a report of two cases. *Forensic. Sci. Med. Pathol.*, 2011;7(3):278-82.

[70] Helling TS. Operative experience and follow-up in a cohort of patients with a BMI > or =70kg/m^2. *Obes. Surg.*, 2005;15(4):482-5.

[71] Hierholzer JC. Adenoviruses. In: Murray PR, Baron EJ, Pfaller MA, Tenover FC, Yolken RH (eds). Manual of Clinical Microbiology, 6th edn. ASM Press: Washington, DC, 1995, pp 947–955.

[72] Higa KD, Ho T, Boone KB. Laparoscopic Roux-en-Y gastric bypass: Technique and 3-year follow-up. *J. Laparoendosc. Adv. Surg. Tech. A,* 2001;11:377–382.

[73] Hultman CS, McPhail LE, Donaldson JH, Wohl DA. Surgical management of HIV-associated lipodystrophy: role of ultrasonic-assisted liposuction and suction-assisted lipectomy in the treatment of lipohypertrophy. *Ann. Plast. Surg.*, 2007;58(3):255-63.

[74] Ives CL, Harrison DK, Stansby GS. Tissue oxygen saturation, measured by near-infrared spectroscopy, and its relationship to surgical-site infections. *Br. J. Surg.*, 2007;94(1):87-91.

[75] Jamal MK, DeMaria EJ, Johnson JM, Carmody BJ, Wolfe LG, Kellum JM, Meador JG. Impact of major co-morbidities on mortality and complications after gastric bypass. *Surg. Obes. Relat. Dis.*, 2005;1(6):511-6.
[76] Jeffery PL, McGuckin MA, Linden SK. Endocrine impact of Helicobacter pylori: Focus on ghrelin and ghrelin o-acyltransferase. *World J. Gastroenterol.*, 2011; 17(10): 1249–1260.
[77] Johnson JA, Heneine W. Characterization of endogenous avian leukosis viruses in chicken embryonic fibroblast substrates used in production of measles and mumps vaccines. *J. Virol.*, 2001;75:3605–3612.
[78] Johnson RT. Prion diseases. *Lancet Neurol.*, 2005; 4: 635–642.
[79] Kakarla VR, Nandipati K, Lalla M, Castro A, Merola S. Are laparoscopic bariatric procedures safe in superobese (BMI ≥50 kg/m2) patients? An NSQIP data analysis. *Surg. Obes. Relat. Dis.*, 2011;7(4):452-8.
[80] Kamimura M, Watanabe K, Kobayakawa M, Mihara F, Edamoto Y, Teruya K, Kikuchi Y, Oka S. Successful absorption of antiretroviral drugs after gastrojejunal bypass surgery following failure of therapy through a jejunal tube. *Intern. Med.*, 2009;48 (12):1103-4.
[81] Kanda T, Takahashi T, Kudo S, Takeda T, Tsugawa H, Takekoshi N. Leptin deficiency enhances myocardial necrosis and lethality in a murine model of viral myocarditis. *Life Sci.*, 2004;75:1435–47.
[82] Karlsson EA, Beck MA. The burden of obesity on infectious disease. *Experimental Biology and Medicine*, 2010;235:1412-1424.
[83] Keats AS. The ASA classification of physical status: A recapitulation. *Anesthesiology,* 1978;49:233–236.
[84] Keithley JK, Duloy AM, Swanson B, Zeller JM. HIV infection and obesity: a review of the evidence. *J. Assoc. Nurses. AIDS Care,* 2009;20(4):260-274.
[85] Khawcharoenporn T, Tice AD, Grandinetti A, Chow D. Risk factors for community-associated methicillin-resistant Staphylococcus aureus cellulitis – and the value of recognition. *Hawai'i medical journal,* 2010;69:232-236.
[86] Kim YS, Carp RI, Callahan SM, Wisniewski HM. Adrenal involvement in scrapie-induced obesity. *Proc. Soc. Exp. Biol. Med.,* 1988; 189: 21–27.
[87] Lancaster RT, Hutter MM. Bands and bypasses: 30-day morbidity and mortality of bariatric surgical procedures as assessed by prospective, multi-center, risk-adjusted ACS-NSQIP data. *Surg. Endosc.*, 2008;22(12):2554–2563.
[88] Lee SK, Yeo SG. Relationship between pediatric obesity and otitis media with effusion. *Curr. Allergy Asthma Rep.*, 2009;9(6):465-472.
[89] Lee WJ, Wang W, Lee YC, Huang MT. Clinical characteristics and outcome of morbidly obese bariatric patients with concurrent hepatitis B viral infection. *Obes. Surg.,* 2008;18(5):589-94.
[90] Loffeld RJ. Helicobacter pylori, obesity and gastro-oesophageal reflux disease. Is there a relation? A personal view. *Neth. J. Med.,* 2005;63(9):344-347.
[91] Lyons MJ, Faust IM, Hemmes RB, Buskirk DR, Hirsch J, Zabriskie JB. A virally induced obesity syndrome in mice. *Science,* 1982; 216: 82–85.
[92] Machado JD, Campos CS, Lopes Dah Silva C, Marques Suen VM, Barbosa Nonino-Borges C, Dos Santos JE, Ceneviva R, Marchini JS. Intestinal bacterial overgrowth after Roux-en-Y gastric bypass. *Obes. Surg.,* 2008;18(1):139-43.

[93] Magee SR, Shih G, Hume A. Malabsorption of oral antibiotics in pregnancy after gastric bypass surgery. *J. Am. Board. Fam. Med.,* 2007;20(3):310-3.

[94] Mancuso P, Gottschalk A, Phare SM, Peters-Golden M, Lukacs NW, Huffnagle GB. Leptin-deficient mice exhibit impaired host defense in gram-negative pneumonia. *J. Immunol.,* 2002;168:4018–24.

[95] Marema RT, Perez M, Buffington CK. Comparison of the benefits and complications between laparoscopic and open Roux-en-Y gastric bypass surgeries. *Surg. Endosc.,* 2005;19:525–530.

[96] Meyers H, Brown-Elliott BA, Moore D, Curry J, Truong C, Zhang Y, Wallace Jr RJ. An outbreak of Mycobacterium chelonae infection following liposuction. *Clin. Infect. Dis.,* 2002;34(11):1500-7.

[97] Miehsler W. Mortality, morbidity and special issues of obese ICU patients. *Wien. Med. Wochenschr.,* 2010;160(5-6):124-128.

[98] Mitra AK, Clarke K. Viral obesity: fact or fiction? *Obes. Rev.,* 2010;11(4):289-296.

[99] Murillo J, Torres J, Bofill L, Ríos-Fabra A, Irausquin E, Istúriz R, Guzmán M, Castro J, Rubino L, Cordido M. Skin and wound infection by rapidly growing mycobacteria: an unexpected complication of liposuction and liposculpture. The Venezuelan Collaborative Infectious and Tropical Diseases Study Group. *Arch. Dermatol.,* 2000;136
(11):1347-52.

[100] Musso G, Gambino R, Cassader M. Interactions between gut microbiota and host metabolism predisposing to obesity and diabetes. *Annu. Rev. Med.,* 2011;62:361-380.

[101] Nagelvoort RW, Hulstaert PF, Kon M, Schuurman AH. Necrotising fasciitis and myositis as serious complications after liposuction. *Ned. Tijdschr. Geneeskd.,* 2002 14;146(50):2430-5.

[102] Newman MI, Camberos AE, Ascherman J. Mycobacteria abscessus outbreak in US patients linked to offshore surgicenter. *Ann. Plast. Surg.,* 2005;55(1):107-10.

[103] Nguyen NT, Paya M, Stevens CM, et al. The relationship between hospital volume and outcome in bariatric surgery at academic medical centers. *Ann. Surg.,* 2004;240:586–593.

[104] Papamichael KX, Papaioannou G, Karga H, Roussos A, Mantzaris GJ. Helicobacter pylori infection and endocrine disorders: Is there a link? *World. J. Gastroenterol.,* 2009;15(22): 2701-2707.

[105] Papanas N, Zissimopoulos A, Maltezos E. The role of nuclear medicine in the diagnosis of common and specific diabetic infections. *Hell J. Nucl. Med.,* 2010;13(2):150-157.

[106] Pasarica M, Dhurandhar NV. Infectobesity: obesity of infectious origin. *Adv. Food Nutr. Res.,* 2007;52:61-102.

[107] Patel S, Szomstein S, Rosenthal RJ. Reasons and outcomes of reoperative bariatric surgery for failed and complicated procedures (excluding adjustable gastric banding). *Obes. Surg.,* 2011;21(8):1209-1219.

[108] Pessaux P, Msika S, Atalla D, et al. Risk factors for postoperative infectious complications in noncolorectal abdominal surgery: A multivariate analysis based on a prospective multicenter study of 4718 patients. *Arch. Surg.,* 2003;138:314–324.

[109] Piliero PJ, Hubbard M, King J, Faragon JJ. Use of ultrasonography-assisted liposuction for the treatment of human immunodeficiency virus-associated enlargement of the dorsocervical fat pad. *Clin. Infect. Dis.,* 2003 15;37(10):1374-7.

[110] Plotkin BJ, Paulson D, Chelich A, Jurak D, Cole J, Kasimos J, Burdick JR, Casteel N. Immune responsiveness in a rat model for type II diabetes (Zucker rat, fa/fa): susceptibility to Candida albicans infection and leucocyte function. *J. Med. Microbiol.,* 1996;44:277–83.

[111] Podnos YD, Jimenez JC, Wilson SE, Stevens CM, Nguyen NT. Complications after laparoscopic gastric bypass: A review of 3464 cases. *Arch. Surg.,* 2003;138:957–961.

[112] Puri P, Sanyal AJ. Role of obesity, insulin resistance, and steatosis in hepatitis C virus infection. *Clin. Liver Dis.,* 2006;10(4):793-819.

[113] Régnier S, Martinez V, Veziris N, Bonvallot T, Meningaud JP, Caumes E. Treatment of cutaneous infections due to Mycobacterium fortuitum: two cases. *Ann. Dermatol. Venereol.,* 2008;135(8-9):591-5.

[114] Reoch J, Mottillo S, Shimony A, Filion KB, Christou NV, Joseph L, Poirier P, Eisenberg MJ. Safety of laparoscopic vs open bariatric surgery: a systematic review and meta-analysis. *Arch. Surg.,* 2011;146(11):1314-22.

[115] Rocha-e-Silva M. Metabolic and infectious pathologies in Brazilian medical literature: a review. *Clinics,* 2010;65(8):809-814.

[116] Rogers PM, Mashtalir N, Rathod MA, Dubuisson O, Wang Z, Dasuri K, Babin S, Gupta A, Markward N, Cefalu WT, Dhurandhar NV. Metabolically favorable remodeling of human adipose tissue by human adenovirus type 36. *Diabetes,* 2008;57(9):2321-31.

[117] Satpathy HK, Fleming A, Frey D, Barsoom M, Satpathy C, Khandalavala J. Maternal. obesity and pregnancy. *Postgrad. Med.,* 2008;120(3):E01-9.

[118] Schaible UE, Kaufmann SHE. Malnutrition and infection: Complex mechanisms and global impacts. *PLoS Med.,* 2007;4(5): e115.

[119] Schauer PR, Ikramuddin S, Gourash W, et al. Outcomes after laparoscopic Roux-en-Y gastric bypass for morbid obesity. *Ann. Surg.,* 2000;232:515–529.

[120] Scher KS. Studies on the duration of antibiotic administration for surgical prophylaxis. *Am. Surg.,* 1997; 63:59–62.

[121] Sehgal R, Berg A, Figueroa R, Poritz LS, McKenna KJ, Stewart DB, Koltun WA. Risk factors for surgical site infections after colorectal resection in diabetic patients. *J. Am. Coll Surg.,* 2011;212(1):29-34.

[122] Sekhar N, Torquati A, Youssef Y, Wright JK, Richards WO. A comparison of 399 open and 568 laparoscopic gastric bypasses performed during a 4-year period. *Surg. Endosc.,* 2007;21(4):665-8.

[123] Selke H, Norris S, Osterholzer D, Fife KH, DeRose B, Gupta SK. Bariatric surgery outcomes in HIV-infected subjects: a case series. *AIDS Patient Care STDS,* 2010;24(9):545-50.

[124] Shope TR, Cooney RN, McLeod J, Miller CA, Haluck RS. Early results after laparoscopic gastric bypass: EEA vs GIA stapled gastrojejunal anastomosis. *Obes. Surg.,* 2003;13(3):355-9.

[125] Smith AG, Sheridan PA, Harp JB, Beck MA. Diet-induced obese mice have increased mortality and altered immune responses when infected with influenza virus. *J. Nutr.,* 2007;137:1236–43.

[126] Stelzmueller I, Hoeller E, Wiesmayr S, Kafka R, Aigner F, Weiss H, Bonatti H. Severe intra-abdominal infection due to Streptococcus Milleri following adjustable gastric banding. *Obes. Surg.,* 2005;15(4):576-9.

[127] Sugerman HJ, Kellum JM Jr, Reines HD, et al. Greater risk of incisional hernia with morbidly obese than steroid-dependent patients and low recurrence with prefascial polypropylene mesh. *Am. J. Surg.,* 1996;171: 80–84.

[128] Sugerman HJ, DeMaria EJ, Kellum JM, Sugerman EL, Meador JG, Wolfe LG. Effects of bariatric surgery in older patients. *Ann. Surg.,* 2004;240(2):243-7.

[129] Sun B, Karin M. Obesity, inflammation, and liver cancer. *Journal of Hepatology,* 2012;56: 704–713.

[130] The Surgeon General's Call to Action to Prevent and Decrease Overweight and Obesity: Washington, D. C. U. S. Department of Health and Human Services. 2001.

[131] Tiktinsky E, Lantsberg S, Agranovich S, Kirshtein B, Lantsberg L. Leukocyte scintigraphy SPECT/CT software fusion diagnosis of infected gastric band. *Obes. Surg.,* 2008;18(7):902-4.

[132] Tipton AM, Cohen SA, Chelmow D. Wound infection in the obese pregnant woman. *Semin. Perinatol.,* 2011;35(6):345-349.

[133] Topaloglu S, Avsar FM, Ozel H, Babacan M, Berkem H, Yildiz Y, Hengirmen S. Comparison of bariatric and non-bariatric elective operations in morbidly obese patients on the basis of wound infection. *Obes. Surg.,* 2005;15(9):1271-6.

[134] Treadwell JR, Sun F, Schoelles K. Systematic review and meta-analysis of bariatric surgery for pediatric obesity. *Ann. Surg.,* 2008;248(5):763-76.

[135] Umeda T, Ohara H, Hayashi O, Ueki M, Hata Y. Toxic shock syndrome after suction lipectomy. *Plast. Reconstr. Surg.,* 2000;106(1):204-9.

[136] Vachharajani V, Vital S. Obesity and sepsis. *J. Intensive Care Med.,* 2006;21(5):287-295.

[137] Vangipuram SD, Sheele J, Atkinson RL, Holland TC, Dhurandhar NV. A human adenovirus enhances preadipocyte differentiation. *Obes. Res.,* 2004; 12: 770–777.

[138] Vangipuram SD, Yu M, Tian J, Stanhope KL, Pasarica M, Havel PJ, et al. Adipogenic human adenovirus-36 reduces leptin expression and secretion and increases glucose uptake by fat cells. *Int. J. Obes.,* 2007;31(1):87-96.

[139] Varela JE, Wilson SE, Nguyen NT. Outcomes of bariatric surgery in the elderly. *Am. Surg.,* 2006;72(10):865-9.

[140] Vasilakopoulou A, le Roux CW. Could a virus contribute to weight gain? *International Journal of Obesity,* 2007;31:1350–1356.

[141] Virji A, Murr MM. Caring for patients after bariatric surgery. *Am. Fam. Physician.,* 2006;73(8):1403-8.

[142] Wang CM, Kaltenboeck B . Exacerbation of chronic inflammatory diseases by infectious agents: Fact or fiction? *World J. Diabetes,* 2010; 1(2): 27–35.

[143] Waisbren E, Rosen H, Bader AM, Lipsitz SR, Rogers SO Jr, Eriksson E. Percent body fat and prediction of surgical site infection. *J. Am. Coll Surg.,* 2010;210(4):381-389.

[144] Waye MM. New insights into how adenovirus might lead to obesity: An oxidative stress theory. *Free Radic. Res.,* 2011;45(8):880-887.

[145] Whigham LD, Israel BA, Atkinson RL. Adipogenic potential of multiple human adenoviruses in vivo and in vitro in animals. *Am. J. Physiol. Regul. Integr. Comp. Physiol.,* 2006; 290: R190–4.

[146] Wieland CW, Florquin S, Chan ED, Leemans JC, Weijer S, Verbon A, Fantuzzi G, van der Poll T. Pulmonary Mycobacterium tuberculosis infection in leptin-deficient ob/ob mice. *Int. Immunol.,* 2005;17:1399–408.

[147] Williams MD, Champion JK. Experience with routine intraabdominal cultures during laparoscopic gastric bypass with implications for antibiotic prophylaxis. *Surg. Endosc.*, 2004;18(5):755-6.
[148] Wittgrove AC, Clark GW. Laparoscopic gastric bypass, Roux-en-Y, in 500 patients: Technique and results, with 3–60 month follow-up. *Obes. Surg.*, 2000;10:233–239.
[149] Wu JC. Does Helicobacter pylori infection protect against esophageal diseases in Asia? *Indian. J. Gastroenterol.*, 2011;30(4):149-153.
[150] Yang CS, Lee WJ, Wang HH, Huang SP, Lin JT, Wu MS. The influence of Helicobacter pylori infection on the development of gastric ulcer in symptomatic patients after bariatric surgery. *Obes. Surg.*, 2006;16(6):735-9.
[151] Zhu Y, Michelle Luo T, Jobin C, Young HA. Gut microbiota and probiotics in colon tumorigenesis. *Cancer Lett.*, 2011;309(2):119-127.

In: Bariatric Surgery
Editor: Christos R. Iavazzo

ISBN: 978-1-62618-995-9

Chapter IX

Anemia after Bariatric Surgery

Silvia Leite Faria[1,2], Orlando Pereira Faria[1], Heloisa Rodrigues de Gouvêa[1] and Mariane de Almeida Cardeal[1,2]
[1]Gastrocirurgia , Brasilia, Brazil
[2]University of Brasília

Abstract

Bariatric surgery is the most effective treatment for morbid obesity, offering satisfactory long-term weight loss and maintenance. It is, however, a procedure susceptible to the development of nutritional deficiencies, i. e. anemia, due to low food intake, the effects of gastric restriction and malabsorption which occurs. Anemic etiology may be due to deficiencies of iron, folate and/or vitamin B_{12}. The risk of iron deficiency anemia is increased after RYGB and may occur because of reduced intake of foods containing organic iron, a lower production of hydrochloric acid and/or the exclusion of the major sites of iron absorption: the duodenum and proximal jejunum. Diagnosis of anemia can be made using a complete blood count. Iron deficiency anemia (hypochromic and microcytic) is characterized by decreased serum ferritin levels (<20ng/ml),associated with increased iron binding capacity, a decrease in hemoglobin concentration and decreased mean corpuscular volume. It is recommended that bariatric patients make daily use of two multivitamins and multiminerals, thus providing for 200% RDA of iron, as a way of preventing iron deficiency anemia. In treating anemia, ferrous sulfate can be used at a dosage of 650mg/d. Thus, in some cases, serum ferritin may be elevated even with low serum iron, characterizing a condition known as anemia of chronic disease, a common framework related to obesity and early post-operative response to surgery. Deficiency of Vitamin B_{12} and folic acid can lead to the development of megaloblastic anemia (macrocytic). Bariatric patients should keep their B_{12} levels above 400ug/dl. With levels between 100 and 400, patients may have subclinical deficiency and supplementation is recommended. The diagnosis of folic acid deficiency can be done using homocysteine and erythrocyte folate tests. Supplementation which aims at preventing folate deficiency must reach 200% of DRIs. Orientation concerning nutritional deficiencies that may result from bariatric surgery are essential to the multidisciplinary team in the post-op phase, in order to maintain the good health and quality of life of patients.

1. Introduction

Bariatric surgery is the most effective treatment for morbid obesity, offering satisfactory long-term weight loss and maintenance [1, 2]. It is, however, a procedure susceptible to the development of nutritional deficiencies due to low food intake, the effects of gastric restriction and malabsorption which occurs following specific procedures, such as Roux-en-Y Gastric Bypass (RYGB) and Biliopancreatic Diversion, with or without Duodenal Switch (BPD / DS) [3], especially in cases where adequate nutritional monitoring is lacking [4]. However, the risk of similar deficiencies occurring in cases of purely restrictive procedures, such as adjustable gastric banding (AGB) or sleeve gastrectomy, should not be disregarded [5].

Since a large number of obese patients referred for bariatric surgery already suffer from vitamin and mineral deficiencies, an increased risk of developing nutritional deficiencies in the postoperative period of bariatric surgery merits attention [6], among which is anemia, one of the major nutritional complications that may follow this form of surgical intervention [7].

Anemia can be defined as a state in which the concentration of hemoglobin in the blood is abnormally low, due to the lack of one or more essential nutrients. This is quite common among patients undergoing bariatric surgery and occurs regardless of the amount of weight lost [8]. Studies have shown that slight post-op reduction in hemoglobin may occur, even in the absence of nutritional deficiencies, and is usually resolved up to 12 weeks post-op. If, after this period, abnormal hemoglobin levels persist, the possibility of nutritional deficiencies should be investigated [9, 10].

Among the studies carried out, the prevalence of anemia after bariatric surgery presents considerable variability due to the difficulty of long-term monitoring of the patients [11]. For this reason in certain studies, anemic prevalence varies from 5-64% after RYGB [11], while in those with more representative sample sizes values range from 20 to 36% among patients one 1 year or more post-op [11, 12, 13].

Anemic etiology varies and may be due to deficiencies of iron, folate and/or vitamin B_{12}. Iron deficiency anemia is the most prevalent, followed by mixed-deficiency anemia (of iron and vitamin B_{12}) [11, 14].

2. Iron Deficiency Anemia

The risk of iron deficiency anemia (iron insufficiency) is increased after RYGB, affecting some 52% of patients [3,14], with a higher prevalence among women of fertile age [11, 13, 15]. CABLE et al. (2011) [11] found that women at this stage are about 60% more likely to develop anemia in relation to postmenopausal women.

Iron deficiency anemia may be associated with any form of bariatric surgery (AGB, Sleeve, RYGB or BPD), showing different causes according to the procedure applied [3, 5]. With respect to RYGB, iron deficiency may occur because of reduced intake of foods containing organic iron (heme iron polypeptide), a lower production of hydrochloric acid and/or the exclusion of the major sites of iron absorption, i. e., the duodenum and proximal jejunum [16]. Furthermore, anemia can develop as a result of surgical complications, namely ulcers, gastritis and/or blood loss [17].

The reduced intake of foods containing iron can be due to the limited size of the gastric pouch after surgery, along with intolerance to foods rich in ferrous iron (heme iron). For this reason, patients with food intolerance to red meat have a higher risk of developing anemia [3, 16, 18]. Such intolerance can reach 50% of the patients in the postoperative period, even up to four years after surgery and may be accompanied by nausea and vomiting. This type of intolerance is more prevalent in patients who have undergone AGB, rather than RYGB [19, 20].

A lower production of hydrochloric acid occurs after RYGB, hindering the reduction of ferric to ferrous iron and its subsequent absorption. It is assumed that after this procedure, a smaller number of receptors are available at the apical membrane of enterocytes (such as duodenal *cytochrome b*). These receptors are also able to reduce ferric iron and, therefore, to execute intracellular transport [21].

In addition to the exclusion of major absorption sites in the duodenum and proximal jejunum resulting from RYGB, malabsorptive procedures cause a slower intestinal transit time of iron and less contact of it with the lumen, but this factor has not been correlated with an increased incidence of iron deficiency anemia, although it results in a greater percentage of excess weight loss [22].

2.1. Diagnosis

Diagnosis of anemia can be made using a complete blood count (CBC), which is available for most patients, despite being a late biochemical marker [3]. Iron deficiency anemia (hypochromic and microcytic) is characterized by decreased serum ferritin levels, associated with increased iron binding capacity, a decrease in hemoglobin concentration and decreased mean corpuscular volume [17].

Serum iron is also a parameter that must be evaluated at recommended intervals: at least six months after bariatric surgery and thereafter annually [3]. The diagnosis of severe anemia is indicated by hemoglobin concentration levels below 10g/dL [18]. The measurement of serum ferritin reflects iron stores, but should not be used as an isolated diagnostic parameter, since it is an acute phase protein, and may vary according to the age of the patient, and the presence of inflammation and/or infection [3].

Thus, in some cases, serum ferritin may be elevated ($\geq$ 200ng/ml), even with low serum iron [13. 23, 24], characterizing a condition known as anemia of chronic disease (ACD), a common framework related to obesity and early post-operative response to surgery. This type of anemia is due to increased hepcidin in the body, a peptide whose production is stimulated by interleukin-6 (IL-6), a pro-inflammatory cytokine. Hepcidin is able to block the intestinal absorption of iron, as well as to block the mobilization of iron stores, thus maintaining high levels of ferritin [25].

In cases of iron deficiency anemia, contrary to what happens in anemia of chronic disease, serum ferritin falls below 40ng/ml. Ferritin should be maintained above 40ng/dL, especially among women of childbearing age who have regular menses [15, 23]. Critical values of iron deficiency anemia are: ferritin ≤ 10ng/ml, serum iron <50ug/ml (for women) and <70ug/ml (for men), TIBC (total iron binding capacity) > 450ug/dL [3, 20]. Transferrin (transferrin binding protein), a protein that maintains iron in soluble form, should also be evaluated. Its normal iron saturation level is 30%. Thus, a saturation level of <16% is indicative of iron deficiency anemia [24].

Clinical signs and symptoms associated with iron deficiency anemia which may help in its diagnosis are fatigue, dizziness, paleness, headache, dyspnea, myasthenia and little disposition for physical activity [3, 17, 20]. Some studies, though, present reference to the correlation between anemia and pica (desire to eat non-food substances) and pagophagia (desire to eat ice) in bariatric patients [26], which can cause irreversible oral lesions, with resolution occurring after the reestablishment of appropriate biochemical parameters through supplementation [27].

2.2. Prevention and Treatment

It is recommended that bariatric patients make daily use of two multivitamins and multiminerals, thus providing for 200% RDA of iron, as a way of preventing iron deficiency anemia [3].

For high-risk populations, such as adolescents, women of childbearing age and patients with occult bleeding, a supplementation of 40 to 65mg of elemental iron and 320mg of fumarate or ferrous gluconate twice daily for the prevention of anemia is recommended [9, 16, 28]. This dosage is not generally found in commercial pluri-vitamins, thus requiring additional supplementation [4]. Only with purely restrictive procedures (e. g. AGB) is this prophylactic supplementation unnecessary.

For more severe cases, the use of contraceptives can be a good alternative, since they are capable of reducing the menstrual flow by about 60% or eliminating it completely, resulting in lower risks of anemia.

As a form of prevention, dosages of elemental iron of up to 300mg per day can be prescribed with the addition of vitamin C supplement for increased absorption of minerals. Vitamin C is necessary to reduce ferric iron (non-heme iron) to ferrous iron (heme iron), since after mixed and malabsorptive procedures there is less production of hydrochloric acid and fewer receptors on the apical membrane of enterocytes, which perform this function [3].

In treating anemia, ferrous sulfate can be used at a dosage of 650mg/d [16]. When ferritin reaches levels below 10ug/dL (indicating severe anemia), intravenous administration of iron, in the form of iron dextran, sucrose gluconato or ferric iron, should be carried out as recommended by the hematologist or clinical staff [3, 9]. This form of administering iron improves the erythrocyte response, energy metabolism and the immune system [18]. In some cases, intravenous transfusion of erythrocytes may be required [17].

Iron supplements and iron-rich foods should be taken at intervals widely spaced from the ingestion of calcium supplements and calcium-rich foods, as well as foods high in caffeine and tannins, since these decrease iron absorption. The intake of foods rich in ferrous iron, such as red meat, should be encouraged [3].

In cases of anemia associated with some chronic diseases, even among post-op patients, iron supplementation has a refractory effect, since the etiology is not from iron deficiency, but from the inflammatory process, which might explain the ineffectiveness of iron supplementation among some bariatric patients (10-15%) [22,28,29]. In this case, any weight loss incurred can improve the inflammatory condition, promoting the bioavailability of iron [4, 13].

3. Anemia from Deficiency of Vitamin B_{12} or Folic Acid

Vitamin B_{12} and folic acid play important roles in human metabolism through their participation in the maturation of erythrocytes. Thus, deficiency of these micronutrients can lead to the development of megaloblastic anemia (macrocytic), characterized by the production of a reduced number of red blood cells, but of greater volume, abnormal shape and immature status, factors which reduce their efficiency in the transport of oxygen throughout the body. Megaloblastic anemia deficiency is related to deficiency of both of these nutrients in about 95% of the cases studied [3]

3.1. Vitamin B_{12}

Vitamin B_{12} deficiency may occur, usually between 1-9 years after RYGB among 12-33% of patients [30]. Despite this occurrence in isolation being uncommon [31], patients undergoing RYGB are at risk of developing disability due to incomplete digestion of food and lower release of vitamin B_{12} from foods providing protein. This last factor is due to reduced production of hydrochloric acid, responsible for transforming pepsinogen into pepsin, which releases vitamin B_{12} from food [23, 32]. In addition, a recent study showed a significant correlation between vitamin B_{12} and dumping syndrome [4], probably due to losses by vomiting and diarrhea.

Intolerance to red meat contributes to reduced availability of vitamin B_{12} in the body, since it is classified as a food source of this nutrient [16]. Another factor that may lead to vitamin B_{12} deficiency and consequently to pernicious anemia is the lower production of the so-called Intrinsic Factor (IF) by the parietal cells of the stomach, since this is responsible for the absorption of vitamin B_{12} in the intestine (terminal ileum) [3, 23].

Given these factors, vitamin B_{12} absorption after RYGB is passive, in most cases, making a specific supplementation of this nutrient necessary, since this absorption route is responsible for only 1% of all vitamin intake in individuals who have not undergone intestinal bypass [3].

Considering the Adjustable Gastric Band (AGB) and Biliopancreatic Diversion (BPD), changes in the exocrine functions of the stomach are insignificant. Thus, the production of hydrochloric acid is hardly affected, and vitamin B_{12} deficiency in such cases is less prevalent [3]. As for the gastric sleeve intervention, a recent study showed that 9% of the patients 1 year post-op showed deficiency of this vitamin due to reduced production of hydrochloric acid by the stomach [5]. A person who has not been operated has a store of about 2mg of vitamin B_{12}, which can last for up to two years when the intake is insufficient. Thus the prevalence of this deficiency may increase over the years, and special attention to this specific case may be necessary [5].

3.1.1. Diagnosis

The monitoring of vitamin B_{12} deficiency can be done by measuring serum concentration of the blood, with serum levels below 200ug/dl (<150pmol/L) indicating disability. In this sense, bariatric patients should keep their B_{12} levels above 400ug/dl. With levels between 100 and 400, patients may have subclinical deficiency and supplementation is recommended. Vitamin B_{12} deficiency with levels below 100 indicates chronic deficiency and treatment should be initiated immediately [3]. However, half of the patients who show signs and symptoms of this deficiency have normal serum levels of this vitamin, so additional tests are necessary for adequate diagnosis, such as the serum level of methymalonic acid and the degree of homocysteine concentration, which are intermediate metabolites of the Vitamin B_{12} path of synthesis [16]. In the diagnose of this deficiency, serum levels of homocysteine should not exceed 13μgmol/L and those of methylmalonic acid should not exceed 0. 4mol/L. However, high levels of homocysteine may be found in cases of folic acid deficiency. Thus, the diagnosis of folic acid deficiency must be excluded before proceeding with the diagnose of vitamin B_{12} [33]. Symptoms related to vitamin B_{12} deficiency include: polyneuropathy, paresthesia and permanent neurological disorders, hallucinations, delusions and even psychosis. If untreated, the patient can develop irreversible neurological damage [3].

3.1.2. Supplementation

As a preventive measure, daily oral supplementation of 350μg of crystalline B_{12} is recommended or intranasal supplementation of 500μg weekly or intramuscular supplementation of 1000μg monthly [3, 16, 9]. With oral dosage, since the passive absorption of this nutrient is only about 1% of intake, on average 3,5μg are absorbed, a level superior to the daily requirement for an adult. A oral dosage of 500μg per day can resolve deficiency symptoms [29].

With sublingual dosages, 2000μg of the vitamin may be administered for 7-12 days. With intramuscular doses, anemia can be treated with 1000μg administered daily for one week, followed by weekly administration for a month and after that, each month for the rest of the patient's life [33, 34].

Patients should be assessed individually before prescribing supplements, as there are various routes (intramuscular, oral, sublingual, nasal), doses and frequency of administration. Supplements should be prescribed in manners that patients can adhere to, since anemia can occur even with supplementation being administered [3]. Studies suggest that oral supplementation in daily megadoses is as effective as intramuscular supplementation. Von Drygalsky (2009) [23] compared two groups of patients receiving supplementation of 2000μg of B_{12} orally in relation to about half of that dose applied intramuscularly during several days after surgery. On the 20th day after surgery, the group that had received oral supplementation of vitamin B_{12} showed serum levels significantly higher than the group supplemented intramuscularly. However, intramuscular doses also appear to be effective, since a dose of 1000μg every three months increases significantly the concentrations of this vitamin to adequate levels, even in late post-op phases [6]. However, in spite of the supplementation administered by both routes being apparently effective, intramuscular doses are to be preferred, since they do not require the discipline of daily intake by the patient, thus reducing the risk of a possible failure due to poor adhesion to ingestion of supplements after surgery [4].

3.2. Folic Acid

Folic acid deficiency is considered rare [31] and less common than vitamin B_{12} deficiency in patients who have undergone RYGB, reaching prevalence levels of 3-65% (BOYLAN et al., 1998; AILLS et al., 2008) ranging from 0 to 38% in the immediate post-op period [23]. Folic acid is considered a marker of intake of pluri-vitamins, so a deficiency can occur due to lack of adherence to this supplementation [4] and also to a lack of food sources in the diet (leafy vegetables, fruits, entrails, liver, dried yeast and fortified foods). This can also occur after RYGB, even with patients who are given a multivitamin supplement, as reported by BOYLAN et al. (1998) [35], showing a prevalence of 47% and 41% after 6 and 12 months after surgery respectively. The normal absorption site of this nutrient is in the duodenum, but patients who have undergone malabsorptive procedures can absorb it all along the intestine as a mechanism of adaptation. As an additional adaptive mechanism, it is suggested that in the post-op phase an endogenous production of folate be produced by bacteria in the initial section of the small intestine, irrespective of the achlorhydria environment resulting from the surgery [36].

3.2.1. Diagnosis

The diagnosis of folic acid deficiency can be done using the following biochemical tests: homocysteine and erythrocyte folate [37].

3.2.2. Supplementation

Supplementation which aims at preventing folate deficiency must reach 200% of IDRs (with the daily ingestion of two multivitamin tablets - 800μg). In treating the deficiency, a daily supplement of 1000mg, which should not be exceeded so as to avoid any masking of a vitamin B_{12} deficiency, can be effective [3].

4. Final Thoughts

Anemia can develop after bariatric surgery, with different etiologies. Deficiency of iron, vitamin B_{12} and folic acid should be investigated for the diagnosis of megaloblastic or iron deficiency anemia. However, nutritional anemia resulting from malabsorptive procedures may involve deficiencies of protein, selenium and copper, which require investigation when screening for iron, vitamin B12 and folic acid present negative results [9].

The diagnosis of anemia should not be restricted to the serum form of nutrients involved. In the case of iron deficiency anemia, for example, it is necessary to investigate the saturation of transferrin, hemoglobin, serum ferritin and TIBC (total iron binding capacity). In cases of megaloblastic anemia, doses of serum homocysteine are recommended. For prevention of anemia, it is necessary to supplement with multivitamins and polyminerals. In some cases, an additional iron supplement is required, for example for women of fertile age. The addition of vitamin B_{12} post bariatric surgery is required for all patients and it may be administered by different routes (oral, intramuscular, sublingual, nasal).

Table 1. Overview of aspects relevant to the diagnosis, prevention and treatment of anemia after bariatric surgery

Etiology	Diagnosis		Prevention	Treatment
	Biochemical	Clinical		
Iron Deficiency	- Ferritin: ≤ 10ng/ml; - Serum iron <50ug/ml (women) and <70ug/ml (men); - TIBC:> 450ug / dL - Transferrin: Saturation <16%	- Fatigue, dizziness, paleness, headache, dyspnea, myasthenia and little disposition for physical activity. - Pica and pagophagia	– Daily use of two multivitamins and multiminerals (providing 200% IDR). - Populations at greatest risk *: supplementation of 40 - 65mg of elemental iron or 320mg of fumarate or ferrous gluconate twice daily or 300mg of elemental iron per day, with the addition of a Vitamin C supplement. - Ingestion of foods high in heme-iron at different times from the intake of food high in calcium and calcium supplements.	- Ferrous sulfate: 650 mg / day - Severe anemia **: Intravenous Administration of iron in the form of iron dextran, ferrous gluconate or ferric sacarose. - Ingestion of foods high in heme-iron at different times from the intake of food high in calcium and calcium supplements.
Chronic (disease) inflammation	- Ferritin: ≥ 200ng/ml - Serum iron: < 50ug/ml	-	-	-
Vitamin B12 deficiency	- Vitamin B12 serum: <200 ug / dl -Homocysteine: <13μgmol / L and - Methylmalonic Acid: <0. 4 mmol / L	- Polyneuropathy, paresthesia, and permanent neurological disorders, hallucinations, delusions, psychosis.		- 500μg orally daily - 2000μg sublingual for 7 to 12 days - 1000μg intramuscularly daily for 1 week, followed by weekly administration for 1 month and thereafter, monthly for the rest of the patient's life.
Folic acid deficiency	- Homocysteine - Erythrocyte folate	-	– Daily ingestion of two multivitamin tablets a day: 800μg (200% of IDRs)	- 1000 mg daily

* Adolescents, women of childbearing age and patients with occult bleeding.

** hemoglobin concentration levels below 10g/dL.

As the occurrence of anemia does not depends on the volume of weight lost, patients who stop losing weight, lose weight improperly or recover part of the weight lost, may believe that supplementation is no longer needed. Another important issue is that patients presenting anemia also present increased needs of protein which is essential for new cell growth. As patients needs are between 60 to 120g/d, supplements may be necessary for these patients. Thus, the need for lifelong adherence to supplementation, independent of weight loss should be emphasized by professionals [8].

Table 1 presents a summary of the most relevant aspects for diagnosis, prevention and treatment of anemia after bariatric surgery considered in this chapter. Orientation on nutritional deficiencies that may result from bariatric surgery are essential to the multidisciplinary team in the post-op phase, in order to maintain the good health and quality of life of patients, since nutritional deficiencies, such as anemia, are eminently predictable, preventable and treatable. Accordingly, the priority of the team should focus on stimulus to good eating habits and adherence by the patient to the program of supplementation, with frequent consultation of the professionals, so as to have adequate clinical and biochemical monitoring, especially in the first two years after surgery [4].

References

[1] Buchwald H, Avidor Y, Braundwald E, et al. Batritric Surgery: a systematic review and meta-analysis. JAMA. 2004;292(14):1724-37. [Review. Erratum in: *JAMA,* 2005; 293(14):1728].

[2] Valezi AC, Junior JM, de Menezes MA. Weight loss outcome after silastic ring Roux-en-Y gastric bypass: 8 years of follow-up. *Obes. Surg.,* 2010;20:1491–5.

[3] Aills L, Blankenship J, Buffington C, et al. ASMBS Allied Health Nutritional Guidelines for the Surgical Weight Loss Patient. *SOARD,* 2008;4(Supp):73S-108S.

[4] Dalcanale L, Oliveira CPMS, Faintuch J, et al. Long-Term Nutritional Outcome After Gastric Bypass. *Obes. Surg.,* 2010 Feb;20(2):181-7.

[5] Arts EO, Janssen IMC, Berends FJ. The Gastric Sleeve: Losing Weight as Fast as Micronutrients? *Obes. Surg.,* 2011 Feb;21(2):207-11.

[6] Aasheim ET, Jonhson LK, Hofso D, et al. Vitamin status after gastric bypass and lifestyle intervention: a comparative prospective study. *Surg. Obes. Relat. Dis.,* 2012 Mar;8(2):169-75.

[7] Faria SL, Faria OP, Gouvêa HR, Melo TR. Nutritional Management of Weight Loss Surgery Complications. *Nutrição em Pauta,* 2011;1:29-33.

[8] Dallal RM, Leighton J, Trang A. Analysis of leucopenia and anemia after gastric bypass surgery. *Surg. Obes. Relat. Dis.,* 2012 Mar;8(2):164-8.

[9] Mechanick JE, Kushner RF, Sugerman HJ, et al. American Association of Clinical Endocrinologists, The Obesity Society, and American Society for Metabolic and Bariatric Surgery Medical Guidelines for Clinical Practice for the Perioperative Nutritional, Metabolic, and Nonsurgical Support of the Bariatric Surgery Patient. *Surg. Obes. Relat. Dis.,* 2008 Sep-Oct;4(5 Suppl):S109-84.

[10] Gasteyger C, Suter M, Calmes JM, Gaillard RC, Giusti V. Changes in body composition, metabolic profile and nutritional status 24 months after gastric banding. *Obes. Surg.*, 2006;16:243–50.

[11] Cable CT, Colbert CY, Showalter T, et al. Prevalence of anemia after Roux-en-Y gastric bypass surgery: what is the right number? *Surg. Obes. Relat. Dis.*, 2011 Mar-Apr;7(2):134-9.

[12] Amaral JF, Thompson WR, Caldwell MD, Martin HF, Randall HT. Prospective hematologic evaluation of gastric exclusion surgery for morbid obesity. *Ann. Surg.*, 1985;201:186 –93.

[13] Drygalsky AV, Andris DA, Nutleman PR, et al. Anemia after bariatric surgery cannot be explained by iron deficiency alone: results of a large cohort study. *Surg. Obes. Relat. Dis.*, 2011 Mar-Apr;7(2):151-6.

[14] Brolin RE, LaMarca LB, Kenler HA, Cody RP. Malabsorptive Gastric Bypass in Patients With Superobesity *J. Gastrointest. Surg.*, 2002;6(2):195-205. A.

[15] Fujioka K. Follow-up of Nutritional and Metabolic Problems After Bariatric Surgery. *Diab. Care,* 2005;28(2):481-4.

[16] Malinowsky SS. Nutritional and Metabolic Complications of Bariatric Surgery. *Am. J. Med. Sci.*, 2006;331(4):. 219-225.

[17] Avgerinos DV, Llaguna OH, Seigerman M, Lefkowitz AJ, Leitman IM. Incidence and risk factors for the development of anemia following gastric bypass surgery. *World J. Gastroenterol.*, 2010;16(15):1867-1870.

[18] Muñoz M, Botella-Romero F, Gómez-Ramírez S, Campos A, García-Erce JA. Iron deficiency and anaemia in bariatric surgical patients: causes, diagnosis and proper management. *Nutr. Hosp.*, 2009;24:640-654.

[19] Avinoah E, Ovnat A, Charuzi I. Nutritional status seven years after Roux-en-Y gastric bypass surgery. *Surgery,* 1992;111:137-142.

[20] Traina F. Deficiência de ferro no paciente submetido à ressecção gástrica ou intestinal: prevalência, causas, repercussões clínicas, abordagem diagnóstica e prevenção. *Rev. Bras. Hematol. Hemoter.*, 2010;32(supl2):78-83.

[21] Wood RJ, Ronnenberg AG. Iron. In: Shils ME, Shike M, Ross AC, Caballero B, Cousins RJ, eds. Modern nutrition in health and disease, 10th ed. Philadelphia: Lippincott Williams and Wilkins, 2006.

[22] Brolin RE, Kenler HA, Gorman JH, Cody RP. Long-limb gastric bypass in the superobese: a prospective randomized study. *Ann. Surg.*, 1992;215:387-395.

[23] Drygalski AV, Andris DA. Anemia After Bariatric Surgery: More Than Just Iron Deficiency. *Nutr. Clin. Pract.*, 2009;24(2):217-226.

[24] Hentze MW, Muckenthaler MU, Galy B, Camaschella C. Two to Tango: Regulation of Mammalian Iron Metabolism. *Cell,* 2010;142:24-38.

[25] Cottam DR, Mattar SG, Barinas-Mitchell E, et al. Chronic inflammatory hypothesis for the morbidity associated with morbid obesity: implications and effects of weight loss. *Obes. Surg.*, 2005;14:589-600.

[26] Kushner RF, Shanta Retelny V. Emergence of pica (ingestion of non-food substances) accompanying iron deficiency anemia after gastric bypass surgery. *Obes. Surg.*, 2005; 15: 1491-1495.

[27] Moizé V, Moizé L, Lacy A and Vidal J. Pica secondary to iron deficiency 1 year after gastric bypass. *Surg. Obes. Relat. Dis.*, 2010 May-Jun;6(3):316-8.

[28] Brolin RE, Gorman JH, Gorman RC, Petschenik AJ, Bradley LB, Kenler HA, Cody RP. Prophylactic iron supplementation after Roux-en-Y gastric bypass: a prospective, doubleblind, randomized study. *Arch. Surg.,* 1998;133:740-744.
[29] Brolin RE, Gorman JH, Gorman RC, et al. Are vitamin B12 and folate deficiency clinically important after Roux-en-Y gastric bypass? *J. Gastrointest. Surg.,* 1998;2:436-442. – b.
[30] Folope V, Coëffier M, Déchelotte P. Nutritional deficiencies associated with bariatric surgery. *Gastroenterol. Clin. Biol.,* 2007;31:369-377.
[31] Brolin RE, Gorman JH, Gorman RC, et al. Are vitamin B12 and folate deficiency clinically important after Roux-en-Y gastric bypass? *J. Gastrointest. Surg.,* 1998;5:436–42.
[32] Ponsky TA, Brody F, Pucci E. Alterations in gastrointestinal physiology after Roux-en-Y gastric bypass. *J. Am. Coll. Surg.,* 2005;201:125–31.
[33] Dali-Youcef N, Andrès E. An update on cobalamin deficiency in adults. *QJM,* 2009;102:17-28.
[34] Andrès E, Vogel T, Federici L, Zimmer J, Kaltenbach G. Update on oral cyanocobalamin (vitamin B12) treatment in elderly patients. *Drugs Aging,* 2008;25:927-932.
[35] Boylan LM, Sugerman HJ, Driskell JA. Vitamin E, vitamin B-6, vitamin B-12, and folate status of gastric bypass surgery patients. *J. Am. Diet. Assoc.,* 1988;88:579–85.
[36] Russel RM, Dhar J, Dutta SK, Rosenberg IH. Influence of intraluminal pH on folate absorption. *J. Lab. Clin. Med.,* 1979;93:428-436.
[37] Carmel R, Green R, Rosenblatt DS, Watkins D. Update on cobalamin, folate, and homocysteine. *Hematology,* 2003:62– 81.

In: Bariatric Surgery
Editor: Christos R. Iavazzo
ISBN: 978-1-62618-995-9

Chapter X

Oral Health after Bariatric Surgery

Mattheos G. Papakiritsis*
Dental Private Practice, Panagouli - Athens, Greece)

Abstract

Overweight and obesity are major risk factors for a number of chronic diseases. Once considered a problem only of high-income countries, obesity rates are rising worldwide and affecting both the developed and developing world.

There are many treatments for obesity such as pharmaceutical and surgical. Anti-obesity drugs may be taken to reduce appetite or inhibit fat absorption. In severe cases, bariatric surgery is performed to reduce stomach volume and/or intestine length, leading to earlier satiation and reduced ability to absorb nutrients from food.

Bariatric surgery (BS) is the only consistently-effective long-term treatment for morbid obesity but some bariatric surgeries can produce adverse effects. The side-effects of bariatric surgery may be reflected in the oral cavity and can cause alterations in oral health.

Patients who have undergone bariatric surgery are seen with increasing frequency in dental offices and dental professionals need to be familiar with the challenges these patients present.

The maintenance of oral health is very important before and after bariatric surgery. Oral health is affected by many factors so dental professionals need to understand the oral implications of obesity, including this population's limited access to care.

To address the many changing oral health needs of patients after bariatric surgery, dental professional should assume the overall medical care while working in close collaboration with the bariatric medical team.

* Corresponding author: Dr. Mattheos G. Papakiritsis,DDS,MSc Dental Private Practice, 67, Panagouli–Athens–14231–Greece. matpapas@gmail.com.

Introduction

The World Health Organization (WHO) defined health as "*a state of complete physical, mental, and social well-being*" and not merely the absence of disease or infirmity [1].

Overweight and obesity are defined as abnormal or excessive fat accumulation that presents a risk to health. Body mass index (BMI) is a simple index of weight-for-height that is commonly used to classify overweight and obesity in adults. It is defined as a person's weight in kilograms divided by the square of his height in meters (kg/m^2).

The WHO definition is:

- a BMI greater than or equal to 25 is overweight
- a BMI greater than or equal to 30 is obesity.

BMI provides the most useful population-level measure of overweight and obesity as it is the same for both sexes and for all ages of adults. However, it should be considered a rough guide because it may not correspond to the same degree of fatness in different individuals.

Overweight and obesity are major risk factors for a number of chronic diseases, including diabetes, cardiovascular diseases and cancer. Once considered a problem only in high income countries, overweight and obesity are now dramatically on the rise in low- and middle-income countries, particularly in urban settings [2,3].

Obesity increases the likelihood of various diseases, particularly heart disease, type 2 diabetes, obstructive sleep apnea, certain types of cancer, and osteoarthritis [4].

Obesity is most commonly caused by a combination of excessive food energy intake, lack of physical activity, and genetic susceptibility, although a few cases are caused primarily by genes, endocrine disorders, medications or psychiatric illness. Evidence to support the view that some obese people eat little yet gain weight due to a slow metabolism is limited; on average obese people have a greater energy expenditure than their thin counterparts due to the energy required to maintain an increased body mass [5,6].

At an individual level, a combination of excessive food energy intake and a lack of physical activity is thought to explain most cases of obesity. A limited number of cases are due primarily to genetics, medical reasons, or psychiatric illness. In contrast, increasing rates of obesity at a societal level are felt to be due to an easily accessible and palatable diet, increased reliance on cars, and mechanized manufacturing [7-11].

Obesity is a leading preventable cause of death worldwide, with increasing prevalence in adults and children, and authorities view it as one of the most serious public health problems of the 21st century [12].

Before the 20th century, obesity was rare [13]. In 1997 the WHO formally recognized obesity as a global epidemic [14]. In 1980, 6% of men and 8% of women in the UK were obese. In 2000, the respective figures had increased to 21% and 21. 4%. About 55% of the adult population is overweight or obese [15,16].

As of 2005 the WHO estimated that at least 400 million adults (9. 8%) were obese, with higher rates among women than men [17].

The rate of obesity also increases with age at least up to 50 or 60 years old and severe obesity in the United States, Australia, and Canada is increasing faster than the overall rate of obesity [18-20].

Once considered a problem only of high-income countries, obesity rates are rising worldwide and affecting both the developed and developing world [21,22].

Obesity Treatment

Dieting and physical exercise are the mainstays of treatment for obesity. Moreover, it is important to improve diet quality by reducing the consumption of energy-dense foods such as those high in fat and sugars, and by increasing the intake of dietary fiber. To supplement this, or in case of failure, anti-obesity drugs may be taken to reduce appetite or inhibit fat absorption. In severe cases, bariatric surgery is performed to reduce stomach volume and/or intestine length, leading to earlier satiation and reduced ability to absorb nutrients from food [23].

Pharmaceutical Therapy

Current drug treatment of obesity is directed at reducing energy/food intake either by an action on the gastrointestinal system or via an action through the central nervous system control of appetite and feeding [24-28].

A. Drugs Acting on the Gastrointestinal System: Pancreatic Lipase Inhibitors

Orlistat (Xenical) the most commonly used medication to treat obesity. This inhibits pancreatic and gastric lipase thereby decreasing ingested triglyceride hydrolysis. It produces a dose-dependent reduction in dietary fat absorption thereby leading to weight loss in obese subjects.

This is current widely available and approved for long term use. Weight loss however is modest with an average of 2.9 kg (6.4 lb) at 1 to 4 years and there is little information on how these drugs affect longer-term complications of obesity [29].

B. Centrally Acting Drugs

Sibutramine promotes a sense of satiety through its central action as a serotonin and norepinephrine re-uptake inhibitor. In addition, it may mitigate against the fall in thermogenesis through stimulation of peripheral norepinephrine receptors [29].

On 26 November 2002, the European Court of First Instance annulled previous European Commission decisions (2000) to withdraw the licences (Marketing Authorisations) for two anorectic agents. In accordance with this, the Medicines Control Agency has reinstated the relevant marketing authorisations for diethylpropion and phentermine, which can now be prescribed [30].

Oral Side Effects due to Medications

The bariatric patient may present with oral side effects related to medication prescribed to treat morbid obesity and comorbidities. The major side effect with the potential to cause oral manifestations is xerostomia. The main symptom of xerostomia is a dry, burning mouth that affects the patient's ability to swallow, taste, speak, and maintain oral tissue integrity. Demineralization of tooth enamel may occur, resulting in the rapid progression of dental caries and overgrowth of candida albicans [31].

The medications used in treating morbid obesity may adversely affect oral health. Direct pharmacological treatment of morbid obesity involves two basic approaches. The first occurs through neurotransmitter medication and the second through impeding the absorption of fats. Medications in the first category are typically either sympathomimetic amines or atypical antidepressants. The sympathomimetic amines work by inhibiting norepinephrine, serotonin, and dopamine as is the case with dibutramine. Diethylpropion is also a sympathomimetic amine that is a partial reuptake blocker of norepinephrine [32].

Most commonly side effects are constipation, anorexia, insomnia; also nausea, tachycardia, palpitations, hypertension, vasodilation, light-headedness, paraesthesia, headache, anxiety, sweating,; rarely, blurred vision [29].

Due to the sympathetic activity of these medications, they all frequently produce xerostomia and taste disturbance. Additionally, sibutamine also produces mouth ulcers in approximately 3% of users [29,33].

Bupropion is an atypical antidepressant useful in appetite suppression. It acts as a weak inhibitor of the reuptake of norepineohrine, serotonin, and dopamine. While not a sympathomimetic amine, bupropion does produce significant sympathetic oral side effects, probably because it is structurally related to phenylethylamines. Among these side effects is a 1% incidence of xerostomia and a 2% incidence of mouth ulcers [34].

The principle agent in medications used to impede the absorption of fats in the treatment of morbid obesity is orlistat. Orlistat is a lipase inhibitor in the lumen of the stomach and in the small intestine. Lipase inhibition obstructs fat digestion and subsequent absorption producing excretion of these substances. Because orlistat is not a sympathomimetic, it typically does not produce xerostomia. It does, however, cause a 4. 3% incidence of carious lesions and a 4. 1% incidence of gingivitis [35].

These effects are probably due to hydrochloric acid regurgitation. A fairly significant number of patients experience nausea and/or vomiting while taking this medication, possibly producing this effect [36].

Morbid obesity creates systemic health problems including hypertension [37],type II diabetes, coronary heart disease, stroke, osteoarthritis, and breast cancer. These conditions are frequently treated with medications that produce oral side effects. Hypertension, coronary heart disease, and stroke are treated with, among other medications, beta blockers, thiazide diuretics, and ACE inhibitors. These commonly cause xerostomia; ACE inhibitors are linked to swelling in the mouth [35]. Strokes are treated with oral anticoagulants, which can produce nausea and vomiting and the attendant oral problems. Type II diabetics frequently take oral hypoglycemics which, in addition to nausea and vomiting, can produce dysgeusia (bad taste in the mouth). Also, the palliative treatment for osteoarthritis, the nonsteroidal anti-inflammatory drugs (NSAIDs), can produce both xerostomia and stomatitis [38].

The risk of breast cancer in a morbidly obese woman is one to five times higher than a normal weight woman [39]. The newer medications used to treat breast cancer—aromatase inhibitors—may cause xerostomia included in their panel of side effects [40].

Anti-Obesity Drugs and Oral Side Effects

Drug	Xerostomia	Oral Ulcers	Oral Swelling	Dysgeusia	Stomatitis	Glositis	Periodontal Diseases
Phentermine	√						
Sibutramine	√	√	√				
Orlistat							√
Bupoprion	√	√	√				
Diethylpropion	√						
Phedimetrazine	√						
B-blockers	√						
Diuretics(Thiazide)	√						
ACE Inhibitors		√	√				
Ca channel blockers	√						
Oral hypoglycemics				√			
NSAIDs	√				√		
Arimidex	√						
Aromasin	√						

Surgical Therapy (Bariatric Surgery)

Bariatric surgery (BS) is the only consistently-effective long-term treatment for morbid obesity [41].

The name 'Bariatric surgery' is derived from the Greek words *baros* and *iatrike* (*bar-iartik*) denoting respectively 'heaviness' and 'medicine'.

Surgery for severe obesity is associated with long-term weight loss and decreased overall mortality. One study found a weight loss of between 14% and 25% (depending on the type of procedure performed) at 10 years, and a 29% reduction in all cause mortality when compared to standard weight loss measures [42].

Preliminary state-level data from the USA cite the number of bariatric surgical procedures at approximately 130,000 in 2005, with a forecast of 218,000 in 2010 [43]. In France, figures from 2008 indicate that the number of bariatric surgical operations (BS) carried out that year was 13,722 [44].

Bariatric surgery includes a variety of procedures and its efficacy is based on both the *restriction* of the quantities of ingested food(Vertical banded gastroplasty, Adjustable gastric band, Sleeve gastrectomy, Intragastric balloon (gastric balloon), Gastric Plication) [and the *malabsorption* of the nutrients through the shunted gut(Biliopancreatic diversion, Endoluminal sleeve) [45-55].

Mixed procedures(Gastric bypass surgery, Sleeve gastrectomy with duodenal switch, apply both techniques simultaneously [49].

According to a new technique(Implantable gastric stimulation),a device similar to a heart pacemaker is implanted by a surgeon, with the electrical leads stimulating the external surface of the stomach. Electrical stimulation is thought to modify the activity of the enteric nervous system of the stomach, which is interpreted by the brain to give a sense of satiety, or fullness. Early evidence suggests that it is less effective than other forms of bariatric surgery [56].

A factor in the success of any bariatric surgery is strict post-surgical adherence to a healthier pattern of eating.

There are some indications of the bariatric surgery [57-60] and the effectiveness [61-71] and complications depends on the technique, the surgeon and experienced or not-experienced hospital units [72-75].

Bariatric Surgery and Oral Health

Some bariatric surgeries can produce adverse effects such as gastroesophageal reflux, nausea, vomiting, malnutrition, anemia, dehydration, vitamin and mineral deficiencies (calcium, iron, folic acid, vitamin B12 and D) among others. This occurs because in most cases there are dysfunctional eating habits, such as overeating, eating too fast, or not chewing food well [76-80].

In around 2% of patients with BPD/DS surgical operation there is severe malabsorption and nutritional deficiency that requires restoration of the normal absorption. The malabsorptive effect of BPD is so potent that those who undergo the procedure must take vitamin and dietary minerals above and beyond that of the normal population. Without these supplements, there is risk of serious deficiency diseases such as anemia and osteoporosis [81].

The side-effects of bariatric surgery may be reflected in the oral cavity and can cause alterations in oral health, such as dental caries, periodontal diseases, xerostomia and dentin hypersensitivity [79,82-84].

The oral condition of obese patients may change after bariatric surgery, because this procedure may have side-effects capable of causing alteration in the oral cavity [79],including nutrient deficiencies impacting healing of oral tissues and gastroesophageal reflux, resulting in tooth erosion. Patients who have undergone bariatric surgery are seen with increasing frequency in dental offices and dental professionals need to be familiar with the challenges these patients present [85].

Dental Caries

Dental caries is a multifactorial disease, whose aetiology is related to the presence of a dental plaque composed by cariogenic bacteria, which can metabolize sugars such as sucrose. As a result of this metabolism, organic acids are produced such as lactic acid, which in turn can induce the demineralization of dental tissues [86,87].

With time, the biofilm becomes saturated regarding minerals that are released from the dental structure, favouring the precipitation and the formation of an initial subsurface carious lesion [88,89].

The early sign of enamel lesion is characterized as white spot (known also as non-cavitated lesion) as consequence of subsurface demineralization. With time and the increase of bacterial metabolism, the intact surface layer can break down leading to formation of cavity, the spread of bacteria and progress of the lesion to dentin. Following exposure of the dentin to the masses of bacteria in the cavity, the most superficial part of dentin will soon be decomposed through the action of acids and proteolytic enzymes. This zone is referred to as the zone of destruction. Beneath this zone, tubular invasion of bacteria is frequently seen. The bacteria invasion has as consequence the pulp inflammation, which may have serious consequences as pain, pulpar necrosis and periapical lesions [90,91].

An increase in dental caries was verified after bariatric surgery [92]. This difference may be related to increased frequency of food ingestion by patients after bariatric surgery, capable of resulting in increased plaque indexes, gingivitis and serious periodontal diseases [59].

Bariatric patients may be at an increased risk for caries due to the need for more frequent and prolonged meals throughout the day. The most significant dietary factor in the etiology of caries is the frequent consumption of sugar and other fermentable carbohydrates [93,94] Although there is not dramatic change in the types of foods consumed before and after the bypass surgery, there is a difference in the pattern of foods/beverages consumed following the procedure. The primary difference included more meals/snacks daily versus main meals. Meals/snacks include cariogenic foods such as bananas, muffins, crackers, potato chips, beer, granola bars, pastries, and chronic sipping of fruit juice [95].

Such foods are reflective of the patient's high average sugar intake (12%). Ingesting more than 10% of calories as sugar and consuming fermentable carbohydrates more than 4 times a day represent an increased risk for dental caries [96].

Since the dietary "rules" for bariatric patients include eating 4 to 6 times per day [97,98] and sipping fluids frequently throughout the day to prevent dehydration, the risk for caries may be increased if fermentable carbohydrates are routinely consumed. Lactose intolerance is a common condition among bariatric patients due to the diminished production of lactase. The dietary recommendations for this condition include avoidance of cow's milk. [97] The intake of dairy products and calcium is low at 30% and 67% of the recommended amounts, respectively. Milk-derived factors such as calcium phosphate and casein are considered anticariogenic since they appear to protect the enamel against demineralization [93]. Reduced exposure to these protective effects may have added to the patient's risk of decalcification.

Dental caries is a multifactorial disease that includes not only dietary factors but also host and bacterial factors [93]. The patient's low salivary production and buffering capacity represent significant risk factors for dental caries [99,100].

Factors that may have contributed to the patient's low salivary production and buffering capacity include low water consumption (60% of recommended), cigarette use [101] and drugs [31-40].

Although it is unclear why patients first recognize the signs of dryness long time after gastric bypass surgery, it is probable that xerostomia contributed to the increased rate of decay due to diminished natural cleansing of the oral cavity and buffering of plaque acids [102].

This risk is compounds by the frequent use of regular cough drops and candy to ease the symptoms of xerostomia. There is also a high plaque index (64%) with high cariogenicity. Cariogenic plaque represents an increased risk for dental caries when the frequency of fermentable carbohydrate consumption is increased [96]. Meals consumed by patients contain more fermentable carbohydrates with 12% of the calories from sucrose. In this case the dental plaque index and cariogenicity are high. Also demonstrated low saliva production with higher viscosity, which has poor buffering capacity [103].

Management of Dental Caries

Dietary recommendations for the patient included reducing sucrose consumption to less than 10% of calories and selecting more nonfermentable carbohydrate snacks [102]. To decrease the patient's risk for caries, recommendations were made to: a) increase complex carbohydrates and reduce the consumption of simple sugars throughout the day [93]; b) include cariostatic food factors such as proteins, cheeses, and phytates (phosphorus-containing compounds found in the outer husks of cereal grains) particularly when consuming acidogenic foods [95]; c)increase water consumption. Water recommends as a substitute to sipping fruit juice to help reduce substrate exposure, increase hydration, and help ease the symptoms of xerostomia [101]. d) stimulate salivary flow via fibrous foods [94]; e) increase the frequency of brushing and flossing after meals/snacks; f) continue the daily use of 1. 1% sodium fluoride and xylitol toothpaste and g) maintain a 4-month recare schedule to monitor for evidence of remineralization or further demineralization [104].

Oral Side Effects due to Dehydration

Saliva has a broad range of protective functions for both oral tissues and the body at large, and contains a wide variety of effective antimicrobial substances against bacteria, viruses and fungi. Saliva also contains other chemoprotective factors that help to neutralize microbial damage and render environmental toxins less harmful [105,106].

Due to reduced gastric capacity dehydration is also a common concern. Inadequate water intake contributes to xerostomia, which can increase caries activity, periodontal disease and tooth wear [77,78].

Saliva flow was reduced in patients before surgery and increased after RYGB, however, the patients continued to experience hyposalivation 3 months after surgery. After 6 months the saliva flow returned to normal. This reduction in salivary flow in patients before surgery and newly operated patients may be associated with the treatment for diabetes in most obese patients [107].

The reduction in the use of medication may have influenced the improvement in salivary flow, such as hyposalivation, that was related to diabetic decompensation and the administration of certain drugs24, 6 months after bariatric surgery [92,108].

At least 5 servings of whole fruit and vegetables were recommended to increase nutrient intake and stimulate salivary flow via fibrous foods [109]

The use of xylitol oral care products (toothpaste, oral rinse, chewing gums, pastiles) recommended to decrease the xerostomia and prevent oral tissue. Saliva substitutes are usefull, too.

Patient's Diet/Poor Oral Health

Another factor related to the development of oral diseases is the patient's diet. Whether the patient has participated in one or more of the behaviors prevalent in eating disorders such as restriction of food, binging and purging of food, or binging without purging, the oral consequences are severe [31]. Poor oral health negatively affects behavioral compliance of the post-operative bariatric surgery patient during the reintroduction of food. The patient is required to cut all food into very small bites and is directed to perform 30 chews per bite. During the postoperative period, chewing is required in order to reduce nausea, vomiting, bloating, and blockage of the stoma [110].

If the patient's oral health is compromised due to untreated dental caries, periodontal disease causing tooth mobility, loss of all or some teeth or an ill fitting denture, the patient may not be able to adequately start the digestion process through the chewing of food [111].

Some surgery failures relate to the inability of the patient to slowly chew food. The patient may experience problems with eating food and turn to high caloric liquid intake and experience a slow or minimal weight loss [112].

International guidelines generally suggest that patient criteria for elective surgery for BS should firstly, include the control of feeding behaviour in order to eat less and more slowly and, secondly, a functional dental status providing good chewing function [113].

This set of conditions was assumed to reduce the prevalence of physiological complications of BS, such as vomiting, diarrhea, pain or dumping syndrome.

Patients scheduled for bariatric surgery (BS) are encouraged to chew slowly in order to optimise the digestion process. The influence of dental status on patients' ability to comply with advice on chewing behaviour is poorly documented.

The relationships between mastication and digestion have previously been investigated in different ways [114].

Increasing mastication shortens the time needed by the stomach to comminute food particles to a diameter small enough to pass through the pylorus [115].

Mastication is also involved in maintaining good motility in the digestive tract by enhancing physiological gastric motion through the activation of parasympathetic nervous activity [116–121].

Moreover, adequate mastication facilitates the initial steps of digestion by stimulating saliva production and activating the cephalic controls that initiate the assimilation of foods [122,123].

Chewing ability in persons with obesity could affect links between nutrition and feeding behaviour. Previous studies on feeding attitudes demonstrated that obese subjects eat faster than their lean peers and suggested that a lack of oral stimulations could be related to energetic metabolism [124,125].

It has been suggested that low activity of the autonomous nervous system explains a decrease in the thermogenic response to food in individuals with obesity [126,127].

It was also shown that the palatability of the meal had an effect on the cephalic phase of dietary thermogenesis and that this effect is significantly decreased in obese subjects compared with non-obese ones [128].

Patients with morbid obesity who have undergone bariatric surgery are thus encouraged to chew slowly in order to slow down food intake and optimize the digestion process. Despite these considerations, BS is often proposed for obese patients whatever their chewing ability.

A study conducted in a group of 44 patients with morbid obesity scheduled for BS, showed that 43% had healthy dental status with at least 7 pairs of functional teeth (Functional Unit: FU), while 23% had 6 FUs, 20% had 5 FUs and 14% wore dentures In this latter study, it was shown that patients with impaired dental status produced a food bolus with a larger particle size than fully dentate patients. [129].

It was not known however whether the patients with impaired dental status were able to comply with advice about increasing chewing and, if such a modification were verified, whether an increase in chewing activity had an impact on the composition of the swallowed bolus. The observations of both the food bolus collected just before swallowing and the kinematic strategy developed to produce this bolus appeared to be good criteria for evaluating mastication [130-132].

It has been demonstrated in healthy adult subjects that the granulometry of the bolus decreases during chewing until reaching a threshold value that corresponds to swallowing [133,134].

This threshold is a constant of each individual and depends on food rheological properties [135,136].

It varies among individuals according to dental status and saliva characteristics and its variability is not affected by gender [137].

In healthy fully dentate subjects, the chewing activity before swallowing differs according to type of food, with more chewing cycles (CC) and longer chewing duration (CT) for hard foods such as carrot and peanuts than for soft foods such as banana and apple, while the chewing frequency (CC/CT) of each individual remains constant [138-141].

Previous studies on the chewing ability of dentally impaired subjects showed that a decrease in the number of functionally paired teeth and oral rehabilitation with removable dentures were linked to a decrease in CT and CC values and to an increased D50 value [129,138].

In obese patients, the impact of potentially increased chewing activity on the granulometry of the pre-swallowed bolus would also depend on dental status.

The influence of dental status on patients' ability to comply with advice on chewing behaviour is poorly documented.

A study concludes that after bariatric surgery, all the obese patients, regardless of dental status modify their chewing kinematics. The effects of this chewing behaviour on bolus granulometry depends on dental status and type of food [142].

Tooth Erosion/Dentin Hypersensitivity

One of the lesions related to the demineralizationis the dental erosion, which is defined as chemical dissolution of dental tissues by a chemical process (acid or chelating agents) without the bacterial involvement [143].

The etiology of erosion is multifactorial and not fully understood. The most important sources of acids are those found in the diet, such as acidic foods and drinks [144] and those originated from the stomach, like gastric acids from regurgitation and reflux disorders. Currently, the increased consumption of acidic foods and soft drinks is becoming an important factor for the development of erosive wear. The acidic attack leads to an irreversible loss of dental hard tissue, which is accompanied by a progressive softening of the surface [145].

This softened zone is more susceptible to mechanical forces, such as abrasion [146] which in turn have little or no effect on sound dental hard tissues [147].

Clinically, early enamel erosion appears as a smooth silky-shining glazed surface. Typical for erosions of the facial aspects of teeth is a ridge of enamel that separates the defect from the marginal gingival(cervical erosion). Occlusal erosion is characterized by rounded cusps and concavities. Further progression of occlusal erosion lead to a distinct grooving of the cusps, and restorations are rising above the level of the adjacent tooth surface. In cases of severe erosion, the whole occlusal or facial morphology disappears. When the dentin is reached, it is common report of hypersensitivity to cold, heat and osmotic pressure. Other consequences of dental erosion are diastema, thin and fractured incisal edges, loss of vertical dimension, opened pseudobite and prominence of aesthetic restorations [148].

Dentine hypersensitivity has been defined as a sharp, short pain arising from exposed dentin in response to stimuli typically thermal, evaporative tactile, osmotic, chemical and which cannot be ascribed to any other form of dental defect or pathology [149].

The short and sharp pain symptoms are thought to be derived from the hydrodynamic challenge. The most affected patients range from 20 to 40 years-old; premolars and incisors tend to be most sensitive teeth, being the pain localized on the facial surface. Sensitive teeth have much greater numbers of open tubules per unit area and the average diameter of tubules is almost 2 times greater than tubules in nonsensitive teeth [150].

Dentine hypersensitivity represents a condition of presumable multifactorial pathology. Two processes are essential for its development:(1) dentin must be exposed through genetic disturbance, enamel defect (lamellae and spindles), loss of enamel (erosion, abrasion, attrition), gingival recession with rapid loss of cementum and (2) the dentin tubules must be open to both the oral cavity and the pulp.

Diagnostic protocol for this condition consisted of Medical, Dental Dietary, Oral Hygiene History and Intra-oral examinations with air indexing method. The treatments in the office can be made with substances that are able to create a smear-layer on dentin surface, occluding dentinal tubules with insoluble precipitates and stimulating the production of reparative dentin and/or sclerotic. This can be achieved chemically with agents like potassium, calcium and fluoride or physically [150,151].

All obese patients had some degree of dental wear, however the severity of dental wear increased with time after bariatric surgery. Statistically significant differences were found between before, 3 months and 6 months after bariatric surgery (p=0. 012). This increased result may be related to chronic vomiting, because any acid below the critical pH of dental enamel (5. 5) can dissolve hydroxyapatite crystals. Vomiting and other gastric disorders are important risk factors for tooth wear, and after bariatric surgery, nausea and vomiting may occur. In most cases dysfunctional eating habits, such as overeating, eating too fast, or not chewing food well may cause these complications [76,78]

The patients show increased vomiting frequencies of at least once a week after RYGB [92]. 37% of the patients who had undergone bariatric surgery had hypersensitive teeth. Hypersensitivity is a complication of dental erosion when there is dentin involvement [79].

Except dental caries, acidic levels in the oral cavity, which are known to be one of the postoperative side-effects of bariatric surgery, directly result in tooth erosion and dentine hypersensitivity. Significant associations were found between reported dental hypersensitivity and vomiting (P=0. 013), and also dental hypersensitivity and indigestion (P=0. 021) [80].

Bariatric Surgery and Periodontal Disease

Obesity is associated with a higher risk of periodontal disease. After bariatric surgery, bone loss frequently occurs because the patients may present metabolic bone disease (osteomalacia and osteoporosis) [17, 18]. Bypassing the antrum and duodenum results in decreased absorption of several nutrients including iron, folate, calcium and vitamin B-12, which can cause bone loss [7, 9]. As a result of this metabolic bone disease, some bariatric patients may present osteoporosis that could influence the bone loss in chronic periodontitis, and may be a co-factor in alveolar bone loss [152-155].

Periodontal disease is an infection of the tissues that hold teeth in place. It's typically caused by poor brushing and flossing habits that allow dental plaque to build up on the teeth and harden. In advanced stages, periodontal disease can lead to sore, bleeding gums; painful chewing problems; and even tooth loss.

The longer plaque and tartar are on teeth, the more harmful they become. The bacteria cause inflammation of the gums that is called gingivitis. In gingivitis, the gums become red, swollen and can bleed easily. Gingivitis is a mild form of gum disease that can usually be reversed with daily brushing and flossing, and regular cleaning by a dentist or dental hygienist. This form of gum disease does not include any loss of bone and tissue that hold teeth in place. When gingivitis is not treated, it can advance to periodontitis. In periodontitis, gums pull away from the teeth and form pockets that become infected. The body's immune system fights the bacteria as the plaque spreads and grows below the gum line. Bacterial toxins and the body's natural response to infection start to break down the bone and connective tissue that hold teeth in place. If not treated, the bones, gums, and tissue that support the teeth are destroyed. The teeth may eventually become loose and have to be removed.

Smoking is one of the most significant risk factors associated with the development of gum disease. Additionally, smoking can lower the chances for successful treatment. Hormonal changes in girls/women. These changes can make gums more sensitive and make it easier for gingivitis to develop. People with diabetes are at higher risk for developing infections, including gum disease. Diseases like cancer or AIDS and their treatments can also negatively affect the health of gums. There are hundreds of prescription and over the counter medications that can reduce the flow of saliva, which has a protective effect on the mouth. Without enough saliva, the mouth is vulnerable to infections such as gum disease. And some medications can cause abnormal overgrowth of the gum tissue; this can make it difficult to keep gums clean. Finally, some people are more prone to severe gum disease than others(genetic susceptibility).

There are two types of periodontal therapy non-surgical and surgical. Some drugs can help but ever in combination with conservative or surgical therapy. Periodontal health should be achieved in the least invasive and most cost-effective manner. This is often accomplished through non-surgical periodontal treatment, including scaling and root planning (a careful cleaning of the root surfaces to remove plaque and calculus from deep periodontal pockets and to smooth the tooth root to remove bacterial toxins), followed by adjunctive therapy such as local delivery antimicrobials and host modulation, as needed on a case-by-case basis. Most periodontists would agree that after scaling and root planning, many patients do not require any further active treatment, including surgical therapy. However, the majority of patients will require ongoing maintenance therapy to sustain health. Non-surgical therapy does have its limitations, however, and when it does not achieve periodontal health, surgery may be indicated to restore periodontal anatomy damaged by periodontal diseases and to facilitate oral hygiene practices. Periodontal surgery is necessary when your periodontist determines that the tissue around your teeth is unhealthy and cannot be repaired with non-surgical treatment. Following are the four types of surgical treatments most commonly prescribed: Pocket Reduction Procedures, Regenerative Procedures, Crown Lengthening and Soft Tissue Grafts [156].

Periodontitis and obesity are both chronic health problems and the literature support an association between the two. Regardless of the type of periodontal surgery , the prevalence of periodontitis proved to be high (81. 45%). There is a statistically significant difference in the prevalence of periodontitis. Differences in periodontal condition were observed in individuals at different times of the bariatric surgery, showing a high prevalence of periodontitis in both pre- and post-operative follow-up [157].

An improved response to non-surgical periodontal therapy is observed in obese patients who had significant weight loss following bariatric surgery compared to obese subject who did not have such a surgery. There is a statistically significant improvement after periodontal therapy in the subjects had previously undergone bariatric surgery compared to the obese group ($P<0.05$) [158].

Patients who have undergone bariatric surgery need to be closely monitored after surgery to prevent the development of oral complications, especially periodontal conditions [159].

People with diabetes are at special risk for periodontal disease. Periodontal disease can lead to painful chewing difficulties and even tooth loss. Xerostomia(dry mouth), often a symptom of undetected diabetes, can cause soreness, ulcers, infections, and tooth decay. Smoking makes these problems worse.

Good blood glucose control is key to controlling and preventing mouth problems. People with poor blood glucose control get gum disease more often and more severely than people whose diabetes is well controlled. Daily brushing and flossing, regular dental check-ups and good blood glucose control are the best defense against the oral complications of diabetes.

Chronic vitamin D deficiency, inadequate calcium intake, and secondary hyperparathyroidism are common in obese individuals, placing them at risk for low bone mass and metabolic bone disease [160].

Vitamin D deficiency is most commonly due to inadequate intake and is present in at least 20% of both obese and nonobese individuals [161,162].

After bariatric surgery, vitamin D deficiency occurs more often in patients who have undergone malabsorptive procedures than in those who had restrictive operations [163,164]. The increased incidence may be due to the length of the jejunoileal common channel [165].

Metabolic bone disease manifesting as osteopenia and secondary hyperparathyroidism have been reported after Roux-en-Y gastric bypass surgery due to reduced calcium absorption. The highest concentration of calcium transporters is in the duodenum. Since the ingested food will not pass through the duodenum after a bypass procedure, calcium levels in the blood may decrease, causing secondary hyperparathyroidism, increase in bone turnover, and a decrease in bone mass. Increased risk of fracture has also been linked to bariatric surgery [166].

Recent studies point to several potentially important periodontal risk indicators. These include the osteopenia [167].

There is increasing evidence that osteoporosis, and the underlying loss of bone mass characteristic of this disease, is associated with periodontal disease and tooth loss. Current evidence including several prospective studies supports an association of osteoporosis with the onset and progression of periodontal disease in humans. The majority of studies have shown low bone mass to be independently associated with loss of alveolar crestal height and tooth loss. However studies that focus on the relation of clinical attachment loss and osteoporosis are less consistent. To date, the majority of studies on the relationship between periodontal disease and osteoporosis have been hindered by small sample sizes, limited control of other potential confounding factors, varying definitions of both periodontal disease and osteoporosis, and few prospective studies where the temporality of the association can be established. Potential mechanisms by which host factors may influence onset and progression of periodontal disease directly or indirectly include underlying low bone density in the oral cavity, bone loss as an inflammatory response to infection, genetic susceptibility, and shared exposure to risk factors. Systemic loss of bone density in osteoporosis, including that of the oral cavity, may provide a host system that is increasingly susceptible to infectious destruction of periodontal tissue [168].

Reduced bone mineral density is a shared risk factor for periodontitis rather than a causal factor. However, more prospective studies are required to fully determine what, if any, relationship truly exists between periodontitis and reduced bone mineral density [169].

After bariatric surgery, patients are at even higher risk, owing to malabsorption and decreased oral intake. Meticulous preoperative screening, judicious use of vitamin and mineral supplements, addressing modifiable risk factors, and monitoring the absorption of key nutrients postoperatively are essential in preventing metabolic bone disease in bariatric surgery patients. Measurement of bone mineral density (BMD) is the best surrogate test for future fractures, in the general population. Metabolic bone disease(osteoporosis) is particularly important in patients about to undergo dental implants placement operation. In this case, dentists have to check calcium levels and bone mass before and after implant surgery.

To help increase the patient's calcium intake, 3 daily servings of dairy products with low lactose (eg, cheese and yogurt) were recommended. An increase in dairy products may contribute to caries protection and also help reduce the risk of osteoporosis, which represents a significant risk among bariatric patients [170].

Nutritional Derangements and Oral Problems

Nutritional derangements due to deficiencies of micronutrients like iron, vitamin B12, fat soluble vitamins(A,D,E,K), thiamine, and folate are especially common after malabsorptive bariatric procedures. Seizures due to hyperinsulinemic hypoglycemia have been reported. Seizures due to hyperinsulinemic hypoglycemia have been reported. Inappropriate insulin secretion secondary to islet cell hyperplasia, called pancreatic nesidioblastosis, might explain this syndrome [171].

Vitamin A help in maintenance of healthy mucous membrane, formation of tooth tissues and maintain salivary flow in the mouth. Vitamin E Help in healing and restoration of damaged oral tissues. Vitamin K may be involved in bone formation and vitamin D related with calcium metabolism, teeth and bone health.

Low serum vitamin D levels are associated with low bone mineral density Supplementation with vitamin D and calcium improves bone mineral density slightly, as well as decreases the risk falls and fractures in certain groups of people [172].

Burning mouth syndrome (BMS) is a painful, complex condition often described as a scalding feeling in the mouth. In addition to pain, dry mouth and a bitter taste may accompany the burning sensation. Symptoms typically worsen throughout the day and into the evening, often subsiding overnight. Although the condition occurs more frequently in women, anyone can be affected. For many people, the exact cause or causes of their burning mouth is elusive. BMS has been associated with a number of conditions, such as hormonal imbalances, oral disorders such as thrush or dry mouth, or damaged nerves (specifically, cranial nerves associated with taste). irritating dentures, or nutritional deficiencies, but their relationship is not clear.

Treatment is tailored to the specific needs of each patient and focuses on the underlying cause(s) of burning mouth if it can be identified, or on the painful symptoms to try to alleviate the discomfort of BMS. Glossodynia or burning mouth syndrome (BMS) (also known as burning tongue [132] and orodynia [173,174].

Iron-deficiency anemia (or iron-deficiency anaemia) is a common anemia that occurs when iron loss (often from intestinal bleeding or menses) occurs, and/or the dietary intake or absorption of iron is insufficient. In iron deficiency, hemoglobin, which contains iron, cannot be formed [175].

Oral symptoms and signs of iron-deficiency anemia include mouth ulcers. Deficiencies in vitamin B12, zinc [138] have been linked to oral ulceration, too [176]. Similarly, ascorbic acid(Vitamin C) deficiencies may lead to scurvy which impairs wound healing, which can contribute to ulcer formation.

Disorders such as iron deficiency anemia and B-vitamin deficiencies could cause glossitis. Especially, Vitamin B9 (Folic acid) and B12 help prevent tongue inflammation, chronic periodontitis and yeast infection. Poor hydration and low saliva in the mouth may allow bacteria to grow more readily and cause glossitis. Also, glossitis could caused by certain blood hypertension medications (ACE inhibitors). Angular cheilitis or angular stomatitis is an inflammatory lesion at the labial commissure, or corner of the mouth, and often occurs bilaterally. The condition manifests as deep cracks or splits. In severe cases, the splits can bleed when the mouth is opened and shallow ulcers or a crust may form [177].

Although the sores of angular cheilitis may become infected by the fungus *Candida albicans* (thrush), or other pathogens, studies have linked the initial onset of angular cheilitis with nutritional deficiencies, namely riboflavin (vitamin B_2) [178] and iron deficiency anemia [179] which in turn may be evidence of poor diets or malnutrition (e. g. celiac disease). Zinc deficiency has also been associated with angular cheilitis [180].

Zinc is absorbed in the duodenum and proximal jejunum, and absorption may be impaired with altered GI tract anatomy. Zinc is lost primarily in the feces, with a small amount excreted in the urine. Therefore, individuals with chronic diarrhea, malabsorption, or steatorrhea are at risk of zinc deficiency. Manifestations of zinc deficiency include impaired immune function (decreased development and activation of T lymphocytes) [181] altered taste and impaired wound healing [182,183].

Pre and Post Surgery Dental Assessment

The maintenance of oral health is very important before and after bariatric surgery, considering that after surgery patients need to chew slowly and for a longer time to prevent adverse effects, such as nausea and vomiting. Therefore oral rehabilitation of patients undergoing bariatric surgery is essential in order to reduce the side-effects after surgery and improve the quality of life of patients before and after the intervention. Patients who have undergone bariatric surgery are seen with increasing frequency in dental offices and dental professionals need to be familiar with the challenges these patients present [184].

Oral health is affected by many factors so dental professionals need to understand the oral implications of obesity, including this population's limited access to care.

In working with obese patients, dental professionals have to collaborate with bariatric doctors. Dental professionals understand the link between oral and systemic health and, thus, all patients considering bariatric surgery should have their oral health status checked before and after bariatric surgery. Oral health also plays a role in surgical outcomes so an operative oral health assessment before and after surgery is critical. The pre-operative assessment survey documents the patient's oral health status and notes any conditions that may affect the surgery. Patients preparing for surgery may present with dental caries, periodontal disease, xerostomia, or oral conditions related to eating disorders. The assessment is important in determining the timeline for surgery, as well as helping insure that the surgery has every chance of producing the desired outcomes.

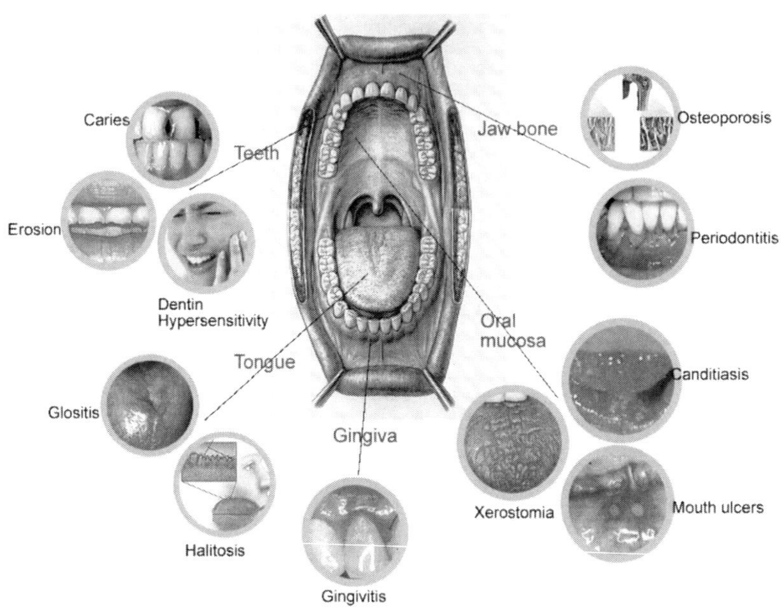

Oral Adverse Effects of Bariatric Surgery.

The oral health assessment survey screens for dental diseases and determines the patient's ability to chew post-operatively. If the assessment indicates poor oral health, the patient should be referred to a dentist for appropriate treatment prior to surgery. The results of the assessment can also be used by the anesthesiologist to prevent dental injuries that may occur during surgical operation. The dental professional can use the assessment inventory to promote post-operative compliance and impact the surgical outcome for the bariatric patient. If the patient reports post-operative problems with side effects from food intake, the screening can be repeated to determine if oral diseases have been treated or if other complications exist affecting the ability to masticate and swallow food.

Another factor that must be taken into consideration is the reduced access of obese individuals in dental care due to lack of transportation and logistical problems. Dental treatment chairs do not support the weight of a patient with a BMI of 40 or more and the supine position required for care is not conducive to adequate respiration or comfort for the morbidly obese [185].

Because the prevalence of extreme obesity continues to increase in, the likelihood that a dental health professional will provide care for patients with a history of bariatric surgery will increase, too [186].

Obese people should be referred to special dental centers that have experience and engineering infrastructure such as transportation and special dental equipment to provide dental services.

Bariatric Patient Pre-/Post-Operative Oral Health Assessment Form		
Patient Name: ____________________ Date:___________ Dentist:_________________________ ID No:__________ Bariatric Surgeon:_______________________________ Anaesthesiologist:_______________________________ Preoperative Alerts:______________________________ ____ ____ Please examine the oral cavity with a dental mirror, explorer and probe and with a light source and interview the patient concerning the following:		
	YES	NO
Does report patient chewing problems?		
Does report patient mouth/facial pain?		
If patient has natural teeth, complete the following section:		
a. Has patient obvious crown caries?		
b. Has patient obvious root caries?		
c. Has patient broken tooth/teeth?		
d. Has patient a loose tooth/teeth?		
e. Has patient calculus(tartar) on the lingual surfaces of the anterior teeth?		
f. Has patient calculus(tartar) on the buccal surface of maxillary molars?		
g. Has patient inflamed or bleeding gingivae?		
h. Has patient periodontal pockets deeper than 3 mm?		

(Continued)

i. Has patient halitosis(bad breath)?		
j. Has patient a grey pseudomembrane?		
k. Has patient thick saliva, full of bubbles?		
l. Has patient dry mouth?		
m. Has patient eroded tooth/teeth?		
n. Has patient conservative restorations, such as fillings that appeared higher than the chewing surface of the teeth?		
o. Is patient palate red and irritated?		
If patient has fixed prosthetic restoration(crown, bridge), complete the following section:		
a. Has patient obvious root caries(underneath the cervical limits of restorations)?		
b. Has patient a problem with fixed restoration such as chipped, broken, loose, uncleanable or missing?		
If patient has artificial teeth(partial/complete denture),complete the following section(remove the appliance before the examination):		
a. Has patient abnormal oral tissue(ulcers, sores, masses, thrush)?		
b. Has patient a problem with partial or complete denture?		
NOTE: If any answers are "YES" the patient should be referred to a dental professional (specialist or not) for further examination and treatment prior the bariatric surgery.		
Referral Date:____________________ Dentist's Name/Facility:____________________ Contact Information:____________________		
Comments:____________________ ____________________ ____________________		

However, as the patient's body mass decreases after bariatric surgery and the ergonomic ability to obtain dental care increases, self-esteem and the desire for good self-care develops, which encourages patients to seek restorative, cosmetic, and preventive dental care.

Health care providers have only recently begun to address the unique needs of the morbidly obese and dental professionals have an important role to play on the bariatric treatment team. The need for pre- and post-operative dental treatment planning is increasing as the number of people seeking bariatric surgery grows. This population's access to oral health care also needs to be increased. Finally, seminars discussing the impact of poor oral health on surgery outcomes and the importance of including a dental health professional on the bariatric treatment team should be developed and presented to bariatric surgery teams [187].

The patient's medical management should be assessed regularly and modified appropriately after surgery because decreased energy intake alone, in addition to weight loss, can rapidly affect medical conditions associated with obesity.

To address the many changing dental needs of patients after bariatric surgery, dental professional should assume the overall medical care while working in close collaboration with the bariatric medical team. Dental professional begin to educate patients pre-operatively and continue their instruction postoperatively.

Dental Follow-up Frequency

We recommend dental evaluations 3 to 4 weeks after surgery, then quarterly for 1 year and annually thereafter or according to the patient's dental needs.

During this re-examination, the dentist will review oral health documenting potential problems, compared with the preoperative state, and will proceed to restore them. It will also inform the patient and emphasize the importance of keeping good oral hygiene. The dentist may need to reassess the type of suggested oral hygiene measures.

In collaboration with the dietitian/nutritionist of the bariatric team will also highlight the importance of selecting appropriate foods, consumption of which promotes oral health.

Obtaining a clinical history is important because persistent nausea, vomiting, diarrhea, or abdominal pain requires evaluation by a physician. These conditions affect total oral health and should take the necessary measures to overcome them.

Oral health recommendations are based on dental post-surgery assessment and should focus on oral hygiene and diet. Rapid weight loss can lead to dehydration. Nausea and occasional vomiting are common in the early post-operative course.

Consuming liquids (water, not acid sugar free fruit juices and milk) for hydration between meals may help avoid common gastrointestinal (GI) symptoms and oral soft tissue dehydration. Attention should be directed toward minimizing unplanned snacking which adversely affects oral health by promoting tooth decay.

Patients should be continually reminded that the primary focus should be healthy lifestyle. medical and dental outcomes rather than weight loss or body weight alone.

The dentist should investigate potential problems of the oral cavity due to certain drugs administered postoperatively to treat certain post-surgical complications, such as NSAID's whose use can cause the creation of oral ulcers.

Additionally, the dental professional as a member of the medical bariatric team should be aware of the deficiency of nutrients such as iron, calcium, water soluble and fat soluble vitamins and trace elements minerals as zinc.

The Greek philosopher Aristotle said, ". . *the alteration of the body causes deterioration of the soul.* " The opposite is also true. Because obese patients also develop psychological problems, the dentist must be in collaboration with the psychologists of the bariatric team. This collaboration will allow the identification of possible psychological problems that affect oral health and early treatment of these problems.

Conclusion

- Bariatric surgery is an important tool in the treatment of extreme obesity.
- Because the prevalence of extreme obesity continues to increase in the United States, the likelihood that a dental health professional will provide care for patients with a history of bariatric surgery will increase too.

- Bariatric patients are at an increased risk for dental caries due to a smaller stomach volume and the need for smaller, more frequent meals/snacks throughout the day.
- Bariatric patients are at an increased risk for dehydration and lactose intolerance that also contribute to caries activity due to the occurrence of xerostomia and reduced exposure to anticariogenic factors in milk.
- Due to poor bibliography, more research is needed with an adequate sample size and controls for multiple risk factors to gain a better understanding of the relationship between recommended meal patterns for bariatric patients and dental caries risk.
- Supportive evidence would stress the need for more preventive dental care among bariatric patients.
- Preoperative nutritional counseling and oral hygiene instruction may prove especially beneficial in helping to reduce the risk of dental caries.
- The delivery of preventive care to help the patient maintain a healthy dentition and good chewing function is especially important in a population already at nutritional risk.

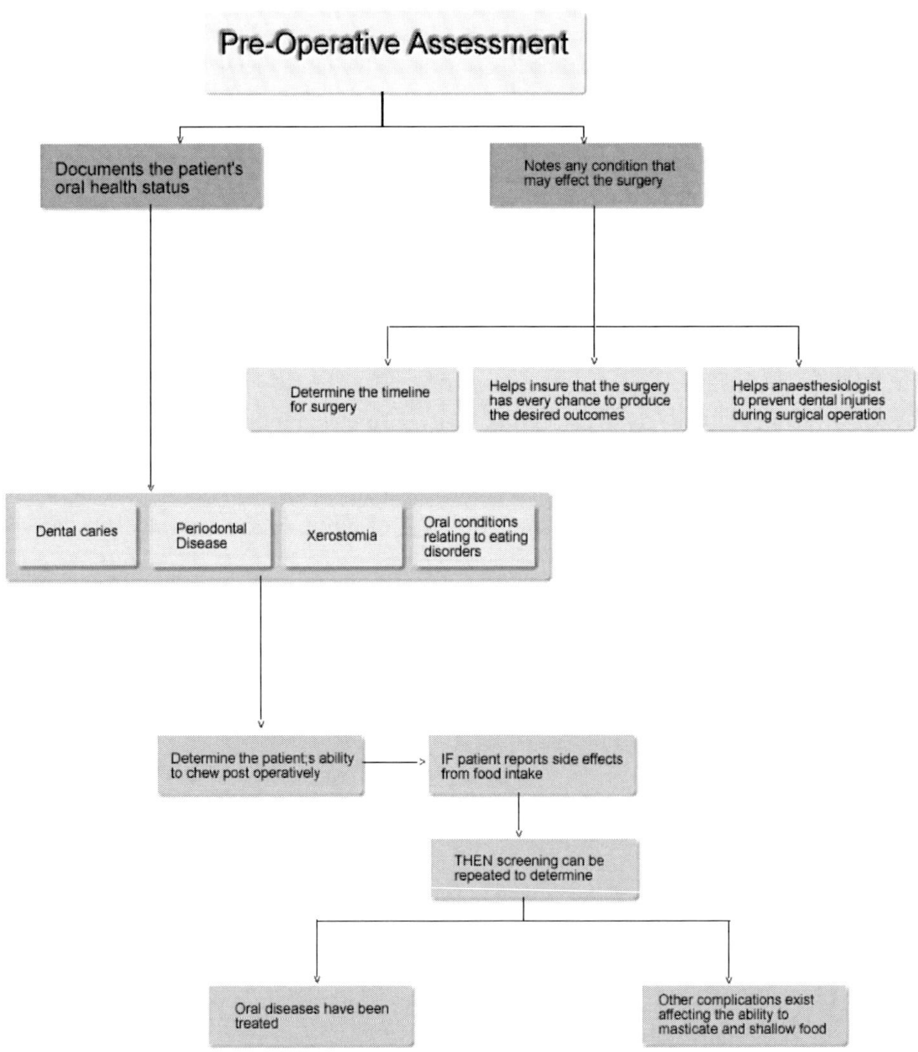

- The medical team needs to relate to potential dental problems after bariatric surgery, and to supply their patients with the appropriate information.
- Instruction regarding oral hygiene maintenance, healthy diet patterns and regular dental health monitoring by a dentist or dental hygienist are of paramount importance.
- Subsequently, there is a need to better understand oral health implications associated with bariatric surgery.
- A comprehensive and team approach provides the best care to this group of patients.

References

[1] World Health Organization. (2006). Constitution of the World Health Organization Basic Documents, Forty-fifth edition, Supplement, October 2006.

[2] http://www. who. int/topics/obesity/en

[3] http://www. who. int/mediacentre/factsheets/fs311/en/

[4] Haslam, DW; James, WP. Obesity. *Lancet*, 2005, 366(9492), 1197–209

[5] Kushner, Robert Treatment of the Obese Patient (Contemporary Endocrinology). Totowa, NJ: 2007, Humana Press. pp. 158

[6] Adams, JP; Murphy, PG. Obesity in anaesthesia and intensive care. *Br J Anaesth*, 2000, 85(1), 91–108.

[7] Lau, DC; et al. 2006 Canadian clinical practice guidelines on the management and prevention of obesity in adults and children summary. *CMAJ*, 2007, 176(8), S1–13.

[8] Bleich, S; et al. Why is the developed world obese? *Annu Rev Public Health,* 2008, 29, 273–95.

[9] Drewnowski, A; Specter, SE. Poverty and obesity: the role of energy density and energy costs. *Am. J. Clin. Nutr.,* 2004, 79(1), 6–16.

[10] Nestle, M; Jacobson, MF. Halting the obesity epidemic: a public health policy approach. *Public Health Rep*, 2000, 115(1), 12–24.

[11] James, WP. The fundamental drivers of the obesity epidemic. *Obes Rev* 2008, 9(1), 6–13.

[12] Barness, LA; Opitz, JM; Gilbert-Barness, E. Obesity: genetic, molecular, and environmental aspects. *Am. J. Med. Genet.,* 2007, 143A(24), 3016–34

[13] Haslam, D. Obesity: a medical history. *Obes Rev*, 2007, 8, Suppl 1, 31–6.

[14] Caballero, B. The global epidemic of obesity: An overview". *Epidemiol Rev*, 2007, 29, 1–5.

[15] Kopelman, PG. Obesity as a medical problem. *Nature*, 2000, 404, 635–43.

[16] Joint Health Survey Health Survey for England, 2001 www. doh. gov. uk/ stats/tables/trendtab06. xls

[17] Obesity and overweight". *World Health Organization*. http: //www. who. int/ mediacentre/factsheets/fs311/en/index. html.

[18] Sturm, R. Increases in morbid obesity in the USA, 2000–2005. *Public Health, 2007,* 121 (7), 492–6.

[19] Howard, Natasha J. et al. Severe obesity, Investigating the socio-demographics within the extremes of body mass index. *Obesity Research &Clinical Practice*, 2008, 2(1), 51–59.
[20] Tjepkema, M. Nutrition, Findings from the Canadian Community Health Survey. Ottawa, Ontario, Statistics Canada. http://www. statcan. gc. ca/ pub/82-620-m/2005001/article/adults-adultes/8060-eng. htm, 2005.
[21] Calle, EE; et al. Body-mass index and mortality in a prospective cohort of U. S. adults. *N. Engl. J. Med*, 1999, 341 (15), 1097–105.
[22] Obesity and overweight. *World Health Organization*. http: // www. who. int/ mediacentre/factsheets/fs311/en/index. html. April 8, 2009.
[23] Imaz, I; et al. Safety and effectiveness of the intragastric balloon for obesity. A meta-analysis. *Obes Surg*, 2008, 18(7), 841–6.
[24] Royal College of Physicians of London. Clinical management of overweight and obese patients with particularreference to the use of drugs. London, RCP, 1998.
[25] National Institutes of Health (NIH), National Heart, Lung and Blood Institute (NLLBI). Clinical guidelines on the identification, evaluation and treatment of overweight and obesity, the evidence report. Washington, US Government Press, 1998.
[26] National Task Force on the Prevention and Treatment of Obesity. Long-term pharmacotherapy in the management of obesity. *JAMA*, 1996, 276, 1907–15.
[27] Haddock, CK; et al. Pharmacotherapy for obesity, a quantitative analysis of four decades of published randomised clinical trials. *Int J Obes*, 2002, 26, 262–73.
[28] Committee on Nutrition, Massachusetts Medical Society. Obesity treatment using drug therapy, White Paper. Waltham MA, The Massachusetts Medical Society, 1998.
[29] Rucker, D; et al. Long term pharmacotherapy for obesity and overweight, updated meta-analysis. *BMJ*, 2007, 335(7631), 1194–99.
[30] Medicines Control Agency statement on European legal action relating to anorectic agents. www. mca. gov. uk/whatsnew/whatsnew_2002. htm#2002
[31] Doniger, S. Saliva and oral health. *RDH.*, 2005, 25(7), 52-55.
[32] Hitner, H; Nagle, B. Battling blubber. *Drug Topics.*, 2005, 149(16), 24-30.
[33] Ahrens, R. Weight matters, the care of overweight and obese patients. CE supplement. *America's Pharmacist*. September, 2003.
[34] Keene, JJ; Jr, Galasko, GT; Land, MF. Antidepressant use in psychiatry and medicine, importance for dental practice. *J Am Dent Assoc.*, 2003, 134, 71-79.
[35] Hitner, H; Nagle, B. *Pharmacology, An Introduction*. New York, McGraw Hill, 2005.
[36] Xenical [package insert]. Nutley, NJ, Roche Laboratories Inc, 2004
[37] Parati, Gianfranco et al. Sleep apnoea and hypertension. Current Opinion in Nephrology & Hypertension, March 2002 - Volume 11 - Issue 2 - 201-214
[38] *Nursing Drug Handbook*. Springhouse, Pa, Springhouse Corp, 2005.
[39] Owens, TM. Morbid obesity, the disease and co-morbidities. *Crit Care Nurs.*, 2003, 26, 162 165.
[40] Arimidex [package insert]. Wilmington, Del, AstraZeneca, 2004.
[41] National Institute of Health (1991) ''Gastrointestinal Surgery for Severe Obesity'' NIH. Consensus Statement Online 1991 March 25-27. Available, http: //consensus. nih. gov/1991/1991GISurgeryObesity084 html. htm.
[42] Sjöström, L; *et al.* Effects of bariatric surgery on mortality in Swedish obese subjects. *N. Engl. J. Med.,* 2007, 357 (8), 741–52.

[43] Santry, HP; Gillen, DL; Lauderdale, DS. Trends in bariatric surgical procedures. *JAMA*. 2005 Oct 19, 294(15), 1909-17.

[44] Buchwald, H; Oien, DM. (2009) Metabolic/bariatric surgery Worldwide, 2008. *Obes Surg*, 19, 1605–1611.

[45] Abell, TL; Minocha, A . Gastrointestinal complications of bariatric surgery, diagnosis and therapy. *Am. J. Med. Sci.,* 2006, 331 (4), 214–8.

[46] Intestinal 'Sleeve' Mimics Effects of Gastric Bypass. HealthDay News 2008, December 4.

[47] http://www. medpagetoday. com/Endocrinology/Diabetes/17008

[48] Schouten, R; *et al.* A multicenter, randomized efficacy study of the EndoBarrier Gastrointestinal Liner for presurgical weight loss prior to bariatric surgery. *Ann. Surg.,* 2010, 251 (2), 236–43.

[49] Stanczyk, M; Martindale, RG; Deveney, C. Bariatric Surgery Overview. In C. D. Berdanier, E. B. Feldman, J. Dwyer. *Handbook of Nutrition and Food*, 2007, Boca Raton, FL, CRC Press. 915–926.

[50] Shikora, SA; Kim, J; Tarnoff, ME. Nutritional and gastrointestinal complications of bariatric surgery. *Nutrition in Clinical Practice*, 2007, 22 (1), 29–40.

[51] Freitas, A; Sweeney, JF. Bariatric Surgery. In B. Banerjee. *Nutritional Management of Digestive Disorders,* 2010, Boca Raton, FL, CRC Press. pp. 327–342.

[52] http://bariatrictimes. com/2009/06/18/laparoscopic-sleeve-gastrectomy/ Bariatrictimes. com.

[53] Mathus-Vliegen, EM. Intragastric balloon treatment for obesity, what does it really offer? *Dig Dis*, 2008, 26(1), 40–4.

[54] Rosenthal, Elisabeth (January 3, 2006). "Europeans Find Extra Options for Staying Slim. *TheNewYorkTimes*. http: //query. nytimes. com/gst/ fullpage. html?res =9400EED61030F930A35752C0A9609C8B63&sec=health&pagewanted=all.

[55] http://thehealthclinic. org. uk/procedures-2/weight-loss-surgery/gastric-balloon

[56] Pardo, JV; *et al.* (November 2007). Weight loss during chronic, cervical vagus nerve stimulation in depressed patients with obesity, an observation. *Int J Obes*, 2007, 31 (11), 1756–9.

[57] Snow, V; et al. Pharmacologic and surgical management of obesity , a clinical practice guideline from the American College of Physicians. *Ann. Intern. Med.,* 2005, 142 (7), 525–31.

[58] Maggard, MA; *et al.* Meta-analysis, surgical treatment of obesity. *Ann. Intern. Med.,* 2005, 142 (7), 547–59.

[59] Fajnwaks, et al. Outcomes of bariatric surgery in patients with BMI less than 35 kg/m2. *Surgery for Obesity and Related Diseases*, 2008, 4 (3), 329·

[60] Robinson, MK. Editorial, Surgical treatment of obesity—weighing the facts. *N. Engl. J. Med.,* 2009, 361 (5), 520–1.

[61] http://www. medscape. com/viewarticle/706394

[62] Maggard, MA; *et al.* (2005). Meta-analysis, surgical treatment of obesity. *Ann. Intern. Med.,* 2005, 142 (7), 547–59.

[63] O'Brien, PE; *et al.* (May 2006). Treatment of mild to moderate obesity with laparoscopic adjustable gastric banding or an intensive medical program, a randomized trial. *Ann. Intern. Med.,* 2006, 144 (9), 625–33.

[64] Sjöström, L; *et al.* Effects of bariatric surgery on mortality in Swedish obese subjects. *N. Engl. J. Med.*, 2007, 357 (8), 741–52.

[65] Adams, TD; *et al.* Long-term mortality after gastric bypass surgery. *N. Engl. J. Med.*, 2007, 357(8), 753–61.

[66] Colquitt, JL; et al. Surgery for obesity. *Cochrane Database Syst Rev,* 2009, (2), CD003641

[67] Sjöström, L; *et al.* Effects of bariatric surgery on mortality in Swedish obese subjects. *N. Engl. J. Med*, 2007, 357 (8), 741–52.

[68] Adams, TD; *et al.* Long-term mortality after gastric bypass surgery. *N. Engl. J. Med.*, 2007, 357 (8), 753–61.

[69] Hazzan, D; *et al.* Laparoscopic bariatric surgery can be safe for treatment of morbid obesity in patients older than 60 years. *Surg Obes Relat Dis*, 2006, 2 (6), 613–6.

[70] Vetter, ML. Mechanisms by which Bariatric Surgerymay Ameliorate Type 2 Diabetes. *CML – Diabete*, 2010, 27(1), 1–12.

[71] Maciejewski, ML; *et al.* Survival among high-risk patients after bariatric surgery. *JAMA*, 2011, 305 (23), 2419–26.

[72] Encinosa, WE; et al. Healthcare utilization and outcomes after bariatric surgery. *Medical care*, 2006, 44 (8), 706–12.

[73] Snow, V; et al. Pharmacologic and surgical management of this is not gastric bypass obesity in primary care, a clinical practice guideline from the American College of Physicians. *Ann. Intern. Med.,* 2005, 142 (7), 525–31.

[74] Flum, DR; *et al.* Perioperative safety in the longitudinal assessment of bariatric surgery. *N. Engl. J. Med.,* 2009, 361(5), 445–54.

[75] Nguyen, NT; *et al.* Result of a national audit of bariatric surgery performed at academic centers, a 2004 University HealthSystem Consortium Benchmarking Project. *Arch Surg*, 2006, 141 (5), 445–9.

[76] Arasaki, CH; et al. Incidence of regurgitation after the banded gastric bypass. *Obes Surg.*, 2005, 15, 1408-17.

[77] Hague, AL; Baechle, M. Advanced caries in a patient with a history of bariatric surgery. *J Dent Hyg.*, 2008, 82, 22-7.

[78] Shikora, SA; Kim, JJ; Tarnoff, ME. Nutrition and gastrointestinal complications of bariatric surgery. *Nutr Clin Pract.*, 2007, 22, 29-40.

[79] Heling, I; et al. Dental complications following gastric restrictive bariatric surgery. *Obes Surg.*, 2006, 16, 1131-4.

[80] Suter, M; et al. European experience with laparoscopic Roux-en-Y gastric bypass in 466 obese patients. *Br J Surg.*, 2006, 93, 726-32.

[81] Abell, TL; Minocha, A. Gastrointestinal complications of bariatric surgery, diagnosis and therapy. *Am. J. Med. Sci.,* 2006, 331 (4), 214–8.

[82] Mandel, L; Da Silva, K. Parotid hypertrophy and bariatric surgery, case report. *J Oral Maxillofac Surg.*, 2008, 66, 572-4.

[83] Archer-Dubon, C; et al. Palatal ulcers due to vomiting after gastric band tightening. *Obes Surg.*, 2007, 17, 556-8.

[84] Greenway, SE; Greenway, FL. Root surface caries, a complication of the jejunoileal bypass. *Obes Surg.*, 2000, 10, 33-6.

[85] Moravec, LJ; Boyd, LD. Bariatric surgery and implications for oral health, a case report. *J Dent Hyg.*, 2011, Summer, 85(3), 166-76. Epub 2011 Aug 8.

[86] Kidd, EA; Fejerskov, O. What constitutes dental caries? Histopathology of carious enamel and dentin related to the action of cariogenic biofilms. *J Dent Res.*, 2004, 83, 35-8.

[87] Takahashi, N; Nyvad, B. Caries ecology revisited, microbial dynamics and the caries process. *Caries Res.*, 2008, 42, 409-18.

[88] Caufield, PW; Griffen, AL. Dental caries, an infectious and transmissible disease. *Pediatr Clin North Am.*, 2000, 47, 1001-19.

[89] Groeneveld, A; Arends, J. Influence of pH and demineralization time on mineral content, thickness of surface layer and depth of artificial caries lesions. *Caries Res.*, 1975, 9, 36-44.

[90] Caufield, PW; Li, Y; Dasanayake, A. Dental caries, an infectious and transmissible disease. *Compend Contin Educ Dent.*, 2005, 26, 10-6.

[91] Kidd, EA; Fejerskov, O. What constitutes dental caries? Histopathology of carious enamel and dentin related to the action of cariogenic biofilms. *J Dent Res.*, 2004, 83, C35-8.

[92] Juliane Avansini Marsicano et al. Interfaces between bariatric surgery and oral health. A longitudinal survey1. *Acta Cirúrgica Brasileira*, 2011, *26 (Suppl. 2), 79*

[93] Moynihan, PJ. Dietary advice in dental practice. *Br Dent J.*, 2002, 193(10), 563-8.

[94] Touger-Decker, R; Mobley, CC. Position of the American Dietetic Association, Oral health and nutrition. *J Am Diet Assoc.*, 2003, 103, 615-25.

[95] Hornick, B. Diet and nutrition implications for oral health. *J Dent Hyg.*, 2002, 76, 67-78.

[96] Sheiham, A. Dietary effects on dental disease. *Public Health Nutr.*, 2001, 4, 569-91.

[97] Parkes, E. Nutritional management of patients after bariatric surgery. *Am J Med Sci.*, 2006, 331(4), 207-13.

[98] Shah, M; Simha, V; Garg, A. Review, Long-term impact of bariatric surgery on body weight, comorbidities, and nutritional status. *J Clin Endocrinol Metab.*, 2006, 91, 4223-31.

[99] Fontana, M; Zero, DT. Assessing patients' caries risk. *J Am Dent Assoc.*, 2006, 137(9), 1231-9.

[100] Sheiham, A. Dietary effects on dental disease. *Public Health Nutr.*, 2001, 4(2B), 569-91.

[101] Trudgill, NJ; et al. Impact of smoking cessation on salivary function in healthy volunteers. *Scand J Gastroenterol.*, 1998, 33, 568-71.

[102] Guggenheimer, J; Moore, PA. Xerostomia Etiology, recognition and treatment. *J Am Dent Assoc.*, 2003, 134, 61-9.

[103] Matsumoto, Y; Yoshii, E. Evaluation of a new plaque acidogencity test. *J Dent Res.*, 2005, 84.

[104] Anusavice, KW. Present and Future Approaches for the Control of Caries. *J Dent Educ.*, 2005, 69(5), 538-54.

[105] Gandara, BK; Truelove, EL. Diagnosis and management of dental erosion. *J Contemp Dent Pract.*, 1999, 1, 16-23.

[106] Turner, MD; Ship, JA. Dry mouth and its effects on the oral health of elderly people. *J Am Dent Assoc.*, 2007, 138, 15-20.

[107] Cercato, C; et al. A randomized double-blind placebocontrolled study of the long-term efficacy and safety of diethylpropion in the treatment of obese subjects. *Int J Obes.*, 2009, 33, 857-65.

[108] von Bültzingslöwen, I; et al. Salivary dysfunction associated with systemic diseases, systematic review and clinical management recommendations. *Oral Surg Oral Med Oral Pathol Oral Radiol Endod.*, 2007, 103, S57 e1-15.

[109] Moynihan, P. Foods and factors that protect against dental caries. *Brit Nutr Found Nutr Bull.*, 2000, 25, 281-6.

[110] Palmer, C. *Diet and Nutrition in Oral Health.* Upper Saddle River, NJ, *Prentice Hall*, 2003.

[111] Boan, J. Postoperative management of the bariatric surgery patient. *Cortlandt Forum.*, 2005, 22, 17-21.

[112] Perugini, RA; Mason, R; Czerniach, DR. Predictors of complications and suboptimal weight loss after laparoscopic Roux-en-Y gastric by pass, a series of 188 patients. *Arch Surg.*, 2003, 138, 541-545.

[113] Agence Nationale d'Accreditation et d'Evaluation en Sante´ (2001) Chirurgie de L'obesite´ morbide de l'adulte. Available, http: //www. has-sante. fr/portail/upload/ docs/application/pdf/chirurgie_obesite_rap. pdf.

[114] N'gom, PI; Woda, A. Influence of impaired mastication on nutrition. *J Prosthet Dent*, 2002, 87, 667–673.

[115] Pera, P; et al. Influence of mastication on gastric emptying. *J Dent Res*, 2002, 81, 179–181.

[116] Lipsitz, LA; et al. Hemodynamic and autonomic nervous system responses to mixed meal ingestion in healthy young and old subjects and dysautonomic patients with postprandial hypotension. *Circulation*, 1993, 87, 391–400.

[117] Kaneko, H; et al. Possibility of postprandial electrogastrography for evaluating vagal/nonvagal cholinergic activity in humans, through simultaneous analysis of postprandial heart rate variability and serum immunoreactive hormone levels. *Am J Gastroenterol*, 1995, 90, 603–609.

[118] Momose, T; et al. Effect of mastication on regional cerebral blood flow in humans examined by positronemission tomography with o-labelled water and magnetic resonance imaging. *Archs Oral Biol*, 1997, 42, 57–61.

[119] Farella, M; et al. Cardiovascular responses in humans to experimental chewing of gums of different consistencies. *Arch Oral Biol*, 1999, 44, 835–842.

[120] De Araujo, IE; Rolls, ET. Representation in the human brain of food texture and oral fat. *J Neurosci*, 2004, 24, 3086–3093.

[121] Hasegawa, Y; et al. Circulatory response and autonomic nervous system activity during gum chewing. *Eur J Oral Sci*, 2009, 117, 470–473.

[122] Mattes, RD. Physiological responses to sensory stimulation by food, nutritional implications. *J Am Diet Assoc*, 1997, 97, 406–410.

[123] Power, ML; Schulkin, J. Anticipatory physiological regulation in feeding biology, cephalic phase responses. *Appetite*, 2008, 50, 194–206.

[124] Bellisle, F; Le Magnen, J. The structure of meals in humans , eating and drinking patterns in lean and obese subjects. *Physiol Behav*, 1981, 27, 649–658.

[125] Bellisle, F; et al. Obesity and food intake in children , evidence for a role of metabolic and/or behavioral daily rythms. *Appetite*, 1988, 11, 111–118.

[126] De Jonge, L; Bray, GA. The thermic effect of food and obesity, a critical review. *Obes Res*, 1997, 5, 622–631.

[127] De Jonge, L; Garrel, DR. Role of the autonomic nervous system in the thermogenic response to food in lean individuals. *Am J Physiol*, 1997, 272, 775–780.

[128] Hashkes, PJ; Gartside, PS; Blondheim, SH. Effect of food palatability on early (cephalic) phase of diet-induced thermogenesis in noobese and obese man. *Int J Obes Relat Metab Disord*, 1997, 21, 608–613.

[129] Veyrune, JL; et al. Impact of morbid obesity on chewing ability. *Obes Surg*, 2008, 18, 1467–1472.

[130] Prinz, JF; Lucas, PW. An optimization model for mastication and swallowing in mammals. *Proc Biol Sci*, 1997, 264, 1715–1721.

[131] van der Bilt, A. Assessment of mastication with implications for oral rehabilitation, areview. *J Oral Rehabil*, 2011, Jan 17. doi, 101111/j.

[132] Woda, A. et al. The masticatory normative indicator. *J Dent Res*, 2010, 89, 281–285.

[133] Mishellany, A; Woda, A; Labas, R; Peyron, MA. The challenge of mastication, preparing a bolus suitable for deglutition. *Dysphagia*, 2006, 21, 87–94.

[134] Woda, A; Mishellany, A; Peyron, MA. The regulation of masticatory function and food bolus formation. *J Oral Rehabil*, 2006a, 33, 840–849.

[135] Agrawal, KR; Lucas, PW; Bruce, IC; Prinz, JF. . Food properties that influence neuromuscular activity during human mastication. *J Dent Res*, 1998, 77, 1931–1938.

[136] Woda, A; et al. Adaptation of healthy mastication pertaining to the individual or to the food. *Physiol Behav*, 2006b, 89, 28–35.

[137] Mishellany-Dutour, A; et al. Is the goal of mastication reached in young dentates, aged dentates, and aged denture wearers? *Brit J Nut*, 2008, 99, 121–128.

[138] Mishellany-Dutour, A; et al. Is the goal of mastication reached in young dentates, aged dentates, and aged denturewearers? *Brit J Nut*, 2008, 99, 121–128.

[139] Slagter, AP; et al. Human jawelevator muscle activity and food comminution in the dentate and edentulous state. *Arch Oral Biol*, 1993, 195-205.

[140] Peyron, MA; Lassauzay, C; Woda, A. Effects of increased hardness on jaw movement and muscle activity during chewing of visco-elastic model foods. *Exp Brain Res*, 2002, 142, 41–51.

[141] Peyron, MA; et al. Influence of age on adaptability of human mastication. *J Neurophysiol*, 2004, 92, 773–9.

[142] Anne Espe´rance Godlewski et al. Effect of Dental Status on Changes in Mastication in Patients with Obesity following Bariatric Surgery. *PLoS ONE*. July, 2011, Volume 6(7), e22324.

[143] Magalhães, AC; et al. Insights into preventive measures for dental erosion. *J Appl Oral Sci.*, 2009, 17, 75-86.

[144] Lussi, A; Jaeggi, T; Zero, D. The role of diet in the etiology of dental erosion. *Caries Res.*, 2004, 38, 34-44.

[145] Lussi, A. Erosive tooth wear - a multifactorial condition of growing concern and increasing knowledge. *Monogr Oral Sci.*, 2006, 20, 1-8.

[146] Rios, D; et al. Influence of toothbrushing on enamel softening and abrasive wear of eroded bovine enamel, an *in situ* study. *Braz Oral Res.*, 2006, 20, 148-54.

[147] Addy, M; Hunter, ML. Can tooth brushing damage your health? Effects on oral and dental tissues. *Int Dent J.*, 2003, 53, 177-86.

[148] Ganss, C; Lussi, A. Diagnosis of erosive tooth wear. *Monogr Oral Sci.*, 2006, 20, 32-43.

[149] Walters, PA. Dentinal hypersensitivity, a review. *J Contemp Dent Pract.*, 2005, 6, 107-17.

[150] West, NX. Dentine hypersensitivity. *Monogr Oral Sci.*, 2006, 20, 173-89.

[151] West, NX. Dentine hypersensitivity, preventive and therapeutic approaches to treatment. *Periodontol*, 2000-2008, 48, 31-41.

[152] Compher, CW; Badellino, KO; Boullata, JI. Vitamin D and the bariatric surgical patient, a review. *Obes Surg.*, 2008, 18, 220-4.

[153] de Prisco, C; Levine, SN. Metabolic bone disease after gastric bypass surgery for obesity. *Am J Med Sci.*, 2005, 329, 57-61.

[154] Nicopoulou-Karayianni, K; et al. Tooth loss and osteoporosis, the OSTEODENT Study. *J Clin Periodontol.*, 2009, 36, 190-7.

[155] Ashley, J; Karels, Brigette, R. Cooper. Obesity and its role in oral health. *IJAHSP*, 2007, 5(1), 2

[156] http: //www. perio. org.

[157] Pataro, AL; et al. Influence of Obesity and Bariatric Surgery on the Periodontal Condition" *J Periodontol.*, 2011, Jul 1.

[158] Lakkis, D; et al. Response to Periodontal Therapy in Subjects Who Had Weight Loss Following Bariatric Surgery and Obese Counterparts, A Pilot Study. *J Periodontol.*, 2011 Oct 20.

[159] de Moura-Grec, PG; et al., Alveolar bone loss and periodontal status in a bariatric patient, a brief review and case report, *Eur J Gastroenterol Hepatol.*, 2012, Jan, 24(1), 84-9.

[160] Williams, SE; et al.l. Perioperative management of bariatric surgery patients, focus on metabolic bone disease. *Cleve Clin J Med.*, 2008, May, 75(5), 333-4, 336, 338

[161] Hamoui, N; Anthone, G; Crookes, PF. Calcium metabolism in the morbidly obese. *Obes Surg.*, 2004, 14, 9-12.

[162] Thomas, MK; Lloyd-Jones, DM; Thadhani, RI; et al. Hypovitaminosis D in medical inpatients. *N Engl J Med.*, 1998, 338, 777-783.

[163] Bloomberg, RD; Fleishman, A; Nalle, JE; Herron DM; Kini, S. Nutritional deficiencies following bariatric surgery, what have we learned? *Obes Surg.*, 2005, 15, 145-154.

[164] Alvarez-Leite, JI. Nutrient deficiencies secondary to bariatric surgery. *Curr Opin Clin Nutr Metab Care.*, 2004, 7, 569-575.

[165] Hamoui, N; Kim, K; Anthone, G; Crookes, PF. The significance of elevated levels of parathyroid hormone in patents with morbid obesity before and after bariatric surgery. *Arch Surg.*, 2003, 138, 891-897.

[166] Bariatric Surgery Linked to Increased Fracture Risk. Science Daily. http: //www. sciencedaily. com/releases/2011/06/110604182010. htm.

[167] Genco, RJ. Current View of Risk Factors for Periodontal Diseases. *J Periodont*, October, 1996, 67,(10), 1041-1049

[168] Wactawski-Wende, J. Periodontal diseases and osteoporosis, association and mechanisms. *Ann Periodontol.*, 2001, 6(1), 197-208.

[169] Megson, E; Kapellas, K; Bartold, PM. Relationship between periodontal disease and osteoporosis. *Int J Evid Based Healthc.*, 2010, 8(3), 129-39.

[170] Malinowski, SS. Nutritional and metabolic complications of bariatric surgery. *Am J Med Sci.*, 2006, 331(4), 219-25.

[171] Chauhan, V; et al. Metabolic, renal, and nutritional consequences of bariatric surgery, implications for the clinician. *South. Med. J.*, 2010, 103(8), 775–785.

[172] Cranney, A; et al. Effectiveness and safety of vitamin D in relation to bone health. *Evidence report/technology assessment*, 2007, (158), 1–235.

[173] James, William, D. et al. *Andrews' Diseases of the Skin, clinical Dermatology*. 2006, Saunders Elsevier. p. 63.

[174] Rapini, Ronald, P; Bolognia, Jean, L; Jorizzo, Joseph, L. *Dermatology, 2-Volume Set*. 2007, St. Louis, Mosby.

[175] Brady, PG. Iron deficiency anemia, a call for aggressive diagnostic evaluation. *South. Med. J.*, 2007, 100(10), 966–7.

[176] Orbak, R; Cicek, Y; Tezel, A; Dogru, Y. Effects of zinc treatment in patients with recurrent aphthous stomatitis. *Dental Materials Journal,*, 2003, 22(1), 21–9.

[177] James, William, D; Berger, Timothy, G; et al. *Andrews' Diseases of the Skin, clinical Dermatology*. 2006, Saunders Elsevier. pp. 60-65. Medline Plus (2005-08-01). Riboflavin (vitamin B_2) deficiency (ariboflavinosis). National Institutes of Health. http: //www. nlm. nih. gov/ medlineplus/druginfo/natural/patient-riboflavin. html.

[179] Lu, S; Wu, H. Initial diagnosis of anemia from sore mouth and improved classification of anemias by MCV and RDW in 30 patients. *Oral Surg Oral Med Oral Pathol Oral Radiol Endod*, 2004, 98(6), 679–85.

[180] Gaveau, D; et al. Cutaneous manifestations of zinc deficiency in ethylic cirrhosis]. ". *Ann Dermatol Venereol.*, 1987, 114 (1), 39–53

[181] Shankar, AH; Prasad, AS. Zinc and immune function, the biological basis of altered resistance to infection. *Am J Clin Nutr.*, 1998, 68(2, suppl), 447S-463S

[182] Fujioka, K. Follow-up of nutritional and metabolic problems after bariatric surgery. *Diabetes Care.*, 2005, 28, 481-484.

[183] Shuster, MH; Vasquez, JA. Nutritional concerns related to Roux-en-Y gastric bypass, what every clinician needs to know. *Crit Care Nurs Q.*, 2005, 28, 227-260.

[184] Moravec, LJ; Boyd, LD. Bariatric surgery and implications for oral health, a case report. *J Dent Hyg.*, 2011, 85(3), 166-76.

[185] Al-Zahrani, MS; Bissada, NF; Borawskit, EA. Obesity and periodontal disease in young, middle-aged, and older adults. *J Periodontol.*, 2003, 74, 610-615.

[186] Santry, HP; Gillen, DL; Lauderdale, DS. Trends in bariatric surgical procedures. *J Am Med Assoc.*, 294, 15, 1909-17.

[187] Dimensions of Dental Hygiene. November, 2006, 4(11), 14-16.

In: Bariatric Surgery
Editor: Christos R. Iavazzo
ISBN: 978-1-62618-995-9

Chapter XI

Diet after Bariatric Surgery

Silvia Leite Faria[1,2], Orlando Pereira Faria[1], Heloisa Rodrigues de Gouvêa[1] and Mariane de Almeida Cardeal[1,2]
[1]Gastrocirurgia de Brasília, Brazil
[2]University of Brasilia, Brazil

Abstract

The part nutrition plays is seen as a vital component for managing post-operative bariatric surgery patients. Nutritional therapy must encompass relevant aspects in weight loss, as well as contribute to maintaining long-term nutritional status. Nutritional care after bariatric surgery does have particular details employed to achieve certain goals. The assessment and monitoring of nutritional status in the postoperative period follows a routine which should occur in an individualized, and prophylactic way for maintaining the health of these patients. In the first postoperative month the use of a multiphase diet is encouraged by many surgical weight loss programs. The role of nutritional education in bariatric surgery continues through the following months as an instrument used to improve the surgical outcome, weight loss and the maintenance of weight loss in the long term. The assessment of weight loss must be carried out every month. In terms of excess weight loss, 70% is expected in the end of the first year. In addition to weight loss and the rate at which it occurs, the quality of weight loss must be monitored. One year after the surgery, patients may be close to a healthy weight. The rate of weight loss and/or weight stabilization has diminished. Two years after the surgery, some patients may present a small weight regain. Nutritional education and advice on how to cut and chew food, along with other eating behavior habits must be given to patients early in the preoperative period to avoid food intolerance. There is a tendency in looking for easy-to-swallow foods instead of protein foods. This may lead the patient to an extensive loss of lean mass and to nutritional deficiencies. Concerning protein consumption, related to bariatric surgery, a minimum of 60 grams per day is recommended. Also, Bariatric patients should consume a low glycemic load diet. Poly-vitamins and polyminerals are routinely prescribed due to three important factors: change in the absorption site, intake restriction and lesser contact of foods with digestive enzymes. Calcium supplementation must be carried out by the use of calcium citrate. Iron supplementation must be carried out in the form of iron with chelated amino acid or in the form of iron fumarate. Nutritional support is indispensable so that this tool may be used successfully, with the aim to achieve a healthy weight loss and maintenance.

1. Introduction

Morbid obesity is a refractory disease related to diets and medication, but which usually responds well to bariatric surgery [1]. Currently, surgical treatment for obesity is divided into two large groups: restrictive surgeries and mixed surgeries, which associate restriction with more or less malabsorptive components [2]. Exclusively malabsorptive surgeries have been abandoned since the 1970s due to high incidence of long-term metabolic and nutritional complications. In the postoperative period, weight loss occurs up to approximately 12 to 18 months after surgery [1]. The consensus about the success criteria is linked to the loss and maintenance of at least 50% of excess weight [3]. Weight loss brings about an improvement in the quality of life of individuals and an improvement or cure of obesity-related co-morbidities. Malnutrition is a risk factor associated with all bariatric procedures [2,4,5]. The consumption restriction imposed by surgical procedures has as consequence a reduced caloric, and macro- and micronutrient intake. The risk of nutritional deficiency varies depending on the degree of restriction or malabsorption brought about by the surgery, as well as on the specific area of the intestine excluded from the digestion process. Besides that, the obese population has a risk factor of being malnourished even prior to bariatric surgery. Four important reasons lead to this condition among the obese population: 1) They usually consume a high caloric diet with a low level of nutrients; 2) They present high prevalence of Eating Disorders (ED); 3) They frequently follow yo-yo diets and fad diets and 4) They present high prevalence of co-morbidities which can lead to a high oxidative stress.

It is essential that any preexisting nutritional deficiency be determined, that an appropriate dietary intervention be elaborated for correction and that an eating plan be created in the postoperative period to help the patient achieve success of the surgery. Anthropometric and biochemical evaluation, prescription of supplemental vitamins, minerals and protein and guidance about the appropriate dietary intake form part of nutritional monitoring in the postoperative period [4]. Thus, the part nutrition plays is seen as a vital component for managing post-operative patients [4]. Nutritional therapy related to bariatric surgery must encompass relevant aspects in weight loss, as well as contribute to maintaining long-term nutritional status.

2. Assessment and Monitoring of Nutritional Status

The assessment and monitoring of nutritional status in the postoperative period follows a routine which should occur in an individualized, and prophylactic way for maintaining the health of these patients. This routine includes appointments with professional dieticians, during which anthropometric, evaluations will be made, i. e., measurements of weight and height, calculation of BMI and of the percentage of excess weight lost along with the assessment of quality weight loss by measuring body composition and assessing, related metabolic and biochemical aspects.

Table 1. Recommendations regarding the frequency of nutritional counseling and the frequency and types of biochemical tests to be carried out during the years after surgery

Type of Nutritional monitoring	Recommended frequency
Appointments with the dietitian	
First six months - With nutritional or metabolic co-morbidities - Without nutritional or metabolic co-morbidities	 Once every 30-60 days Once every 30-60 days
Second semester - With nutritional or metabolic co-morbidities - Without nutritional or metabolic co-morbidities	 Every 3 – 6 months Only once
Second year - With nutritional or metabolic co-morbidities - Without nutritional or metabolic co-morbidities	 Every six months Every six months
Thereafter	Annually
Biochemical exams	During the first year: once or twice a semester. Thereafter: Annually *Dual-energy x-ray absorptiometry* should be performed annually to monitor bone density.
- Complete Blood count: platelets	
- Electrolytes	
- Glucose in fasting period	
- Ferritin, transferrin and serum iron	
- Vitamin B12	
- Liver Function	
- Protein (total and fractions)	
- Serum vitamin A	
- Ionic calcium	
- Serum magnesium	
- Creatinine	
- Urea	
- Serum Zinc	
- 25-hydroxyvitamin D	
Optionall: - Intact PTH - Thiamine - RBC folate	

Source: Rhode and MacLean (2000) [10] and Heber et al. (2010) [5].
PTH = parathyroid hormone; RBC = red blood cell.

Table 1 shows the recommendation on the frequency of appointments and biochemical tests that should be carried out during the years after surgery. Bioimpedance analysis is a fast, noninvasive, and relatively cheap method for assessing body composition. A low-level electrical current passes through the patient's body, and impedance (opposition to the flow of current) is measured with a bioimpedance analyzer. There are validated formulas for assessing body composition in obese patients [6]. Such an assessment must be made starting from the first phase of evaluation, so the evolution of weight loss quality can be followed.

Another good device to evaluate body composition is DXA, very precise but more expensive than Bioelectrical impedance. Another exam that may be used, in the post-operative moment is indirect calorimetry (IC), to evaluate the resting metabolic rate (RMR). The RMR value is positively related to the amount of lean mass and its increase is related to a lower possibility of weight regain [7]. In cases when the professional doesn´t have IC available to measure RMR, Mifflin´s formula can be used with good results.

3. Postoperative – 1st Month (RYGB)

Nutritional care after bariatric surgery does have particular details employed to achieve certain goals: to ensure adequate energy intake and nutrients required to support tissue healing after surgery; to support the preservation of lean body mass during extreme weight loss; to minimize reflux, early satiety, and dumping syndrome while maximizing weight loss and, ultimately, weight maintenance [4]. The diet in this first fifteen days must be of liquid consistency in order not to disrupt the healing period, which requires the protection of anastomoses' integrity [2, 6]. It is important to maintain relative gastric rest. Any solids or larger pieces of food may increase the intragastric pressure, which increases the tension in surgical anastomoses. There are two stages of liquid diets. Table 2 shows these stages with their respective characteristics. The use of straws for consuming liquids should be avoided in all stages since this habit favors aerophagia and worsens the occurrence of gas in the postoperative period, in which the patient may experience gas as a result of air inflated by the surgeon into the torso to provide greater mobility within the abdomen in cases of laparoscopic surgery. After RYGB, the new gastric pouch holds up to 20 ml to 30 ml [8]. In the first and second day (first stage), the diet to be prescribed must be a clear liquid diet, left to the surgeon's discretion. The patient is, thus, guided to consume small, frequent sips of liquids (20 ml every 3 minutes). Liquids allowed are: water, teas, coconut water, isotonic drinks, diet or light gelatin and strained soup broth. The patient must avoid drinks with some sort of secretagogue — such as mate tea, black tea, chocolate flavored drinks and coffee — since they increase the production of stomach acid, which could disrupt a relative gastric rest that is important for healing. It is important that the patient consume two liters of liquids every day, being one of water and one of other liquids, thus avoiding dehydration. Extreme temperatures—i. e. very hot or very cold liquids—are not well tolerated. After two days (second stage), the diet must be a full liquid diet with two oral supplements included: one of vitamins and minerals and the other of proteins. The goal is to avoid precocious nutritional deficiencies and/or extensive loss of lean mass. Since the use of pills must be avoided in the first two months, the poly-vitamin supplement prescribed in this stage must be in liquid or chewable form and the protein supplement must be dissolved in water, milk or soy extract without sugar. Soy extract is preferred to skim milk because patients may develop lactose intolerance, abdominal distension and flatulence in the first post-operative month. Liquids should be without sugar to prevent the occurrence of *dumping syndrome*. In this stage the patient can include milk and alternatives, artificially sweetened yogurt, strained cream soups, cream cereals, and sugar-free puddings.

Table 2. Liquid and pureed diet stages in the 1st postoperative month with respective duration and characteristics

Period	Type of diet and duration	Characteristics
First stage	Clear liquid Duration: 1-2 days	Composed of clear liquids. Includes: water, teas without caffeine, coconut water, isotonic drinks, diet or light gelatin, and strained soup broth.
Second stage	Full liquid Duration: 10-14 days	Milk and alternatives, artificially sweetened yogurt, strained cream soups, cream cereals, and sugar-free puddings and protein supplement dissolved in water or soy extract without sugar.
Third stage	Pureed diet Duration:10- 14 days	Scrambled eggs and egg substitute, pureed meat, flaked fish and meat alternatives, pureed fruits and vegetables, soft cheeses, and hot cereal.

The consumption of water, coconut water, teas, and isotonic drinks is maintained. In this stage , the patient can begin to control the size of each sip, which must remain small, and its frequency. It is important, though, to achieve a minimum of at least two liters of total liquids and always to seek to increase water consumption in order to avoid dehydration. A daily poly-vitamin supplement that meets the Dietary Reference Intake (DRI) should be used. A nutritional deficiency of complex B vitamins may occur, mainly of thiamin after ten days postoperative [9]. Therefore, at this moment, complex B vitamins are also prescribed in a liquid form—100 times the Recommended Dietary Allowance (RDA) [10]. Protein in form of food supplement must be prescribed to be taken at least once a day, supplying 10 grams of protein at least. There are several types of supplement in the market and the nutritionist must calculate the quantity of powder to be dissolved daily. After an average of two weeks post-surgery, is prescribed a pureed diet (third stage). This phase consists of foods that have been blended or liquefied with adequate fluid, resulting in foods that range from milkshake to pudding to mash potato consistency. In addition, foods, such as scrambled eggs and canned fish (tuna or salmon), can be incorporated into the diet [4]. However, the pureed diet has some disadvantages that we should consider: in cases where the patient becomes used to having puree-like food after one month post-op, this habit does not teach the patient to chew efficiently. The introduction of meat and raw vegetables is harder in this case. And besides that, these foods do not help in the sensation of satiety and can present a high caloric value, which could be detrimental to weight loss. Table 2 shows the duration of each phase of this routine. After one month patients should be encouraged to eat solid food, which can contribute to satiety sensation.

In cases of patients submitted to gastric banding, a restrictive procedure, the diet evolution is faster than the one described above, which is usually applied to patients submitted to Roux-en-Y Gastric Bypass (RYGB). The sample liquid phase is not necessary, the clear liquid stage has a duration of 2 days, the full liquid stage must last 13 days and, thereafter, the patient starts a diet with solid foods.

Some surgical weight loss programs present other types of consistency evolution in the first postoperative month. Some services suggest 1 month of liquid diet. To sum up, there are different ways of prescribing a diet after bariatric surgery. However, the use of a multiphase diet is encouraged by many surgical weight loss programs [4].

4. Postoperative between 2nd and 12th Months (RYGB)

The role of nutritional education in bariatric surgery continues through the following months as an instrument used to improve the surgical outcome, weight loss and the maintenance of weight loss in the long term [4]. It is known that frequent nutritional assessment and dietary management has correlated significantly with the success of the surgery [11].

Thus, the nutritional follow-up must include a routine of:

- Food intake analysis (emphasis on the quantity of daily proteins).
- Analysis of percentage of excess weight loss.
- Analysis of quality of weight loss (lean mass x body fat).
- Clinical-nutritional exams (signs and symptoms of nutritional deficiencies).
- Analysis of possible surgical complications related to food intake (dumping, food being cramped, vomiting, reflux.).
- Prescription of daily vitamin and mineral supplementation.
- Protein supplementation.
- Lab tests must be solicited every three months.

Solid foods are included in the diet after one month postoperative, in cases of RYGB procedure [12]. The food volume consumed reaches 50 to 80 grams and increases gradually. In the first 15 days of solid food consumption, the preparations with drier, hard meats (such as beef jerky) and insoluble fiber (raw salad and fruit peels) should be avoided. Oil must be restricted to 1 tablespoon a day in this period. This phase allows the intake of foods which will theoretically pass easily from the gastric pouch through the gastrojejunostomy into the jejunum or through the adjustable gastric band [4].

After this adaptation period, all foods are allowed, following the orientations of a healthy post-bariatric diet: Promote anti-obesity foods containing omega-3 fatty acids; high fiber; lean quality protein sources; whole fruits and vegetables; foods rich in phytochemicals and antioxidants; and low-fat dairy (calcium). Dietitians must also discourage pro-obesity processed foods containing refined carbohydrates as well as trans and saturated fatty acids [4, 13, 14]. During the second post-operative month, patients must maintain the poly-vitamin supplement and they should increase their protein supplement to a level of 20 grams a day.

In the sixth month, the patient consumes around 120 to 200 grams per meal, taking more than 20 minutes for each. By the end of the first year, most patients consume around 200 to

250 grams per meal. In general, intake revolves around 1,000 kcal in the first year [15]. The quantity of foods consumed depends on the duration of the meal, on chewing, on the consistency of food—liquid and pasty foods empty the gastric pouch faster—and on the type of food—those foods that crumble in the mouth are more rapidly consumed (crackers, peanuts, cashew nuts, etc.).

Weight Loss during the First Postoperative Year

The results of weight loss after bariatric surgery are to be expressed in percentage of excess weight loss [16]. The assessment of weight loss must be carried out every month. In terms of excess weight loss, 20% is expected in the 1st month, 30% in the 2nd, 50% in the 6th, and 70% by the end of the first year.

Most patients have unreal expectations concerning weight loss in the postoperative period [17]. In general, they expect to lose more weight than desirable. The first step is to demystify the treatment. For that reason, precise, clearly founded information on the treatment must be provided, stressing that there is no "magic;" the success in the loss of excess weight and maintenance of healthy weight requires behavioral changes that contribute to a reasonable weight, one which is compatible with reality.

In addition to weight loss and the rate at which it occurs, the quality of weight loss must be monitored. A patient is expected to lose up to 80% of body fat and 20% of lean mass. When the patient loses more than 20% of lean mass, it may be an indicator of malnutrition. The patient may recover lost lean mass in this first year through a hyperproteic diet (usually based on protein supplements) and regular physical activity. Since weight loss in this period is fast and calorie intake is low, protein supplementation in this first year is mandatory.

5. Orientations of How to Optimize Food Intake

Nutritional education and advice on how to cut and chew food, along with other eating behavior habits must be given to patients early in the preoperative period to avoid food intolerance. A classic example is meat intake, that requires a lot of chewing and special cuts, i. e., in small pieces and against the fiber, so that the meat can be well chewed and swallowed.

All patients undergoing RYGB must receive orientation for efficient chewing. The patient must take more than 30 minutes in each meal [8] and chew foods exhaustively—20 to 25 times for each bite. In order to reduce the food intake speed, patients must be oriented using techniques having cognitive and behavioral bases, such as resting flatware between bites. Vomiting may occur due to lack of time for an efficient chewing and is one of the ten most common nutritional complications after bariatric surgery [18]. Patients must be advised not to drink any liquid during meals and to chew every piece of food exhaustively, efficiently and slowly [18, 19]. They must also avoid placing a large amount of food in the mouth at the same time. If the patients prefer, they are also encouraged to make use of dessert flatware during meals.

6. Macronutrient Intake

Protein - Due to a necessary adaptation to chewing efficiency and gastric capacity, a stage of low protein intake occurs in the first postoperative year [15]. In this stage, the nutritionist must make an effort towards teaching the patient to consume the proper daily quantity of protein, in association with the protein supplement intake, to reach protein requirements [15]. There is a tendency in looking for easy-to-swallow foods (pasta, crackers, purees, juices) instead of protein foods. This may lead the patient to an extensive loss of lean mass and to nutritional deficiencies, usually manifested as anemia and alopecia. A greater loss of lean mass may influence weight loss, since a reasonable quantity of muscle favors higher energy expenditure. It is known that 500 grams of muscle "burn" 40 kcal and 500 grams of fat "burn" 6 kcal. A 5 kg lean mass loss reflects a reduction of 400 kcal in the basal energy expenditure and a 5 kg fat loss reflects a 72 kcal reduction in the basal energy expenditure of an individual.

Concerning protein consumption, related to bariatric surgery, a minimum consumption of 60 grams per day is recommended [5, 8, 20]' and the ideal values are 80 grams per day for women and 100 grams per day for men[21]. There is also a recommendation based on body weight of 1. 5 grams of protein per ideal body weight [15]. We must emphasize the consumption of proteins of high biological value (animal origin proteins), since due to the gastric restriction, foods that contain all essential amino acids in a small portion are to be prioritized [20]. Patients must be oriented to consume first animal protein. Thereafter, they consume cereals, grains, fruits and vegetables. The emphasis on food consumption is no longer on caloric value, but on the quantity of protein and quality of the menu. A protein rich diet helps by inducing satiety, stimulating weight loss, improving body composition, maintaining FFM, regulating blood glucose levels, and reducing the level of serum triglycerides [20].

Carbohydrates and Fats - Recently, Moize et al. (2010) [22], proposed a food pyramid model for bariatric surgery, in which a carbohydrates (CHO) intake of between 40-45% of daily Total Energy Intake (TEI) was recommended. Considering their caloric intake, such a recommendation represents an absolute CHO value of between 100 to 130g/d, adhering to the minimum amount recommended by the DRI [23] and American Diabetes Association (ADA) [24].

Another important factor related to CHO intake is the glycemic index of foods and glycemic load (GL) of meals, since these variables can hinder weight loss of RYGB patients in a later postoperative period [25]. These findings highlight the importance not only of the quantity, but also the quality of CHO to be consumed by the bariatric population.

Considering that patients, six months after surgery, can ingest, on average, 850 kcal / day [26, 27] and following the recommendation of a minimum of 60g of protein per day [5, 8, 20], they should consume about 40-45% of CHO, which represents an average consumption of 90 grams.

After the first year, when TEI nears 1300 kcal/day [13, 27], protein consumption levels should be increased. We can, therefore, establish that 40% of their diet should be supplied by CHO, reflecting a diet of nearly 120 g /d of CHO. Also, bariatric patients should consume a low GL diet.

As for fat, considering the priority of protein consumption and the care related to CHO consumption, recommendations related to fat must complete the remainder of calories supplied by these macronutrients. Findings in the literature show that RYGB patients usually consume about 30% of lipids [13, 27]. This usual level of consumption is seen to be suitable, since the recommended protein intake would supply 30% and CHO would supply 40% of TEI, as recommended in the preceding paragraphs.

7. Micronutrient Supplementation

Poly-vitamins and polyminerals are routinely prescribed due to three important factors: change in the absorption site, intake restriction—which leads to lesser consumption of foods and consequent reduction in nutrient intake—and lesser contact of foods with digestive enzymes, which also leads to malabsorption of vitamins and minerals, as shown in figure 1.

Vitamin B_{12} is administered in a 100 μg to 350 μg daily dose of crystalline B_{12} taken orally or in three doses of 5,000 μg every six months or 1000 μg every month taken intramuscularly [4, 10]. This via is preferred because RYGB patients have a significant decrease of hydrochloric acid production and pepsinogen which is necessary for the pepsin production and the release of vitamin B_{12} from protein. Moreover, they have decreased availability of intrinsic factor, which is necessary to absorb vitamin B_{12} in the terminal ileum [4]. It is known that daily intake of a poly-vitamin and polymineral that meet 200% of DRI corrects most nutritional deficiencies, except for those that had their absorption site changed. These need exceeded doses [10] and need a supplementation apart. Table 3 shows recommended supplementation for bariatric patients. Calcium supplementation must be carried out by the use of calcium citrate and its doses must be divided twice a day (i. e. 750 mg twice a day). This supplementation should be divided twice a day to avoid the occurrence of kidney stones. A dose of vitamin D_3 (800 UI daily) should be added.

Nutrients that have changed the absorption site	**Food restriction**		**Reduction in contact with digestive secretions**	
Vitamin A	↓	Protein	↓	absorption of vitamin A
Iron	↓	Zinc	↓	absorption of vitamin K
Calcium	↓	Iron	↓	absorption of vitamin E
Vitamins B	↓	Calcium	↓	absorption of vitamin D
	↓	Magnesium	↓	absorption of folic acid
	↓	Vitamins B	↓	absorption of iron
			↓	absorption of calcium
Absence of contact with **intrinsic factor** – leads to malabsorption of vitamin B_{12}				

Source: Rhode, 2000 [10].

Figure 1. Causes of nutritional deficiency in the postoperative period of bariatric surgery.

Table 3. Nutrient supplementation after bariatric surgery

Nutrient	AGB	RYGB	Comment
Multivitamin-mineral supplement	100% of DRI	200% of DRI/d	
B_{12}	-	1000 μg/m	Intramuscular injection
		350-500μg/d	Oral tablet (crystalline form)
B complex	B-50 dosage/d	B-50 dosage/d	
Calcium	1500mg	1500-2000mg/d	(calcium citrate with vitamin D_3)
Vitamin D_3		800UI/d	
		50000UI/w	In cases of deficiency
Iron	-	18-27mg/d 50-100mg/d (menstruating women)	Elemental iron. To be taken with a vitamin C supplement
Vit. C		500mg	With iron supplement
		150-300mg/d	Fumarate
Fat soluble vitamin	-	-	
B_1		20-30mg/d	Oral doses. Early neuropathy
		50-100mg/d	Intravenous. Protracted vomiting
Essential fatty acids	1g/d	1g/d	In the form of flaxseed oil

Source: Rhode and MacLean (2000) [10]; Aills et al. (2008) [4].

Table 4. Signs and symptoms related to nutritional deficiency in bariatric surgery patients

Body region	Signs and symptoms	Related nutrients
Hair	Loss of gloss, dryness, brittleness, easily plucked	Protein and Zinc
Face	Nasolabial seborrhea, facial edema	B_2, Iron and Protein
Eyes	Conjunctival pallor	Iron
Tongue	Glossitis, magenta tongue, atrophy of the papillae	B_2, B_3, B_{12}
Nails	Koilonychias, brittleness	Iron
Nervous system	Psychomotor changes, formication of hands and feet	B_1, B_6 and B_{12}

Adapted from: Duarte, 2002.

In cases of vitamin D deficiency, 50,000 IU ergocalciferol should be taken orally, once weekly, for 8 weeks [4]. In women of fertile age, ferritin levels must not continue below40 μg/dl [12]. Iron supplementation must be carried out in the form of iron with chelated amino acid or in the form of iron fumarate to enhance the absorption in the absence of hydrochloric acid.

The intake must reach 10 times the Recommended Dietary Allowance (RDA) (150 mg/day), and can reach up to 300 mg/day in the cases of iron deficiency. The concurrent intake of vitamin C (500 mg/day) helps in the absorption of this mineral. In the case of ferritin levels below 10 μg/dl, it may be necessary to prescribe intravenous supplementation of iron. Moreover, the nutritionist must pay attention to signs and symptoms of nutritional deficiencies and also to the quality of weight loss (fat and lean mass).

Table 4 shows the main signs and symptoms of nutritional deficiencies found in bariatric surgery patients during the postoperative period. Lab tests in the first year are important instruments for monitoring the nutritional status. They must be done every three months and must include CBC, protein (total and fractions), transferrin, ferritin, serum iron, parathormone, serum vitamin A, serum 1. 25 cholecalciferol, serum vitamin B_1, serum vitamin B_{12}, ionic calcium, serum magnesium, serum zinc, urea, creatinine, and glycaemia [10] (Table 1).

8. Nutritional Complications after Bariatric Surgery

Hair loss - A common complaint among patients in the first postoperative year is alopecia. It usually occurs after the third postoperative month and may be associated with deficiency of protein, iron, vitamin A, zinc, selenium, essential fatty acids, and biotin [28]. Protein intake must be monitored and supplementation for zinc, selenium, and vitamin A must be given in order to achieve bariatric requirements (200% of DRI)[4]. Essential fatty acids supplementation must be carried out with one capsule of flaxseed oil taken daily [10]. Biotin supplementation must be carried out through a daily dose of 2. 5 mg [28].

Dumping Syndrome - Moreover, people with preference for sweets, who have undergone RYGB may more frequently present the dumping syndrome, which is defined as a series of symptoms — sweating, tachycardia, tremors, diarrhea — which may occur after consumption of highly caloric meals. In surgeries with a higher malabsorptive component (Scopinaro or Duodenal-Switch), patients may present unsatisfactory weight loss.

Therefore, to avoid dumping syndrome, patients should avoid sugar intake, have frequent and small meals with a low glycemic index and have an adequate fiber intake. The soluble fiber form gels with carbohydrates, delay glucose absorption and prolong the intestinal transit time.

There is also the case of late postprandial dumping, occurring with reactive hypoglycemia due to the large amount of insulin released. To avoid it, hypoglycemic foods, such as those high in caffeine (tea, coffee and soft drinks) as well as wine, beer and alcoholic beverages, in general should be avoided [18, 29].

9. Long-Term Postoperative Procedures – After 12 Months Postoperative (RYGB)

One year after the surgery, patients may be close to a healthy weight. The rate of weight loss and/or weight stabilization has diminished. According to a meta-analysis on results of bariatric surgery, RYGB patients showed an average excess weight loss (EWL) of 61. 6% up to 2 years after the surgery1. It is, therefore, important to help patients to cultivate habits that favor reaching or maintaining a healthy weight [31].

Two years after the surgery, some patients may present a small weight regain (2 kg to 7 kg). This condition may cause distress to some patients. The patient must be informed that this small regain is normal and may be controlled with proper diet orientation and practice of regular physical activity.

Possible causes of weight regain are: anatomical and physiological adaptations that take place over time after the surgery (gastric pouch dilatation) causing part of the early satiation triggered by the stomach's reduced volume to be lost; inadequate eating habits (consumption of highly caloric liquids and the presence of abnormal eating patterns, such as binge-eating and snack-eating patterns); progressive increase in the diet's total calorie intake.

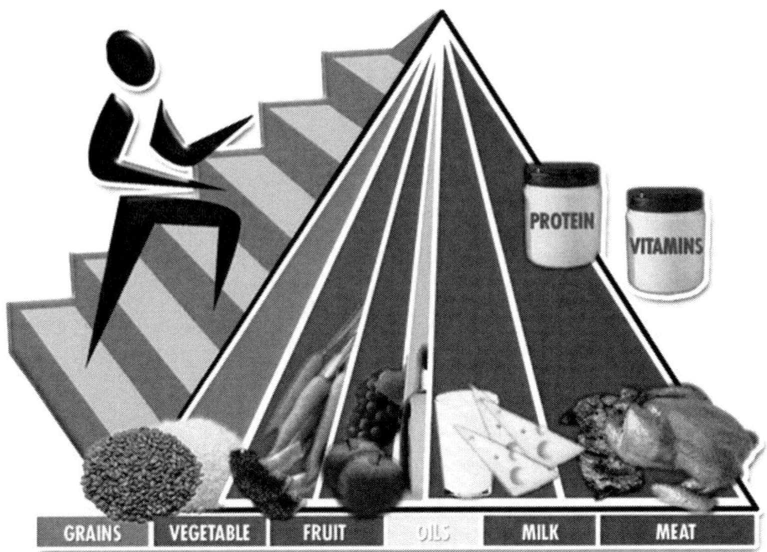

Grains	Vegetables	Fruits	Oils	Dairy	Meat
½ a roll o f salted bread 2 slices of whole wheat 2 tablespoons of rice (=85 grs)	4 tablespoons of vegetables (=60 grs.)	apple and a slice of melon) (=220 grs	4 teaspoons (=20 grs)	1 glass of milk + 2 slices of cheese (=250 grs)	1 medium-sized steak and 1 filet of of fish (=250 grs)

Figure 2. Adaptation of the food pyramid for RYGB patients, one year after surgery.

A diet with low glycemic load, rich in protein food sources, fiber supplement (15g a day) and dairy products (high calcium content) and omega-3 supplementation may prevent weight regain and promote weight loss [18]. However, the literature shows that patients may not tolerate well fibrous, dry and fatty foods (e. g., meat), and raw vegetables [31], which may lead to a reduced protein and fiber intake.

Patients must not reduce the consumption of proteic foods, to avoid the risk of nutritional deficiency. There is also a tendency for patients to consume large quantities of carbohydrates, a behavior that is associated with minor sensation of satiety [30].

It is estimated that a percentage of body fat, from 24% to 31% for women and from 16% to 24% for men, is healthy for this population. A lesser percentage of lean mass is associated to lesser energy expenditure, which makes it difficult to maintain weight in the long term.

Figure 2 shows an adaptation made of the pyramid published by the U. S. Department of Agriculture (2005) [32]. It was an adaptation for post-bariatric patients. The main modifications in the pyramid for the general population proposed here take into account the fact that bariatric patients require more proteins, regular use of vitamin, mineral and protein supplementation, and a limitation imposed by gastric restriction concerning food intake [8].

Figure 2 shows food consumption in household measures and the sum, in grams, of foods in each group. The patients must meet with their nutritionist every three months and the routine blood tests must be carried out every six months as of the second postoperative year.

In order to guide protein consumption, patients may be provided with a table of foods that are a protein source of high biological value (animal protein: groups of meats and dairy products). A portion of proteic food must contain at least 7 to 10 grams of protein. This table may be calculated and provided to the patient aiming to facilitate the intake of daily protein quota. Patients themselves may calculate how many portions they have consumed and whether it is necessary to take a protein supplement each day. Average protein intake among RYGB patients one year after surgery ranges from 50 to 60 grams a day. If a patient consumes 2 slices of cheese (30 g), 1 pot of yoghurt (200 ml), 1 medium steak (100 g), and 1 boiled egg (60 g), this patient will have consumed 53 grams of protein. Since the ideal is 80–100 grams every day, this patient must take some supplement that will provide the necessary amount of protein so the proper intake of this nutrient is reached. The nutritionist must help their patients in choosing the supplement (form and flavor) and the recommended daily dose.

10. Abnormal Eating Patterns

It is common to find some sort of change in the eating patterns among patients after bariatric surgery. This fact may be related to the deliberate use of fad diets, to the use of medications and formulas for weight loss, as well as to environmental and genetic factors. Among the obese population, there is prevalence of change in the eating patterns reaching from 65% to 85%.

There is no consensus but some papers show that the eating patterns may interfere in weight loss in the postoperative period. After bariatric surgery, patients generally improve their eating habits (increasing the number of meals, reducing the consumption of snacks, increasing the consumption of meals of low caloric value and decreasing their "nibbling" between meals), however, over time, poor eating habits can appear again [33].

We know the snack-eating pattern may present slower or unsatisfactory weight loss when compared to a normal eating pattern [34]. This occurs because the snack-eating pattern presents higher calorie intake, due to the consumption of foods that do provide satiety, reaching almost two times the energy intake of a person who presents a normal eating pattern [30, 34]. This pattern is found, according to the literature, in an individual who consumes salty snacks—crackers, packaged snack foods, peanuts—between meals, twice a week or more, in portions that add up to 150 kcal or more [27].

The cross-sectional study written by Larsen et al. [35] found that the prevalence of binge eating (usually, more than two times a week, with a fast bulky intake of food and no compensatory actions) was significantly lower in bariatric groups when compared with pre-op groups. Scholtz et al. [36] found that subjects who developed an eating disorder (including binge eating disorder - BED) postoperatively were more likely not to succeed after RYGB surgery, presenting a loss of excess weight of less than 40%.

11. Surgeries with a Higher Malabsorptive Component

In surgeries with a higher malabsorptive component, the evolution in the first postoperative month follows the same pattern seen among RYGB patients, but since gastric restriction is not so intense, the intake volume may be increased to 50 ml in the first days. Due to the malabsorption, fits of diarrhea may occur, which are handled with a low-residue, hypolipidic diet. The high consumption of greasy foods may increase the incidence of diarrhea and flatulence. Larger fecal losses of protein, along with some vitamins and minerals, occur [37]. Table 5 shows the daily absorption of calories, fats, nitrogen, and calcium after Scopinaro surgery. Due to losses related to this type of operation, protein intake in Scopinaro or Duodenal-Switch surgery patients must be higher than among those who underwent RYGB surgery. The daily recommendation is at least 90 grams of protein [37]. Concerning calcium, a daily supplementation of 2 grams of calcium citrate must take place. Excess weight loss in malabsorptive surgeries reaches 80% of this value in long term (more than five postoperative years). Nutritional assessments and lab tests must be performed following the same procedure as in RYGB. Vitamin and mineral supplementation must be taken throughout the patient's whole life [17].

Table 5. Consumption of calories, fats, nitrogen, and calcium and average daily absorption in Scopinaro surgery patients

Nutrient	Average consumption	Average absorption
Calories in 24h	3,070	58%
Fat (g/24h)	130	28%
Nitrogen (g/24h)	27	57%
Calcium (mg/24h)	1,994	26%

Source: Scopinaro (2000) [37].

Conclusion

Bariatric surgery is the only efficient treatment for severe obesity nowadays. Nutritional support is indispensable so that this tool may be used successfully, with the aim to achieve a healthy weight loss. Nutritional follow-up in bariatric surgery must begin from the preoperative period, contemplating changes in eating habits.

Diet prescription should be personalized . Diet therapy adherence will depend on the ability of the professional nutritionist to adapt recommendations related to bariatric surgery to the individual's lifestyle and preferences. The use of protein, vitamin and mineral supplementation is essential in maintaining a healthy weight loss.

A fundamental dietary factor for healthy weight loss in bariatric surgery is a proper consumption of proteins of high biological value. An inadequate protein intake is associated with lean mass loss and malnutrition. These factors influence in long-term weight maintenance and in the quality of life of these patients.

References

[1] Buchwald H, Avidor Y, Braundwald E, et al. Batritric surgery: a systematic review and metaanalysis. *JAMA*, 2004;292(14):1724 37.

[2] Elliot K. Nutritional Consideration After Bariatric Surgery. *Crit. Care Nurs. Q*, 2003;26(2):133 - 138.

[3] Brolin, RE, Robertson LB, Kenler, H, Cody, R. Weight Loss and Dietary Intake After Vertical Banded Gastroplasty and Roux-en-Y Gastric Bypass. *Annals of Surgery*, 1994;220:782-790.

[4] Aills L, Blankenship J, Buffington C, et al. ASMBS allied health nutritional guidelines for the surgical weight loss patient. *Surg. Obes. Relat. Dis.*, 2008;4(Supp):73-108.

[5] Heber D, Greenway FL, Kaplan LM, et al. Endocrine and nutritional management of the post-bariatric surgery patient: na Endocrine Society Clinical Practice Guideline. *J. Clin. Endocrinol. Metab.*, 2010;95(11):4823–43.

[6] Kushner RF, Kunigk A, Alspaugh M, Andronis PT, Leitch CA e Schoeller D. Validation of bioeletrictrial-impedance analysis as measurement of change in body composition in obesity. *Am. J. Clin. Nutr.*, 1990;52:219-23.

[7] Faria SL, Kelly E, Faria OP. Energy expenditure and weight regain in patients submitted to Roux-en Y gastric bypass. *Obes. Surg.*, 2009 Jul;19(7):856-9. Epub 2009 Apr 28.

[8] Marcason, W. What are the Dietary Guidelines Following Bariatric Surgery? Question of the month. *Journal of the American Dietetic Association*, 2004;104: 487-488.

[9] Maclean LD, Rhode BM, Shizgal, HM. Nutrition following gastric operations for mordid obesity. *Ann. Surg.*, 1983;198(3):347-55.

[10] Rhode, BM, Maclean LD. Vitamin and Mineral Supplementation after Gastric Bypass. In: Up date: Surgery for the morbidly obese patient. 1[a] ed, FD – Communications Inc., Toronto: 161-170, 2000.

[11] Cottam DR, Atkinson JA, Anderson A, Grace B, Fisher B. A case-controlled matched-pair cohort study of laparoscopic Rouxen-Y gastric bypass and Lap-Band® patients in a single U. S. Center with three-year follow-up. *Obes. Surg.*, 2006;16:534–40.

[12] Kushner RF. Managing the obese patient after bariatric surgery: a case report of severe malnutrition and review of the literature. *Journal of Parenteral and Enteral Nutrition*, 2000;24 (2):126-32.

[13] Faria SL, Faria OP, Lopes TC, Galvão MV, Kelly EO, Ito MK. Relation Between Carbohydrate Intake and Weight Loss After Bariatric Surgery. *Obes. Surg.*, 2009b;19:708-16.
[14] Faria SL, Kelly EO, Lins RD, Faria OP. Nutritional Management of Weight Regain After Bariatric Surgery. *Obes. Surg.*, 2010b;20:135-139.
[15] Moize V, Geliebter A, Gluck ME, *et al.* Obese Patients Have Inadequate Protein Intake Related to Protein Intolerance Up to 1 Year Following Roux-en-Y Gastric Bypass. *Obes. Surg.*, 2003;13:23-8.
[16] Standard Committee. Guidelines for Reporting Results in Bariatric Surgery. *Obes Surg.*, 1997;7:521-522.
[17] Stocker DJ. Management of bariatric surgery patient. *Endocrinololy and Metabolism Clinics North America,* 2003;32:437-457.
[18] Faria SL, Faria OP, Gouvêa HR, Melo TR. Nutritional Management of Weight Loss Surgery Complications. *Nutrição em Pauta,* 2011;1:29-33.
[19] Jones D. Weight LOss surgery: A Multidisciplinary approach. Pennsylvania: Matrix Medical Communications, 2008.
[20] Faria, SL, Faria OP, Buffington C, Cardeal MA, Ito MK. Dietary Protein Intake and Bariatric Surgery Patients: A Review. *Obes. Surg.*, 2011b;21(11):1798-805.
[21] Woodward, BG. The surgical Experience. In: A complete guide to obesity surgery 1[a] ed Trafford Publishing, *Victoria,* 82:115, 2001.
[22] Moize VL, Pi-Sunyer X, Mochari H, et al. Nutritional Pyramid for Post-gastric Bypass Patients. *Obes. Surg.,* 2010;20(8):1133-41.
[23] DRI. Institute of Medicine, Food and Nutrition Board, Dietary Reference Intakes: energy, carbohydrate, fiber, fat, fatty acids, cholesterol, protein and amino acids. Washington: The National Academy; 2005.
[24] Diabetes Care. American Diabetes Association - ADA. Clinical Practice Recommedation. 2011. 4. Avaliable in:http://care. diabetesjournals. org/content/34 /Supplement_1#Introduction.
[25] Faria SL, Faria OP, Lopes TC, et al. Relation between carbohydrate intake and weight loss after bariatric surgery. *Obes. Surg.*, 2008;19(6):708–16.
[26] Scruggs DM, Cowan GS, Klesges L, et al. Weight Loss and Calorie Intake after Regular and Extended Gastric Bypass. *Obes. Surg.,* 1993;3:233-8.
[27] Brolin RE, Robertson LB, Kenler HA, et al. Weight Loss and Dietary Intake After Vertical Banded Gastroplasty and Roux-en-Y Gastric Bypass. *Ann. Surg.,* 1994;220(6):782-90.
[28] Faria SL, Faria OP, Lins RD, Gouvêa HR. Hair Loss Among Bariatric Patients. *Bariatric Times,* 2010;7(11):18-20.
[29] Goldemberg, L. Hyperinsulinemic Hypoglycemia Following Weight Loss Surgery. In: Rosenthal RJ, Jones DB (Eds.). Weight Loss Surgery: A Multidisciplinary Approach. Edgemont: Ed. MMC (Matrix Medical Communications), 2008. p. 407-412.
[30] Hsu LKG, Benotti PN, Dwyer J, Roberts S, Saltzman E, Shikora S *et al.* Nonsurgical Factors That Influence the Outcome of Bariatric Surgery : A Review. *Psychosomatic Medicine,* 1998;60:338-346.
[31] Valezi AC, de Brito SJ, Junior JM, de Brito EM. Late meal pattern in obese people after banded Roux-en-Y gastric bypass: comparision between male and female. *Rev. Col. Bras. Cir.,* 2008;35(6):387-91.

[32] Department of Health and Human Services (HHS); Department of Agriculture (USDA). Food Guide Pyramide (2005). 2005. Disponivel em http://www. sne. org /myplate/index. php.

[33] Lang T, Hauser R, Buddeberg C, Klaghofer R. Impact of gastric banding on eating behavior and weight. *Obes. Surg.*, 2002;12:100 – 7.

[34] Faria SL, Kelly EO, Faria OP, Ito MK. Snack-Eating Patients Experience Lesser Weight Loss After Roux-En-Y Gastric Bypass Surgery. *Obes. Surg.,* 2009;19:1293-1296.

[35] Larsen JK, van Ramshorst B, Geenen R, Brand N, Stroebe W, van Doornen LJ. Binge eating and its relationship to outcome after laparoscopic adjustable gastric banding. *Obes. Surg.,* 2004 Sep;14(8):1111-7.

[36] Scholtz S, Bidlake L, Morgan J, Fiennes A, El-Etar A, Lacey JH. Long-term outcomes following laparoscopic adjustable gastric banding: postoperative psychological sequelae predict outcome at 5-year follow-up. *Obes. Surg.,* 2007;17:1220 – 5.

[37] Scopinaro N, Adami GF, Marinari GM, Traverso E, Papadia F e Camerini G. Biliopancreatic Diversion: Two Decades of Experience. In: Update: Surgery for the morbidly obese patient. 1[a] ed, FD – Communications Inc., Toronto: 227-258, 2000.

In: Bariatric Surgery
Editor: Christos R. Iavazzo
ISBN: 978-1-62618-995-9

Chapter XII

Bariatric and Metabolic Revisionary Surgery

W. Konrad Karcz and Simon Kuesters
Centre for Obesity and Metabolic Surgery,
University of Freiburg, Germany

Abstract

The number of bariatric operations performed each year is growing continuously, and it is to be assumed that this trend will continue in the coming years. Furthermore, we will probably experience a lot of metabolic operations in the near future. Surgical procedures for type II diabetes alone may lead to a dramatic extension of this field. In the past, not all of our procedures for treating obesity were well chosen. Some of them were not adequate for the patient needs, behaviour or metabolic disease. Over time, there has been growing need for re-operations to improve outcome. We do not know how many patients have undergone redo bariatric and metabolic surgery worldwide. Each clinic has its own percentage of re-operations, and it is said to be between 2 and 20%. In our clinic, there is a growing number of patients who need revisionary surgery due to poor weight loss after the primary operation. Patients in need of redo bariatric surgery usually come to a reference metabolic centre. The development and improvement of diagnostic procedures and guidelines prior to redo surgery is still one of our main objectives. The problem of choosing the right revisionary procedure and discussing it with the patient is of highest importance.

Introduction

Primary bariatric operations are relatively safe; a meta analysis reports mortality rates of 0. 02-1% [1]. However, the re-operation rate has been as high as 56% in some series and bariatric redo-operations are technically demanding [2]. The real number of reoperations is not known. Revisionary operations within 30 days after primary surgery are mostly caused by technical problems and should be treated according to general surgical principals. It must be mentioned that clinical diagnosis of in intra abdominal complications is more difficult in obese patients. In case of any suspect early diagnosis using abdominal computed tomography and if necessary diagnostic re-laparoscopy must be achieved. The most common indications for late re-operation are metabolic indications: insufficient weight loss, weight regain or recurrence of obesity-related comorbidities [2, 3]. Nevertheless, some patients come with chronic abdominal symptoms like pain, symptoms of stenosis or dumping syndrome. Thirdly, there is a group of patients that suffers from overly "effective" operation results, e. g. extreme gastric restriction or malabsorption. In this chapter we present various options for redo surgery and guidelines that should be considered when choosing the procedure.

Indications for Redo Surgery

Indications for revisionary operations can be divided into two categories: early and late postoperative complications. The first group includes haemorrhage (intraluminal, intra abdominal and others), suture insufficiency (pouch, remnant stomach, duodenum, intestine, GEA, DIA, JJA and JIA), early herniations (mostly Littre`s hernia), ileus, primary implant problems, wound infections, intra abdominal abscess etc. These complications should be promptly and consistently solved according to general surgical principals. The second group can be divided into three different clusters: implant-related, alimentary tract-related and metabolic recurrence or aggravation-related problems.

Implant-related complications are directly associated with gastric banding, Endo Barrier, rings and bandings [4-6]. The three most common problems associated with implants are migration, dislocation and infection. Also common are port disorders in cases of adjustable gastric banding [5].

Alimentary tract-related complications usually lead to general and unspecific symptoms like: recurrent emesis, abdominal pain, pyrosis or diarrhoea. Correlating morphologic diagnoses include stenosis (GEE, JJE), oesophageal dilatation, biliary or acid reflux, ulcerations (pouch, remnant stomach, duodenum, GEA), bowel obstruction and others. The most interesting group of late surgical complications includes appearance, recurrence or persistence of metabolic disorders. Here we include inadequate weight loss, weight regain, dumping syndrome [early and late], extensive malabsorption, problems related to malabsorption of medication [7], persistence and recurrence of obesity-related diseases (recurrence of isolated diabetes [insulin required, oral drugs required], recurrence of metabolic syndrome or dyslipidemia, etc.). Up to now, the most common cause for reoperations following bariatric surgery is insufficient weight loss or weight regain. However, the current changes and extension of indications for primary operations will probably lead to changes of redo-surgery in this field [2, 3, 8-10].

We have identified several important indications for revisionary surgery after bariatric and metabolic operations:

- Emergency operations – according to general surgical principles.
- Weight regain – more than 2 kg per month for longer than 3 months,

- Insufficient restriction – dilatation of GE, pouch or sleeve, dysfunction of lower oesophageal sphincter, band slippage.
- Insufficient weight control – BMI >40 kg/m^2 2 years after the primary procedure.
- Poor quality of life - BAROS Score < 3 with accordant complaints [11]
- Recurrence or persistence of obesity-related diseases one year after primary surgery
- intestinal tract-related problems.

Contraindications of Revisionary Surgery

Two main principals should be considered: patients without a follow up history ought to undergo 3 to 6-month observation in a reference centre before redo surgery. Detailed evaluation and adequate diagnostics performed in the reference centre are absolutely necessary. In our opinion, contraindications for a redo procedure are: lack of full diagnostic evaluation, lack of approval from the associated consultants on a metabolic board, lack of sports activity and lack of compliance. We are also using practical metabolic redo principles: avoid combining a strong restriction with malabsoption, do not reduce the gastric pouch volume to fewer than 10 ml and do not shorten the common channel under 50 cm. Ignoring these principles leads to late complications and further reoperations.

Diagnostics before Revision

The patient's eating habits is one of the most important factors which should be evaluated in detail. Eating protocols are very useful and should be analyzed by a professional dietician and a psychologist specialized in eating disorders. All questions concerning volume and frequency of meals are important for the surgeon, since they provide information about the functional stomach volume. In practice, we use the so-called Pizza-question, which gives approximate information about the gastric pouch volume. If the patient is able to eat more than half of a medium pizza, the restriction is no longer sufficient. Other tests, like the cottage cheese probe described by Flanagan are also useful [12]. The second important factor is the patient's physical activity which should be assessed with objective measurements, for instance resting energy expenditure (REE) or calorimetry to objectify the muscle condition [13]. Unfortunately, the information given by the patients is always subjective. Prior to a revisionary operation, the surgeon needs objective and detailed information about the stomach pouch volume. As a standard method, a two dimensional X-ray with contrast medium is used to estimate the stomach pouch volume and its function [14-18].

However, the volume of the pouch is reduced to two dimensional areas which are measured semi-quantitatively. Furthermore, images can often only be taken in one plane due to the obese patient's body dimensions. It is also possible that different parts of the stomach pouch or sleeve are not placed in an optimal position – which results in an over-projection, especially if the pouch or sleeve is voluminous. The development of the stomach pouch volumetry using multislice computed tomography scans (MSCT) and special software for 3D-rendering allows precise estimation of pouch and sleeve volumes and also evaluation of related anatomical structures [19]. It also allows exact measurement of anastomoses, their shapes and positions after gastric bypass surgery (Figure 1).

This directly influences redo surgery. Furthermore, other pathologies like fistulas or internal herniations can be evaluated.

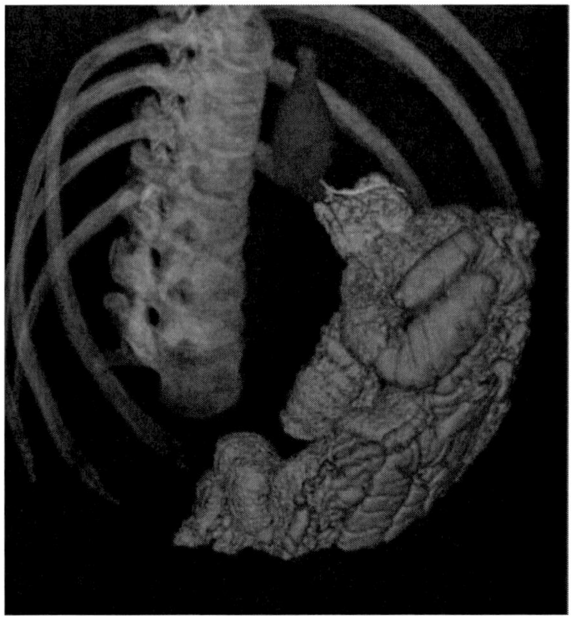

Figure 1. 3D volume rendering reconstruction of abdominal MSCT showing a dilatation of the stomach pouch ($55cm^3$) and GE anastomosis (Diameter 4. 2 cm, area 12. $2cm^2$). Manual and semi-automatic segmentation techniques are applied to show the pouch (orange), the Roux-limb (green), and the staple sutures (white).

Another essential examination is upper endoscopy with morphological inspection of the oesophagus, the lower oesophageal sphincter, the stomach pouch, anastomoses and the upper intestine [20, 21]. All pathological changes should undergo histopathological inspection. The Helicobacter pylori test (f. i. HUT) needs to be performed prior to each redo surgery procedure [22].

There is another group of functional examinations that can deliver useful information: Oesophageal and stomach pouch / sleeve 24h manometry, pH-metry and NMR Dynamic Stomach Movement (NMR-DSM) are the most important ones [23-25]. The lower oesophageal sphincter (LES) is responsible for keeping the pouch closed. After food enters into the stomach, the region of the cardia is stretched, resulting in a feeling of satiety. An insufficient LES is responsible for gastroesophageal reflux after sleeve gastrectomy, partly for a lack of satiety as well as oesophagus dilatation after gastric banding, VBG, sleeve or bypass procedures.

The peristaltic NMR-DMS is able to recognize the speed of stomach emptying and peristaltic wave after sleeve gastrectomy and the function of the pylorus. In the future, these examinations could influence the selection of the procedure if metabolic redo surgery is needed [25]. Blood tests can objectify the patient's response to oral vitamin and microelement supplementation. Results should influence the selection of redo surgery.

Redo Surgery Following Obsolete Bariatric Operations

There are still patients who received jejunoileal bypasses (JIB) in the past and should undergo redo surgery. In the past, we performed such revisions mainly in open technique. The laparoscopic approach can be very difficult because of intestinal adhesions which can lead to long operation time and intestinal lesions [26]. Almost all bariatric operations, from physiological reconstruction to the Scopinaro-operation, were performed after JIB [27-30]. Concerning the choice of the revisionary operation, the patient's BMI, the time of follow-up, and individual patient needs ought to be considered. The most conservative option is to transform the JIB into a BPD or BPD-DS. This can be done easily as an open procedure under the following conditions: the patient has no diarrhoea, no hypoproteinemia, no liver disorder and no deficiency of lipid-soluble vitamins. From the technical point of view, the procedure itself could be performed as a hybrid operation with the upper part done laparoscopically at the beginning (almost no adhesions there) and the intestinal part with open access through the old cicatrix. In our opinion, the conversion should be performed if 20 min of laparoscopic operation do not lead to progress.

The conventional proximal gastric bypass is a good option especially for patients with malnutrition, severe flatulence and diarrhoea. Another popular procedure is the physiological reconstruction of the intestine followed by sleeve gastrectomy to prevent weight regain. Isolated reconstruction of the intestine was mostly done in patients with extreme malabsorption.

Patients after Vertical Banded Gastroplasty (VBG) are still seen in clinical practice. Today, the VBG is rarely performed due to disappointing long-term results and a variety of alternative metabolic operations [2, 31]. Frequent complications with the band and the vertical stapling line lead to a high re-operation rate after VBG [2, 32]. In the past, a common redo operation was restapling of the vertical suture or the complete separation of the pouch and remnant stomach with a GIA stapler. After VBG, we found two main groups of patients: patients with strong restriction (vomiting more than once every day) and without any restriction (mostly due to vertical stapling rupture and gastro-gastric fistula).

The anatomical and functional status of the stomach should be evaluated with gastroscopy, contrast medium or if possible 3D MSCT. If the patient regains weight or in cases of aggravation or recurrence of associated comorbidities, it might be necessary to perform a conventional Roux-en-Y gastric Bypass (CRYGB) as a revisionary operation [2, 31, 33-35] (Figure 2). In patients scheduled for CRYGB after VBG, Fobi at al. left the pouch and band in place and performed the bypass distal to the VGB-banding. This led to the development of the primary Banded Roux-en-Y gastric bypass procedure [36, 37]. Nowadays, patients who don't suffer from strong restriction after VBG can be operated with a Banded Gastric Bypass (BRYGB), but with formation of a completely new pouch.

The first reoperations after VBG were done in open fashion. Now, we prefer to perform the operation laparoscopically. After adhaesiolysis, dissection of the greater curvature and the opening of the bursa omentalis should be performed.

The whole fundus should then be separated from the omentum majus with cutting of the short gastric vessels. The whole fundus should then be separated from the omentum majus with cutting of the short gastric vessels. The adhesions in the bursa omentalis are then much easier to identify and to separate, the banding is easier to identify, and the vertical stapler line is clearer to see. Afterwards, the stomach should be horizontally dissected under the banding using a vertical linear stapler. Preparation of the lesser curvature and the left diaphragm crus is then easy to perform. Afterwards, the formation of the stomach pouch with a partial resection of the old dilated VBG pouch, the fundus and banding can be done. Weiner et al. proposed performing the Scopinaro procedure after VBG under three conditions: The distal stomach with the banding should be resected, the rejunction of the vertical VGB separation ought to be performed, and the patient's BMI has to be over 50 kg/m^2 [35, 38].

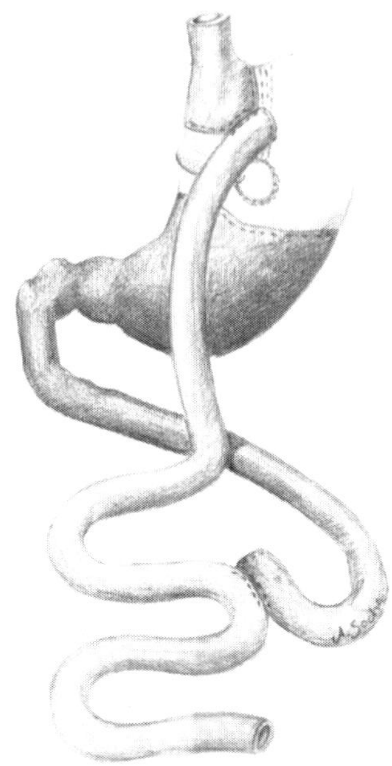

Figure 2. Conventional Roux-en-Y Gastric Bypass after Vertical Banded Gastroplasty.

Several types of operations can be performed to re-establish sufficient restriction. Indications are: vertical staple line rupture, a good toleration of restriction, and relatively slow weight regain. There are several options: introduction of gastric banding or the sleeve gastrectomy with or without resection of the band [39]. The B2 – gastric bypass, also called the Minibypass might lead to biliary reflux if it is performed as a one anastomosis bypass without the Braun's anastomosis. Furthermore, stomach pouch and GEA dilatation are frequent because of the pouch formation technique, and the incidence of Petersen herniation is higher than after the RnYGB. The size of the stomach pouch should be carefully evaluated before redo surgery. The transformation into RYGB or BRYGB is normally combined with a pouch reduction, a translocation of the biliopancreatic limb 80 to 100 cm below the GEA and closing of the Petersen and Y apertures. Those reoperations usually lead to weight stabilization and improvement of the local mucosa status. The procedure can be easily performed laparoscopically. The adhesions are normally not severe, and identification of anatomical structures is possible. When the patient gains weight prior to the revision and the pouch is bigger than 150 ml, it is possible to perform a biliopancreatic diversion with a common channel (CC) of 75 to 100 cm. To perform a Scopinaro-standard CC, the stomach pouch has to be bigger than 200 ml and the patient's BMI has to be >45 kg/m^2. If these conditions are not fulfilled, the standard BPD-S operation with a short CC should not be performed.

Revisionary Operations after Restrictive Surgery

Almost all bariatric procedures include gastric restriction either by building a small pouch a sleeve or upper stomach formation. The mechanical control and the neural sensation of satiety are the two main components of gastric restriction. In cases of insufficient weight loss or recurrent metabolic comorbidities, the anatomic aspects of stomach pouch or sleeve inlet, outlet and volume have to be evaluated [40]. Many revisionary operations focus on the stomach pouch and its outlet but in the case of LES dysfunction, there will be no success if the revision is limited to the pouch size and pouch outlet.

The most popular metabolic operations based on restriction are the Laparoscopic Adjustable Gastric Banding (LAGB), the Laparoscopic Sleeve Gastrectomy (LSG) and the Laparoscopic Roux-en-Y Gastric Bypass, if it is not performed as a distal bypass. If there is pouch dilation, the re-establishment of restriction leads to weight reduction and improvement of the metabolic disorders in most cases [18, 41].

Introduction of Malabsorption

Insufficient restriction quickly leads to metabolic disturbances, weight regain and recurrence of associated diseases, especially in procedures based solely on food limitation. It is not easy to decide which method ought to be chosen in these cases. It is also not easy to decide in favour of a revisionary malabsorptive surgery.

The most important question that has to be answered is: Is the patient capable of accepting the disadvantages of malabsorption? Artificially shortening of the intestine leads to chronic physiological changes. The recovery of sufficient restriction should therefore be considered first. An accurate diagnostic investigation may help to understand the mechanical situation of the intestinal tract, but is it a sufficient argument for introducing a malabsorptive component? All patients, who qualify for malabsorptive surgery, ought to be discussed by an interdisciplinary board following independent psychological, dietetic and metabolic consultation. After patient education concerning the disadvantages of malabsorption, preoperative diagnostics and interdisciplinary consensus, the indication for malabsorptive surgery can be made.

It has to be noted that there are clear contraindications of secondary malabsorptive operations, such as a BMI under 35 after the primary metabolic procedure, a pre-existing malabsorptive state, malnutrition in vegetarians, pre-existing diarrhoea, psychiatric diseases, and apparent lack of compliance. All patients with a history of major abdominal surgery with consecutive malabsorption, like after ileum or colon resections for any reason, history of drug or alcohol abuse, history of recent or chronic steroid medication, autoimmune disease, inflammatory bowel disease, liver cirrhosis (CHILD B + C), serious active viral or bacterial diseases (e. g. HIV, Hepatitis B and C, Tbc etc), pregnancy, history of any neoplasms in the last five years, need of long-term anticoagulation for any reason and immunosuppression should be excluded from this type of treatment. Proper selection of patients for malabsorptive procedures is a fundamental principle.

The amount of malabsorption is directly associated with the length of the common channel (CC). The standard malabsorptive operations, i. e. the Scopinaro procedure and the duodenal switch (DS), have a CC of 50 and 75-100cm [42, 43]. The incidence of malabsorptive complications is higher in patients with lower compliance. In all redo procedures, one should attempt a laparoscopic approach.

Revisions after Gastric Banding

The LABG was a favoured bariatric operation due to its low invasiveness and complete reversibility. But long-term observation showed a high rate of reoperations and an explantation rate of up to 40% [44-47]. Suter et al. reported a 33% complication and 20% revision rate [48]. These results demonstrate that correct implantation of the band is not an easy task. Regaining weight after LAGB is mostly caused by dislocation, migration and pouch dilation. However some patients show a substantial weight regain with the band still remaining in its correct position. In some cases further blocking of the band will lead to vomiting while leaving it with no further blocking will result in weight regain.

Other common problems are infection and port-related problems like infection, dislocation, or disconnection [5]. There are a lot of possibilities for re-establishing restriction after gastric banding. Re-banding is possible, but an even higher failure rate is reported after re-banding [49-52]. It is also possible to perform a sleeve gastrectomy after removal of the band. The results published by Frezza et al. show that SG after LAGB is a real alternative to RYGB [52]. It is important to completely remove adhesions and sutures in the area where the band was placed so that the gastric wall is completely unfolded. Otherwise a stapling of the still doubled gastric wall might occur, leading to a leakage.

The option of a gastric bypass should be strongly considered for patients with persistent or recurrent metabolic diseases [49, 50]. In our opinion the band should be removed and the bypass should be created as a two-step procedure. The two-step procedure (band removal as a first and bypass formation as a second operation) could reduce the risk of leakage caused by muscular atrophy underneath the band or doubling of the stomach wall in the staple line. Differences of thickness of the stomach wall might also lead to stapler line insufficiencies. In our opinion, it is important to restore the anatomy by removing the band and performing the secondary operation two or more months later.

There are a lot of clinics that perform the Scopinaro procedure after gastric banding. The advantage of this technique is that it involves another "operating region" and a completely different mechanism of action. This option seems to be very good for patients with stress eating habits and a BMI over 50kg/m^2. The BPD-DS is not always easy to perform after LAGB because the sleeve resection involves the band adhesion area which can lead to local stapler insufficiencies and thus significantly influence the risk for complications. There is also the option of introducing malabsorption with a 100cm CC as an isolated duodenal switch. The band has to be completely opened or better explanted during the procedure; a gastric resection is not made. Such a procedure leads to roughly 60% of EWL [53].

Revisions after Sleeve Gastrectomy

The sleeve gastrectomy was first performed in the context of BPD-DS [42;54]. The volume of the remaining gastric tube should be roughly 100 -120 ml. This can be controlled by using a calibration tube during the procedure [55, 56]. Nowadays, most bariatric surgeons use a 32 or 34 F Bogie to form a proper-sized sleeve [56, 57]. A larger gastric tube seems to correlate with a higher risk of weight regain and sleeve dilatation [55]. We do not have long term results yet, but it is already known that 50% of all patients after SG undergo a secondary operation. Nocca et al. reported a 6% rate of weight regain 2 years after SG [58]. We recommend performing a stomach 3D MSCT with volumetry before reoperations [19].

Restoring restriction with a re-sleeve-operation could lead to dysfunction of stomach motility, stenosis, and reflux with emesis or dysphagia. Such complications have to be treated with myotomy or resection of a stenosis [59 [. Re-sleeve gastrectomy is therefore only recommended in cases of large sleeve dilations with a sleeve volume >500 ml [60]. There are two main causes for dilation after SG: an operative technique with a primary sleeve greater than 200 ml and patients who keep or relapse into volume eating habits [58]. The re-sleeve operation can be used safely for patients who still have a BMI over 50-60 and a volume of the primary sleeve > 400ml. In these cases it is also possible to place a ring (banded sleeve gastrectomy) around the upper part of the sleeve (approx. 6 cm below the cardia) to reduce the risc of a re-dilatation [61]. In case of a sleeve dilation of 250-400 ml, where a re-sleeve-resection should not be performed, duplication of the gastric wall using an extraluminal running suture will reduce the sleeve volume and can lead to a sufficient restriction [62].

Another option for restoring restriction is the conversion into a gastric bypass. It is easy to transform the sleeve into a conventional or banded gastric bypass. The conventional gastric bypass does not lead to large weight changes, but the influence on metabolic disorders is greater compared to the SG [63;64]. The gastric bypass operation can also be performed in case of a localized stricture of the sleeve, if the stricture is located distally enough to create the pouch for the gastric bypass.

Since the sleeve gastrectomy was first performed only in the context of BPD-DS, the consequent secondary malabsorptive procedure after sleeve gastrectomy is the BPD with duodenal switch. At about one third of patients after sleeve gastrectomy receive secondary BPD in our series. The introduction of malabsorption with a CC of 75 -100cm (longer CC in case of stronger restriction / smaller sleeve volume) with DS is an effective method. In our series, almost all patients with super-obesity weighed less than 100kg one year after DS performed as a second-step operation, and a mean BMI reduction of 12 points is seen in our patients [65]. However, the indication for a second step BPD should be considered carefully, as BPD might lead to severe complications like malnutrition and hypovitaminosis. It is also possible to perform a single anastomosis duodeno-ileal omega bypass after the LSG (SADI-S) [66]. The advantage of this procedure is the fact that only one anastomosis is needed and the common channel is longer than after BPD-DS, which might reduce the risk of malabsorption syndrome. However, long term results of the SADIS-S operation still have to be evaluated.

Acid reflux and eosophagitis is commonly seen after sleeve gastrectomy. However, the data in the literature differs concerning the question if reflux symptoms after sleeve gastrectomy get worse or get better. In our experience an aggravation of reflux occurs in some patients, probably due to a partial migration of the sleeve into the thorax, thus weakening the LES and a poor peristalsis in the sleeve itself [67]. We therefore usually perform a "sleevepexie", suturing the upper end of the sleeve to the left crus of the diaphragm to prevent thoraxic migration. In case of severe reflux symptoms and eosophagitis after sleeve gastrectomy we would fist initiate a consequent protone pump inhibitor therapy. The next step would be a laparoscopic hiatoplastic and sleevopexie or a revision in to a gastric bypass. This normally solves all reflux symptoms, but takes the passibility to perform a BPD-DS or SADIS-S as a second step in case of weight regain.

Revisions after Gastric Bypass Surgery

The gastric bypass, the gold standard of bariatric surgery, leads to regain of weight in up to 40% of patients in the long term follow up [68], but the redo surgery rate is still lower than after VBG [2]. The long-term results presented by Chistou et al. show that 35% of patients after RYGB still have a BMI >35 kg/m^2 [69]. Other authors report better results (70, 71). It is unclear how many patients suffer from pouch dilatation or what the prevalence of GE dilatation is. The volume of the gastric pouch should be between 15 and 30 ml [71]. Larger pouch volumes can be caused by inappropriate operating techniques or secondarily by eating habits. The width of the GEA also plays an important role: if it is too small, it can lead to stenosis and impaired emptying of the pouch, but if it is too large, a dilation of the first jejununal loop can result [15]. In this case the first jejunum loop can contribute to the functional stomach volume and thus enlarge it [72].

The precise evaluation of the diameter and area of the anastomosis allows the surgeon to choose the best redo strategy for the patient. It is known that GE anastomosis dilation can lead to insufficient weight control [73]. If the patient tolerates restriction, there are several options for redo surgery. Endoscopic suturing to tighten a dilated gastric pouch is technically feasible and safe with Stomafix as NOS (Natural Orifice Surgery), and may lead to weight loss for certain patients [74]. Another logical option is to implant a GaBP Ring in a redo operation with or without resizing of the pouch, thus creating a banded bypass [37]. An analogous procedure with gastric banding in addition to the RnYGB was proposed by Bessler et al. [75]. It might be an easy and effective way to control the volume and outlet of the pouch. We recommend using rings of at least 6. 5 cm length in primary and 7. 0 cm in redo operations [76, 77]. Some studies report a better weight reduction after banded bypasses. The banded bypass causes satiety and reduces caloric intake by delaying gastric emptying, even with low food intake. After 2 years, the percentage of EWL ranged around 80%, and at 5-year follow-up, the EWL was roughly 75%. Only a slight weight regain of 2. 5% or 5% is observed between the second and fifth postoperative year, whereas weight regain following LCRYGB is reported to be over 10% in the same period [78]. A gastro-gastric fistula can also lead to weight regain, patients normally report a lack of satiety and bigger meals. Normally a fistula can be diagnosed in radiological examination (contrast swallow / MSCT). However, in some cases the fistula might not be seen radiologically but then be diagnosed intraoperatively. Remarkably there is a big difference in the frequency of gastro-gastral fistulas after gastric bypass reaching from a few up to 40% in the literature [79, 80]. The dissection of the fistula, normally with a linear stapler will lead to further weight loss.

It is also possible but not uncritical to introduce malabsorption after gastric bypass surgery. In our opinion, a patient scheduled for reoperation should have a BMI > 40kg/m^2, a tendency of gaining weight or recurrence of associated morbidities to qualify for redo malabsorption. The size of the stomach pouch must be measured before the operation. The knowledge of the pouch volume allows the surgeon to choose the redo strategy and offers a criterion for introducing malabsorption.

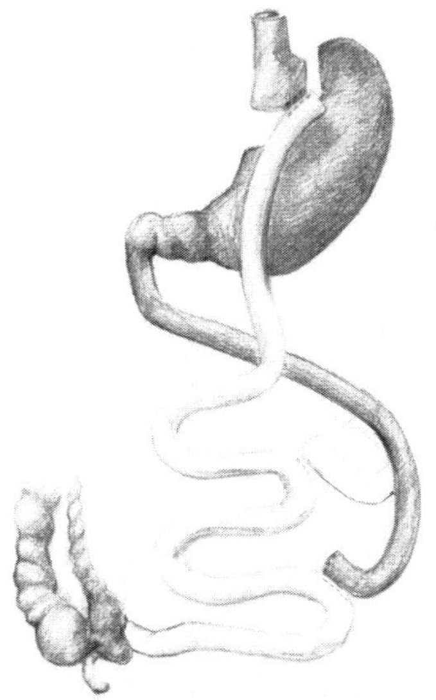

Figure 3. Biliopancreatic limb distalisation after conventional Roux-en-Y Gastric Bypass [conditions see the text] (Sugarman Procedure).

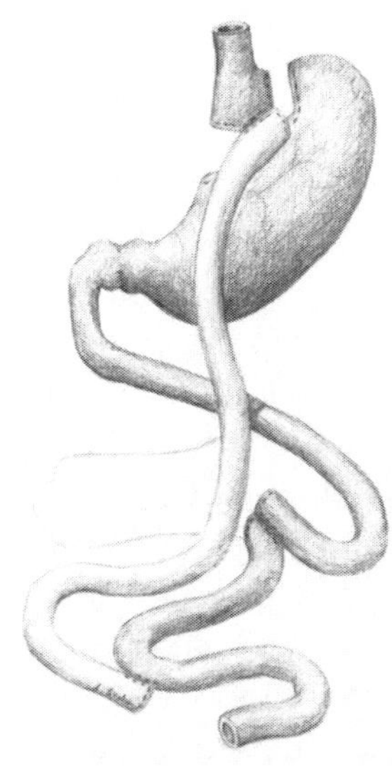

Figure 4. Alimentary limb distalisation after conventional Roux-en-Y Gastric Bypass [conditions see the text] (Himpens-Lemmens Procedure).

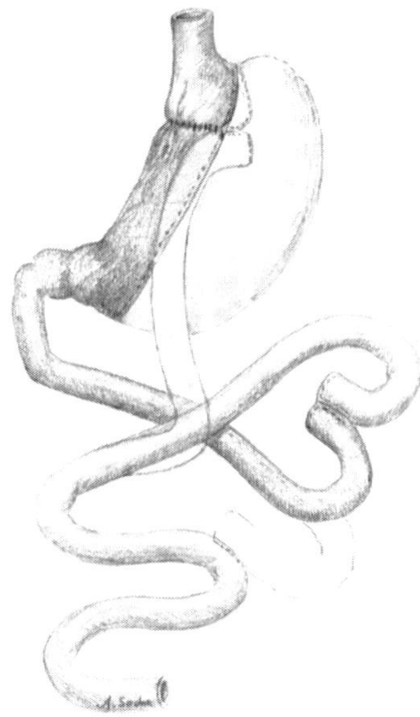

Figure 5. Roux-en-Y Gastric Bypass transformed into Sleeve gastrectomy with reconstruction of the intestinal tract.

When the functional stomach volume is bigger than 200ml (summary of stomach pouch and first jejunal loop when the anastomosis is bigger than 2. 5 cm), it is possible to perform the Sugerman operation with distalisation of the biliopancreatic loop or the relocation of the alimentary loop at about 100cm from Bauhin's Valve thus performing a distal gastric bypass (81;82)(Figure 3,4). Both of these operations are relatively easy to perform laparoscopically. The most difficult part is to disconnect the Roux-Y-anastomosis which can lead to stenosis or leakage. The ends of the trans positioned loops should always be resected to avoid suturing of the anastomosis in the scar tissue. Both operations lead to weight reduction and improvement of the metabolic situation. In case of a small functional gastric volume severe malnutrition symptoms can occur if malabsorption is added.

In this case another option, proposed by Gagner et al., is to change the RnYGB into a biliopancreatic diversion with duodenal switch [83] (Figure 5, 6). Gagner published a 40 % failure rate after RnYGB; these patients were successfully treated with a BPD-DS [68].

The transformation to a duodenal switch is technically difficult and has many potential complications. The reconstruction of the bypassed stomach with a gastro-gastrostomy and the following sleeve resection are the most difficult parts of the operation. The second half is very similar to the standard duodenal switch procedure. Performing the whole transformation during one operation is sometimes very difficult and leads to very long operating times [68, 83]. We have introduced a straight-forward criterion for when to perform a one-step operation: if the reconstruction of the stomach and the sleeve resection takes less than 120 min, we perform the whole operation at once. Usually, it is easier to divide the operation into two separate parts. This reduces the complication rate. The recovery of restriction and introduction of malabsorption usually lead to an improvement of weight loss and metabolic status in a short time [68].

Revisions after the Biliopancreatic Diversion

There are patients who underwent BPD-DS procedures without the use of gastric tubes for sleeve calibration. Many of these patients now suffer from considerable stomach dilatation with ensuing recurrence of metabolic disorders or weight regain in cases where the common channel is > 100cm.

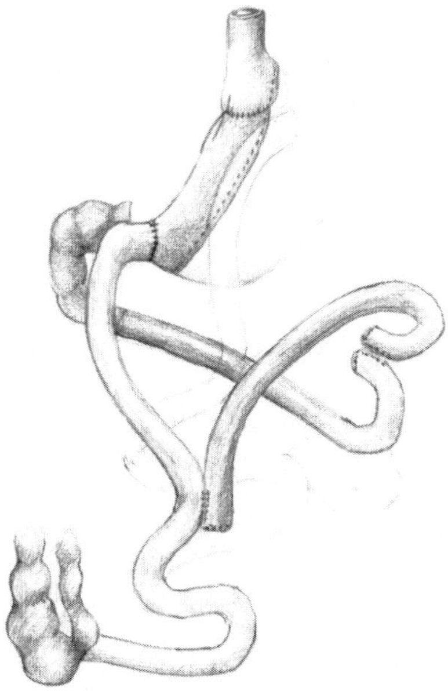

Figure 6. Roux-en-Y Gastric Bypass transformed procedure into Biliopancreatic Diversion with Duodenal Switch.

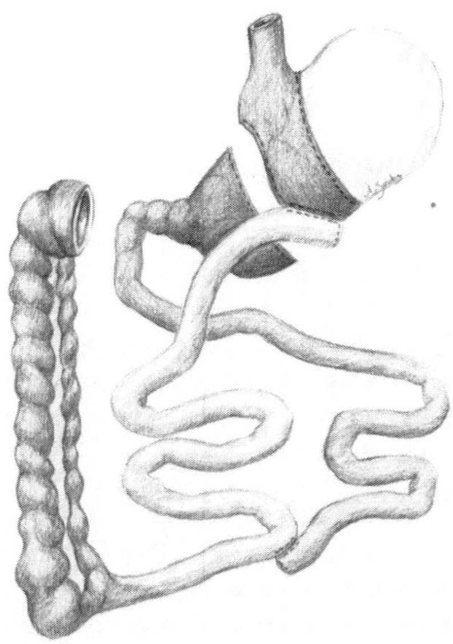

Figure 7. Biliopancreatic Diversion with additional stomach fundus resection.

The stomach volume should then be reduced to about 200ml to evoke a feeling of satiety again [60]. A similar constellation can be observed in a small group of BPD patients who present an upper stomach dilatation which can be treated with a fundus resection when necessary, thus reducing the stomach pouch to 150 – 200 ml. In our series a gastric re-resection after BPD leads to a mean reduction of 8 BMI points [65] (Figure 7).

In case of malnutritive symptoms with severe hypoalbuminemia, liver dysfunction, severe diarrhoeas, flatulence and in cases where the patient is not able to supplement adequately, it may be necessary to reduce malabsorption but preserve restriction. The introduction of the restriction with reduction of malabsoption is possible by transforming the BPD into the conventional or Banded Gastric Bypass. Analogous procedures are BPD-DS to C- or B-RYGB transformations. The transformation of BPD to BPD-DS is technically possible under the condition that the distal gastrectomy was not performed.

Conclusion

There is a variety of possible secondary operations after all bariatric operations. It may be a big challenge for the surgeon to choose the right revisionary procedure in case of insufficient weight loss. Detailed anamnesis and diagnostics are needed. If the wrong procedure is chosen, the patient might not lose further weight or suffer from severe complications.

However, if the right procedure is chosen there is a good chance for significant weight loss. In our series of reoperations due to poor weight loss or weight regain a mean loss of 10 BMI points is seen one year after the revision [65].

In our opinion, the artificial control of satiety is at least partly associated with the pouch volume. Hormonal and neural mechanisms also play an important role. Each year, several new hormonal or neurogenic active intestinal peptides are identified. Also, the electrical stimulation alone of vagal nerves, pylorus stimulation or stimulation of the duodenum leads to significant changes in the intestinal tract and body homeostasis [84]. In the future, restrictive surgery may be influenced by biologically active implants that react to physiological impulses from the IT and communicate directly or indirectly with central hunger regulation areas.

Prospective randomized trials are needed to compare different procedures. The group of patients with a revisionary operation due to recurrent or persistent metabolic disorders is growing. Reasons might be the limited spectrum of primary bariatric and metabolic procedures performed in some clinics and the lack of good indication guidelines. A systematic analysis of indications for different metabolic procedures needs to be discussed. This could probably lead to a lower reoperation rate. At the moment, there seems to be no golden standard operation in the growing area of metabolic surgery.

There are many new procedures, e. g. the duodenal bypass, the loop duodenal switch, the ileal transposition, the banded sleeve resection and the vertical stomach separation. Vagus-, stomach- or duodenal pacemakers and the Endo-Barrier are currently performed in small series or are still in the process of development [84-87]

Certainly, there will be different types of new primary and revisionary operations as a result of better understanding of the pathophysiology of metabolic processes. Furthermore, new methods implementing bioactive implants, genetically modified "simbionts", gene therapy, or new drugs will undoubtedly have a significant impact on primary and revisionary metabolic surgery in the future.

References

[1] Maggard MA, Shugarman LR, Suttorp M, Maglione M, Sugerman HJ, Livingston EH, et al. Meta-analysis: surgical treatment of obesity. *Ann. Intern. Med.,* 2005 Apr 5;142(7):547-59.

[2] van Gemert WG, van Wersch MM, Greve JW, Soeters PB. Revisional surgery after failed vertical banded gastroplasty: restoration of vertical banded gastroplasty or conversion to gastric bypass. *Obes. Surg.,* 1998 Feb;8(1):21-8.

[3] Gawdat K. Bariatric re-operations: are they preventable? *Obes. Surg.,* 2000 Dec;10(6):525-9.

[4] Fobi M, Lee H, Igwe D, Felahy B, James E, Stanczyk M, et al. Band erosion: incidence, etiology, management and outcome after banded vertical gastric bypass. *Obes. Surg.,* 2001 Dec;11(6):699-707.

[5] Weiss HG, Kirchmayr W, Klaus A, Bonatti H, Muhlmann G, Nehoda H, et al. Surgical revision after failure of laparoscopic adjustable gastric banding. *Br. J. Surg.,* 2004 Feb;91(2):235-41.

[6] Fishman E, Melanson D, Lamport R, Levine A. A novel endoscopic delivery system for placement of a duodenal-jejunal implant for the treatment of obesity and type 2 diabetes. *Conf. Proc. IEEE Eng. Med. Biol. Soc.,* 2008;2008:2501-3.

[7] Padwal R, Brocks D, Sharma AM. A systematic review of drug absorption following bariatric surgery and its theoretical implications. *Obes. Rev.,* 2009 Jun 1.

[8] Martin MJ, Bennett S. Pretransplant bariatric surgery: a new indication? *Surg. Obes. Relat. Dis.,* 2007 Nov;3(6):648-51.

[9] Pillai AA, Rinella ME. Non-alcoholic fatty liver disease: is bariatric surgery the answer? *Clin. Liver Dis.,* 2009 Nov;13(4):689-710.

[10] Schulman AP, Del GF, Sinha N, Rubino F. Metabolic Surgery for the Treatment of Type 2 Diabetes. *Endocr. Pract.,* 2009 Jul 20;1-24.

[11] Oria HE, Moorehead MK. Bariatric analysis and reporting outcome system (BAROS). *Obes. Surg.,* 1998 Oct;8(5):487-99.

[12] Flanagan L. Measurement of Functional Pouch Volume following the Gastric Bypass Procedure. *Obes. Surg.,* 1996 Feb;6(1):38-43.

[13] de Castro CM, de Lima Montebelo MI, Rasera I, Jr., de OA, Jr., Gomes Gonelli PR, Aparecida CG. Effects of Roux-en-Y gastric bypass on resting energy expenditure in women. *Obes. Surg.,* 2008 Nov;18(11):1376-80.

[14] Nishie A, Brown B, Barloon T, Kuehn D, Samuel I. Comparison of size of proximal gastric pouch and short-term weight loss following routine upper gastrointestinal contrast study after laparoscopic Roux-en-Y gastric bypass. *Obes. Surg.,* 2007 Sep;17(9):1183-8.

[15] Roberts K, Duffy A, Kaufman J, Burrell M, Dziura J, Bell R. Size matters: gastric pouch size correlates with weight loss after laparoscopic Roux-en-Y gastric bypass. *Surg. Endosc.*, 2007 Aug;21(8):1397-402.
[16] Madan AK, Tichansky DS, Phillips JC. Does pouch size matter? *Obes. Surg.*, 2007 Mar;17(3):317-20.
[17] Forsell P, Hellers G, Laveskog U, Westman L. Validation of Pouch Size Measurement Following the Swedish Adjustable Gastric Banding Using Endoscopy, MRI and Barium Swallow. *Obes. Surg.*, 1996 Dec;6(6):463-7.
[18] Langer FB, Bohdjalian A, Felberbauer FX, Fleischmann E, Reza Hoda MA, Ludvik B, et al. Does gastric dilatation limit the success of sleeve gastrectomy as a sole operation for morbid obesity? *Obes. Surg.*, 2006 Feb;16(2):166-71.
[19] Karcz WK, Kuesters S, Marjanovic G, Suesslin D, Kotter E, Thomusch O, et al. 3D-MSCT gastric pouch volumetry in bariatric surgery-preliminary clinical results. *Obes. Surg.*, 2009 Apr;19(4):508-16.
[20] Munoz R, Ibanez L, Salinas J, Escalona A, Perez G, Pimentel F, et al. Importance of routine preoperative upper GI endoscopy: why all patients should be evaluated? *Obes. Surg.*, 2009 Apr;19(4):427-31.
[21] de Moura AA, Cotrim HP, Santos AS, Bitencourt AG, Barbosa DB, Lobo AP, et al. Preoperative upper gastrointestinal endoscopy in obese patients undergoing bariatric surgery: is it necessary? *Surg. Obes. Relat. Dis.*, 2008 Mar;4(2):144-9.
[22] Hartin CW, Jr., Remine DS, Lucktong TA. Preoperative bariatric screening and treatment of Helicobacter pylori. *Surg. Endosc.*, 2009 May 15.
[23] Klaus A, Weiss H. Is preoperative manometry in restrictive bariatric procedures necessary? *Obes. Surg.*, 2008 Aug;18(8):1039-42.
[24] Merrouche M, Sabate JM, Jouet P, Harnois F, Scaringi S, Coffin B, et al. Gastro-esophageal reflux and esophageal motility disorders in morbidly obese patients before and after bariatric surgery. *Obes. Surg.*, 2007 Jul;17(7):894-900.
[25] Baumann T, Kuesters S, Grueneberger J, Marjanovic G, Zimmermann L, Schaefer AO, et al. Time-resolved MRI after ingestion of liquids reveals motility changes after laparoscopic sleeve gastrectomy--preliminary results. *Obes. Surg.*, 2011 Jan;21(1):95-101.
[26] Gentileschi P, Lirosi F, Benavoli D, Sica G, Di LN, Venza M, et al. Laparoscopic reoperative approach after open bariatric surgery. *Chir. Ital.*, 2009 Mar;61(2):137-41.
[27] Raftopoulos I, Courcoulas AP. Revision of jejunoileal bypass to Roux-en-Y gastric bypass: technical considerations and outcomes from 2 cases. *Surg. Obes. Relat. Dis.*, 2008 Mar;4(2):198-201.
[28] Hanni CL, Pool LR, Dean RE, Cronquist JC. Treatment of jejunoileal bypass failure by reanastomosis and gastroplasty in a single-stage procedure. Review of 47 cases. *Am. Surg.*, 1984 Jul;50(7):354-7.
[29] Junker K, Jensen JB, Jensen HE. Simultaneous small-intestinal reconstruction and gastric partitioning as treatment for complications after jejunoileal bypass for morbid obesity. *Scand. J. Gastroenterol.*, 1981 Apr;16(3):433-6.
[30] LaFave JW, Alden JF. Gastric bypass in the operative revision of the failed jejunoileal bypass. *Arch. Surg.*, 1979 Apr;114(4):438-44.
[31] Schouten R, van Dielen FM, van Gemert WG, Greve JW. Conversion of vertical banded gastroplasty to Roux-en-Y gastric bypass results in restoration of the positive

effect on weight loss and co-morbidities: evaluation of 101 patients. *Obes. Surg.,* 2007 May;17(5):622-30.

[32] Marsk R, Jonas E, Gartzios H, Stockeld D, Granstrom L, Freedman J. High revision rates after laparoscopic vertical banded gastroplasty. *Surg. Obes. Relat. Dis.,* 2009 Jan;5(1):94-8.

[33] Behrns KE, Smith CD, Kelly KA, Sarr MG. Reoperative bariatric surgery. Lessons learned to improve patient selection and results. *Ann. Surg.,* 1993 Nov;218(5):646-53.

[34] Sanchez H, Cabrera A, Cabrera K, Zerrweck C, Mosti M, Sierra M, et al. Laparoscopic Roux-en-Y Gastric Bypass as a Revision Procedure after Restrictive Bariatric Surgery. *Obes. Surg.,* 2008 Dec;18(12):1539-43.

[35] Daskalakis M, Scheffel O, Theodoridou S, Weiner RA. Conversion of Failed Vertical Banded Gastroplasty to Biliopancreatic Diversion, a Wise Option. *Obes. Surg.,* 2009 Aug 29.

[36] Fobi MA, Lee H. The surgical technique of the Fobi-Pouch operation for obesity (the transected silastic vertical gastric bypass). *Obes. Surg.,* 1998 Jun;8(3):283-8.

[37] Fobi MA. Placement of the GaBP ring system in the banded gastric bypass operation. *Obes. Surg.,* 2005 Sep;15(8):1196-201.

[38] Menon T, Quaddus S, Cohen L. Revision of failed vertical banded gastroplasty to non-resectional Scopinaro biliopancreatic diversion: early experience. *Obes. Surg.,* 2006 Nov;16(11):1420-4.

[39] Elazary R, Hazzan D, Appelbaum L, Rivkind AI, Keidar A. Feasibility of Sleeve Gastrectomy as a Revision Operation for Failed Silastic Ring Vertical Gastroplasty. *Obes. Surg.,* 2008 Oct 7.

[40] Kuesters S, Marjanovic G, Karcz WK. [Redo operations after bariatric and metabolic surgery]. *Zentralbl. Chir.,* 2009 Feb;134(1):50-6.

[41] Muller MK, Wildi S, Scholz T, Clavien PA, Weber M. Laparoscopic pouch resizing and redo of gastro-jejunal anastomosis for pouch dilatation following gastric bypass. *Obes. Surg.,* 2005 Sep;15(8):1089-95.

[42] Hess DS, Hess DW, Oakley RS. The biliopancreatic diversion with the duodenal switch: results beyond 10 years. *Obes. Surg.,* 2005 Mar;15(3):408-16.

[43] Marceau P, Hould FS, Potvin M, Lebel S, Biron S. Biliopancreatic diversion (doudenal switch procedure). *Eur. J. Gastroenterol. Hepatol.,* 1999 Feb;11(2):99-103.

[44] DeMaria EJ, Sugerman HJ, Meador JG, Doty JM, Kellum JM, Wolfe L, et al. High failure rate after laparoscopic adjustable silicone gastric banding for treatment of morbid obesity. *Ann. Surg.,* 2001 Jun;233(6):809-18.

[45] Angrisani L, Furbetta F, Doldi SB, Basso N, Lucchese M, Giacomelli M, et al. Results of the Italian multicenter study on 239 super-obese patients treated by adjustable gastric banding. *Obes. Surg.,* 2002 Dec;12(6):846-50.

[46] O'Brien PE, Dixon JB. Lap-band: outcomes and results. *J. Laparoendosc. Adv. Surg. Tech. A,* 2003 Aug;13(4):265-70.

[47] Weiner R, Blanco-Engert R, Weiner S, Matkowitz R, Schaefer L, Pomhoff I. Outcome after laparoscopic adjustable gastric banding - 8 years experience. *Obes. Surg.,* 2003 Jun;13(3):427-34.

[48] Suter M, Calmes JM, Paroz A, Giusti V. A 10-year experience with laparoscopic gastric banding for morbid obesity: high long-term complication and failure rates. *Obes. Surg.,* 2006 Jul;16(7):829-35.

[49] Weber M, Muller MK, Michel JM, Belal R, Horber F, Hauser R, et al. Laparoscopic Roux-en-Y gastric bypass, but not rebanding, should be proposed as rescue procedure for patients with failed laparoscopic gastric banding. *Ann. Surg.,* 2003 Dec;238(6):827-33.

[50] Lanthaler M, Mittermair R, Erne B, Weiss H, Aigner F, Nehoda H. Laparoscopic gastric re-banding versus laparoscopic gastric bypass as a rescue operation for patients with pouch dilatation. *Obes. Surg.,* 2006 Apr;16(4):484-7.

[51] Acholonu E, McBean E, Court I, Bellorin O, Szomstein S, Rosenthal RJ. Safety and short-term outcomes of laparoscopic sleeve gastrectomy as a revisional approach for failed laparoscopic adjustable gastric banding in the treatment of morbid obesity. *Obes. Surg.,* 2009 Dec;19(12):1612-6.

[52] Frezza EE, Torre EJ, Enriquez C, Gee L, Wachtel M, Corvala JA. Laparoscopic Sleeve Gastrectomy After Gastric Banding Removal: A Feasibility Study. Surg Innov 2008 Dec 12.

[53] Slater GH, Fielding GA. Combining laparoscopic adjustable gastric banding and biliopancreatic diversion after failed bariatric surgery. *Obes. Surg.,* 2004 May;14(5): 677-82.

[54] Johnston D, Dachtler J, Sue-Ling HM, King RF, Martin G. The Magenstrasse and Mill operation for morbid obesity. *Obes. Surg.,* 2003 Feb;13(1):10-6.

[55] Weiner RA, Weiner S, Pomhoff I, Jacobi C, Makarewicz W, Weigand G. Laparoscopic sleeve gastrectomy--influence of sleeve size and resected gastric volume. *Obes. Surg.,* 2007 Oct;17(10):1297-305.

[56] Deitel M, Crosby RD, Gagner M. The First International Consensus Summit for Sleeve Gastrectomy (SG), New York City, October 25-27, 2007. *Obes. Surg.,* 2008 Mar 21.

[57] Baltasar A, Serra C, Perez N, Bou R, Bengochea M, Ferri L. Laparoscopic sleeve gastrectomy: a multi-purpose bariatric operation. *Obes. Surg.,* 2005 Sep;15(8):1124-8.

[58] Nocca D, Krawczykowsky D, Bomans B, Noel P, Picot MC, Blanc PM, et al. A Prospective Multicenter Study of 163 Sleeve Gastrectomies: Results at 1 and 2 Years. *Obes. Surg.,* 2008 Mar 4.

[59] Dapri G, Cadiere GB, Himpens J. Laparoscopic seromyotomy for long stenosis after sleeve gastrectomy with or without duodenal switch. *Obes. Surg.,* 2009 Apr;19(4):495-9.

[60] Gagner M, Rogula T. Laparoscopic reoperative sleeve gastrectomy for poor weight loss after biliopancreatic diversion with duodenal switch. *Obes. Surg.,* 2003 Aug;13(4):649-54.

[61] Karcz WK, Marjanovic G, Grueneberger J, Baumann T, Bukhari W, Krawczykowski D, et al. Banded sleeve gastrectomy using the GaBP ring--surgical technique. *Obes. Facts,* 2011;4(1):77-80.

[62] Brethauer SA, Harris JL, Kroh M, Schauer PR. Laparoscopic gastric plication for treatment of severe obesity. *Surg. Obes. Relat. Dis.,* 2011 Jan;7(1):15-22.

[63] Rosenthal R, Li X, Samuel S, Martinez P, Zheng C. Effect of sleeve gastrectomy on patients with diabetes mellitus. *Surg. Obes. Relat. Dis.,* 2009 Jul;5(4):429-34.

[64] Pories WJ, Swanson MS, MacDonald KG, Long SB, Morris PG, Brown BM, et al. Who would have thought it? An operation proves to be the most effective therapy for adult-onset diabetes mellitus. *Ann. Surg.,* 1995 Sep;222(3):339-50.

[65] Kuesters S, Grueneberger JM, Baumann T, Bukhari W, Daoud M, Hopt UT, et al. Revisionary bariatric surgery: indications and outcome of 100 consecutive operations at a single center. *Surg. Endosc.,* 2011 Dec 22.

[66] Sanchez-Pernaute A, Herrera MA, Perez-Aguirre ME, Talavera P, Cabrerizo L, Matia P, et al. Single anastomosis duodeno-ileal bypass with sleeve gastrectomy (SADI-S). One to three-year follow-up. *Obes. Surg.,* 2010 Dec;20(12):1720-6.

[67] Baumann T, Grueneberger J, Pache G, Kuesters S, Marjanovic G, Kulemann B, et al. Three-dimensional stomach analysis with computed tomography after laparoscopic sleeve gastrectomy: sleeve dilation and thoracic migration. *Surg. Endosc.,* 2011 Jul;25(7):2323-9.

[68] Trelles N, Gagner M. Revision bariatric surgery: laparoscopic conversion of failed gastric bypass to biliopancreatic diversion with duodenal switch. *Minerva Chir.,* 2009 Jun;64(3):277-84.

[69] Christou NV, Look D, Maclean LD. Weight gain after short- and long-limb gastric bypass in patients followed for longer than 10 years. *Ann. Surg.,* 2006 Nov;244(5):734-40.

[70] Fobi M, Lee H, Igwe D, Felahy B, James E, Stanczyk M, et al. Gastric bypass in patients with BMI < 40 but > 32 without life-threatening co-morbidities: preliminary report. *Obes. Surg.,* 2002 Feb;12(1):52-6.

[71] Madan AK, Harper JL, Tichansky DS. Techniques of laparoscopic gastric bypass: on-line survey of American Society for Bariatric Surgery practicing surgeons. *Surg. Obes. Relat. Dis.,* 2008 Mar;4(2):166-72.

[72] Karcz WK, Kuesters S, Marjanovic G, Suesslin D, Kotter E, Thomusch O, et al. 3D-MSCT Gastric Pouch Volumetry in Bariatric Surgery-Preliminary Clinical Results. *Obes. Surg.,* 2008 Dec 18.

[73] Naslund I. A method for measuring the size of the gastric outlet in obesity surgery. *Acta. Chir. Scand.,* 1984;150(5):399-404.

[74] Thompson CC, Slattery J, Bundga ME, Lautz DB. Peroral endoscopic reduction of dilated gastrojejunal anastomosis after Roux-en-Y gastric bypass: a possible new option for patients with weight regain. *Surg. Endosc.,* 2006 Nov;20(11):1744-8.

[75] Gumbs AA, Margolis B, Bessler M. Laparoscopic banded-Roux-en-Y gastric bypass. *Surg. Obes. Relat. Dis.,* 2006 May;2(3):408-9.

[76] Crampton NA, Izvornikov V, Stubbs RS. Silastic ring gastric bypass: a comparison of two ring sizes: a preliminary report. *Obes. Surg.,* 1997 Dec;7(6):495-9.

[77] Stubbs RS, O'brien I, Jurikova L. What ring size should be used in association with vertical gastric bypass? *Obes. Surg.,* 2006 Oct;16(10):1298-303.

[78] Fobi MA, Lee H, Felahy B, Che K, Ako P, Fobi N. Choosing an operation for weight control, and the transected banded gastric bypass. *Obes. Surg.,* 2005 Jan;15(1):114-21.

[79] Patel S, Szomstein S, Rosenthal RJ. Reasons and Outcomes of Reoperative Bariatric Surgery for Failed and Complicated Procedures (Excluding Adjustable Gastric Banding). *Obes. Surg.,* 2010 Jul 30.

[80] Fronza JS, Prystowsky JB, Hungness ES, Nagle AP. Revisional bariatric surgery at a single institution. *Am. J. Surg.,* 2010 Nov;200(5):651-4.

[81] Sugerman HJ, Kellum JM, DeMaria EJ. Conversion of proximal to distal gastric bypass for failed gastric bypass for superobesity. *J. Gastrointest. Surg.,* 1997 Nov;1(6):517-24.

[82] Fobi MA, Lee H, Igwe D, Jr., Felahy B, James E, Stanczyk M, et al. Revision of failed gastric bypass to distal Roux-en-Y gastric bypass: a review of 65 cases. *Obes. Surg.*, 2001 Apr;11(2):190-5.

[83] Parikh M, Pomp A, Gagner M. Laparoscopic conversion of failed gastric bypass to duodenal switch: technical considerations and preliminary outcomes. *Surg. Obes. Relat. Dis.*, 2007 Nov;3(6):611-8.

[84] Wang TT, Hu SY, Gao HD, Zhang GY, Liu CZ, Feng JB, et al. Ileal transposition controls diabetes as well as modified duodenal jejunal bypass with better lipid lowering in a nonobese rat model of type II diabetes by increasing GLP-1. *Ann. Surg.*, 2008 Jun;247(6):968-75.

[85] Mason EE. Ileal [correction of ilial] transposition and enteroglucagon/GLP-1 in obesity (and diabetic?) surgery. *Obes. Surg.*, 1999 Jun;9(3):223-8.

[86] Salvi PF, Brescia A, Cosenza UM, D'Urso R, Cardelli P, Badiali M. [Gastric pacing to treat morbid obesity: two years experience in four patients]. *Ann. Ital. Chir.*, 2009 Jan;80(1):25-8.

[87] Miller K, Hoeller E, Aigner F. The Implantable Gastric Stimulator for Obesity : An Update of the European Experience in the LOSS (Laparoscopic Obesity Stimulation Survey) Study. *Treat Endocrinol.*, 2006;5(1):53-8.

In: Bariatric Surgery
Editor: Christos R. Iavazzo

ISBN: 978-1-62618-995-9

Chapter XIII

Body-Contouring after Bariatric Surgery

Franco Migliori
EURAPS (European Association of Plastic Surgeons);
ASPS (American Society of Plastic Surgeons);
ISAPS (International Society of Aesthetic Plastic Surgery);
IFSO (International Federation for the Surgery of Obesity);
SICPRE (Italian Society of Plastic, Reconstructive and Aesthetic Surgery);
SICOB (Italian Society of Obesity Surgery);
SIUST (Italian Burns Society)

Abstract

In the last decades the rising demand for bariatric procedures worldwide has exponentially increased the need of post-bariatric plastic surgery. Accordingly a new chapter of plastic surgery has been born, since the standard technique usually performed in body-contouring wasn't perfectly suited for post-bariatric tissues due to the different tissue structures of post-bariatric patients. The anatomical areas most frequently treated are limbs, breast and trunk. In this chapter, the leading strategies for any of these areas, with the main attention kept on general concepts, technical aspects and patient management, are summarized. This field of the plastic surgery is not an easy one; it requires good surgical experience, as well as organized and dedicated teams because it can't be managed by a single professional. Respecting these rules leads to great results and great patient satisfaction.

Introduction

The increase of body-contouring (BC) procedures after massive weight loss (MWL) following bariatric surgery (BS) is astonishing: in the U. S. A in 2004, almost 56. 000 out of

140. 000 bariatric patients underwent BC surgery, in 2005 100. 000 out of 250. 000 [1]. Even a neologism has been proposed: “Bariplasty [2]”. The expectations are increasing numbers for at least the next two decades. This wide horizon should propose (as it already does in fact) an integrated treatment approach [3] (bariatric surgery, plastic surgery, motivation for physical activity, and psychological support) for the years to come. BS effects are more and more perceived by patients as an intermediate stage quite unsatisfactory. BS dramatically reduces weight and normalizes body-mass, but enhances dismorphisms and creates new problems such as skin redundancy and flabbiness, sweating and eczemas, general aesthetical uneasiness, low self-esteem: BC completes therapeutical course restoring body shape and solving these problems. BC after BS is mainly performed on 4 anatomical areas:

Arms	7 %
Breast	38 %
Torso	40 %
Legs	15 %

Bariatric Surgery Sequelae Influencing Body-Contouring

Among thousands of “pros and cons” described, after BS procedures, the following are those mainly conditioning plastic surgeons performing BC.

Clinical Consequences

Significant *advantages* of BS are:

a) the extreme weight loss (up to 80-100 kg) within an average time interval of 12-18 months;
b) normalization of hyperglycemia and hypercholesterolemia.

Challenging associated *complications*, mainly in malabsorptive procedures, are:

1) Fe^{++}malabsorption with sideropenic anemia;
2) Ca^{++}malabsorption with bone demineralization;
3) in 5%of patients, protein malnutrition.

Morphological Consequences

The clinical evidenced disadvantage following BS is the inefficacy of the soft tissue scar retraction, probably due to histological alterations, causing an overall non-esthetic aspect. The inelastic and atrophic tissues result in deep folds and creases. The main aspects are large dermo-adiposal folds in the arms, abdomen and inner thighs, and medium-to-severebreast ptosis in women.

Anatomo-Surgical Consequences

The preoperative and intraoperative challenge of BC after BS is the reduced vascular perfusion of the tissues, mainly in the dermis, which appears thinner, and in the fat, which appear shy potrophic, "pale" or even "gray". The presence of BS scars in the abdominal wall causes reduced elasticity in that specific area and a compromised dermal plexus, both enhancing specific complications.

Histological Consequences

A personal histologic study on post-BS dermis and fat is running nowadays. Preliminary reports, comparing post-BS tissues with healthy tissues, demonstrates:

a) in the *Fat*: presence of collapsed adipocytes with thicker membranes, prominent nuclei (usually not visible) and thickened intracellular fibrous septa (Figure 1).
b) in the *Dermis*: thickening of the fibrous net and the hypertrophy of the vascular net. A reduction of elastic fibers is supposed, but results of histochemical and EM study are awaited (Figure 2).

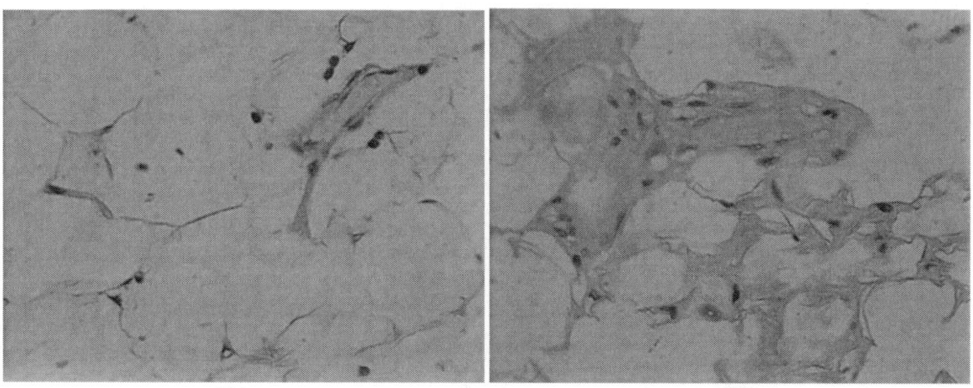

(A) **(B)**

Figure 1. a) Normal Fat Tissue; b) Post-bariatric Fat Tissue.

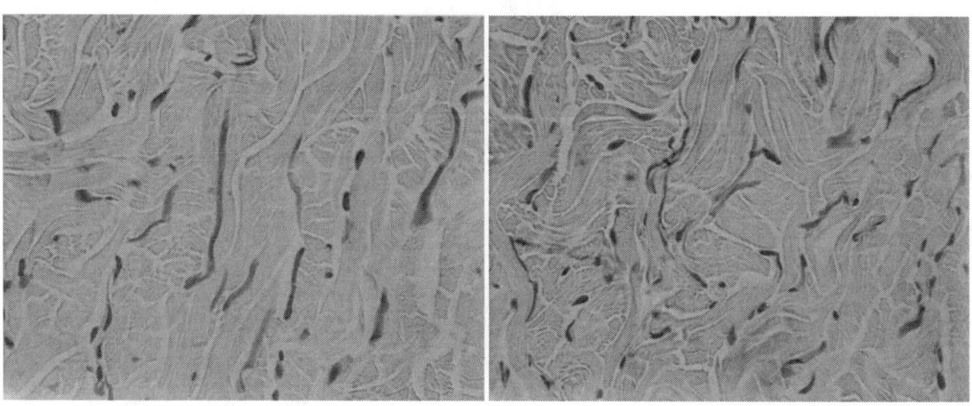

(A) **(B)**

Figure 2. a) Normal Dermal Tissue; b) Post-bariatric Dermal Tissue.

General Surgical Strategies

Plastic surgery is a science, and Body-Contouring is a scientific art. This means that, despite any surgical algorithm, there is no "perfect shape" to aim to: there can be, for each body district, some key points to respect; but the main key point remains the patient's "body image" as a whole. This concept includes subjective and objective evaluations, which differ from patient to patient. The only general rule we always follow for female figure (♀ are 80-85 % of all BC after BS) is the "silhouette" image (Figure 3): prominent breast and buttocks, narrow waist and ankles, can reasonably be considered as good-looking for every woman.

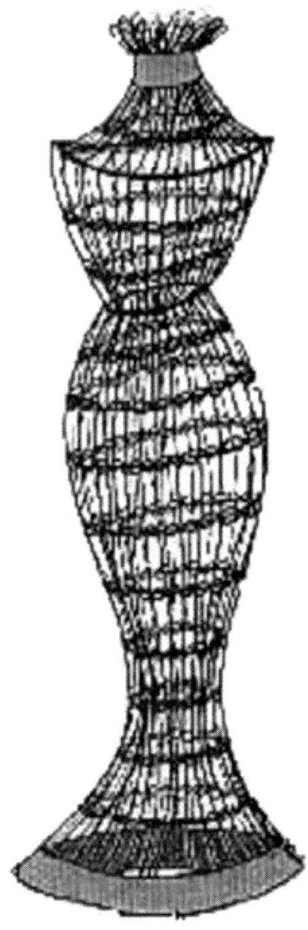

Figure 3. "Silhouette" model profile.

In our experience 67% of post-bariatric patients underwent to multiple BC procedures (from 2 to 4 operations): there is no algorithm that determines the timing and suitability of one procedure rather than another. Among every consideration, the psychological impact on the patient should be considered, trying to choose more effective one as starting procedure.

As usually happens in plastic surgery procedures, the surgeon main aim is to find the right compromise between maximal reduction of excess tissue and maximal reduction of scar length. Moreover, BC is quite an aggressive surgeryand the risk/benefit rate is important to be well evaluated and understood: the same operations could fit a patient but not another.

BC procedures are not novelties in plastic surgery: some of them have been described one century ago, most of them several decades ago ('60 and '70), all of them far before BS was born and set its wide success. When liposuction came in fashion ('80) the initial euphoria let al.l plastic surgeons believe that traditional BC would have been dismissed. As euphoria subsided and BS and MWL grew up, BC could slowly taste its cold revenge: it's today well accepted that liposuction is not a substitute for BC, and that both represent different solutions for different cases in different stages [4]. The anatomo-surgical and histological features of post-BS patients confer to their tissues an "anergic behavior", meaning a poor or absent scar retraction. Because of that, the surgical techniques mainly suggested are those removing all exceeding tissue. Thus liposuction, where results depend on scar retraction, cannot be utilized except as an ancillary technique, in rare selected cases. BC techniques of decades ago, of course, have taken benefits by all technical and knowledge advances and have "changed their suit": in these pages a summary of old concepts and new criteria is proposed, looking for maximal reshaping and minimal visible scars.

General Management

On complication of BS (mainly gastric bypass and biliopancreatic diversion) can be vitamin B_{12} and Fe^{++}malabsorption, with consequent anemia [5]. Therefore, these levels need to be checked, because major reconstruction will result in blood loss. In those cases, auto-transfusion should be considered. However, auto transfusion can be performed only with a hemoglobin rate > 11. 5, which in post-BS patient is not so frequent. Therefore, we always perform infiltration of all the tissues to be excised with a diluted solution of adrenaline (1 cc. /500 cc. NaCl) at least 20' before cutting: this procedure allows a great amount of circulating mass to be squeezed off, significantly reducing blood losses.

Another major risk in BC is deep venous thrombosis [6], with blood clots and pulmonary embolism. We always perform prophylaxis with antiembolic compressive stockings and low-molecular weight heparin (4000/6. 000 U. I. 12 hour before surgery, continued daily for two weeks).

Seromas and liponecrosis can be challenging complications. There are two rules to reduce their incidence:

- avoiding any cutting device but blade: no other known instrument is less tissue-damaging;
- limiting undermining.

The extension of scars can be overwhelming in many procedures. Extreme accuracy in suture technique and material choice can make the difference, reducing hypertrophies and keloids occurrence. Only deep, dermal and intradermal suture should be utilized, with no cutaneous stitch. Specific plastic surgery dedicated threads and needles have been conceived, and it is advisable to use them in BC.

Techniques

Arms

Within BC procedures performed on BS patients, brachioplasty appears to be very exclusive, since the request is definitely lower than for other districts.

Reviewing literature [7,8,9,10,11,12,13,14] modest results are usually found, due to modest improvement of the morphological defect, together with remarkable scars and important complication risks.

In this particular anatomical district, the best possible result should be pursued, optimizing cost/benefit ratio in terms of *maximal correction/less visible scars*. If this strategy cannot be applied, brachioplasty should be discouraged.

A technique has therefore been developed, based on a linear scar programmed to be hidden in the medial bicipital groove, and aiming to obtain the best possible morphological correction. This doesn't mean passing from a "batwing" effect to a "sweater sleeve" effect, but to a normal arm profile. A stigmata of this "normality" should be represented by a slight concavity in the lower arm profile proximal to the elbow.

Patients are grouped according with Strauch [8] 4-class classification of defects: post-BS patients usually belong to classes 3 and 4. The anatomical districts interested by surgery were area 3 (forearm) and area 4 (axilla), according with Strauch[8] anatomical scheme.

Pre-Operative Markings

Special care is taken in evaluating the amount of tissue to be excided. Only the anterior aspect of the excision is normally drawn, and the actual quantity of skin to be dismissed intraoperatively determined. This algorithm is operator-dependent and the compulsory rule is that markings must be drawn by the first surgeon.

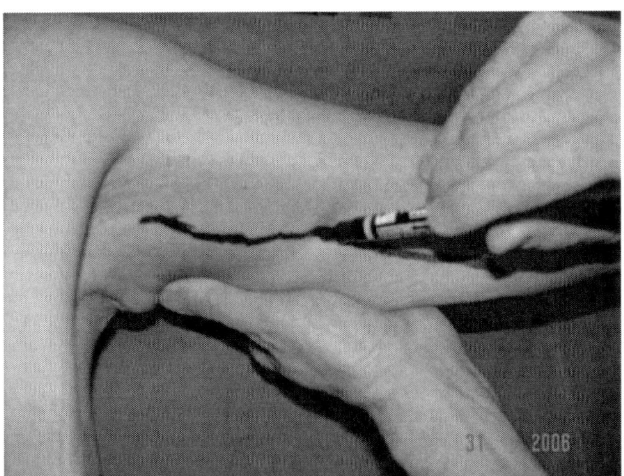

Figure 4. Brachioplasty: drawing with manual tension.

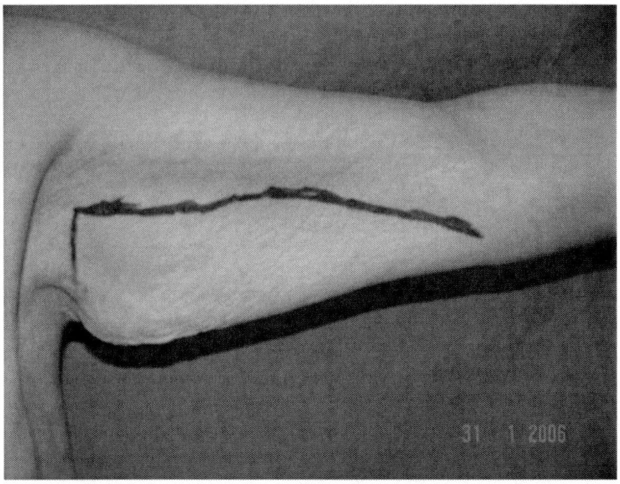

Figure 5. Brachioplasty: final drawing.

With the patient standing in a frontal view, arms abducted at shoulder level and forearms proned ("crucifix" position), the incision line is drawn within the medial bicipital groove, while applying with counterlateral hand a slight antero-posterior tension on the medial face of the arm (the same tension will be applied during surgery) (Figure 4). This line continues on the posterior axillary pillar, gently curving at 90° and becoming vertical, just posterior to and extending as axillary hair (4-5 cm.) (Figure 5).

Surgical Technique

After a wide literature review, proposing any kind of incision shape, no acceptable demonstration is found that linear incision (from medial epicondyle to axilla along medial bicipital groove) is worse than other ones. A deep incision is done on that line, directly on the muscular fascia, preserving it.

An antero-posterior undermining is gently performed with the tip of a blade, following fascia surface for almost half circumference of the arm. All perforating vessels and nerves long enough to be let loose are preserved until exceeding tissue extension is determined (Figure 6).

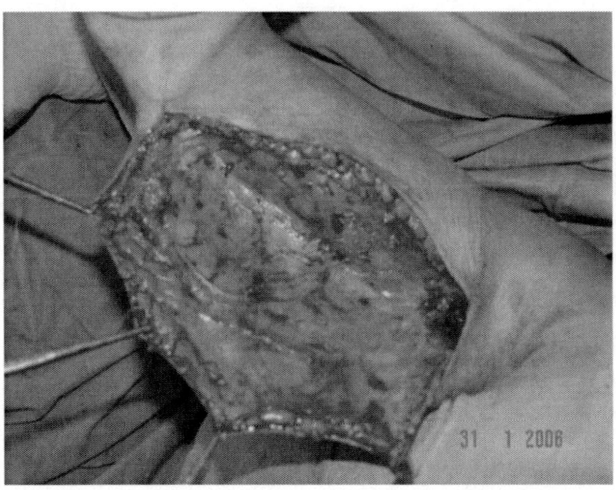

Figure 6. Brachioplasty: suprafascial undermining.

As the undermining is completed, an overcorrective tension is applied to the anterior edge of incision and to the undermined flap, similar to that one applied while marking. The flap is overlapped to incision edge, whose superficial projection is spot-marked with 3-4 transfixed needles and completed with a straight line joining front incision tips. A back incision is then performed obtaining, in this way, an excided tissue extension always rather abundant: only perforating vessels and nerves feeding this area are tied and cut (Figure 7).

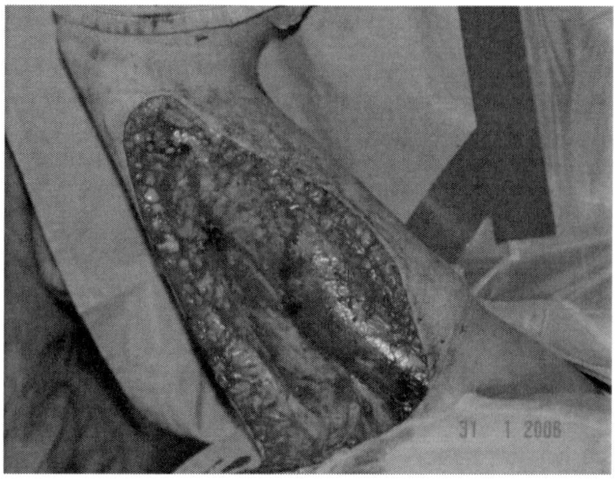

Figure 7. Brachioplasty: tissue excision completed.

Suture is evidently performed under tension, so great care is spent to provide precise and tight edges fitting, through at least two suture layers. First stitch must fix a posterior flap whose medial length is determined by the axillary incision angle (Figure 8). Suction drains are placed and maintained 1-2 days post-op.

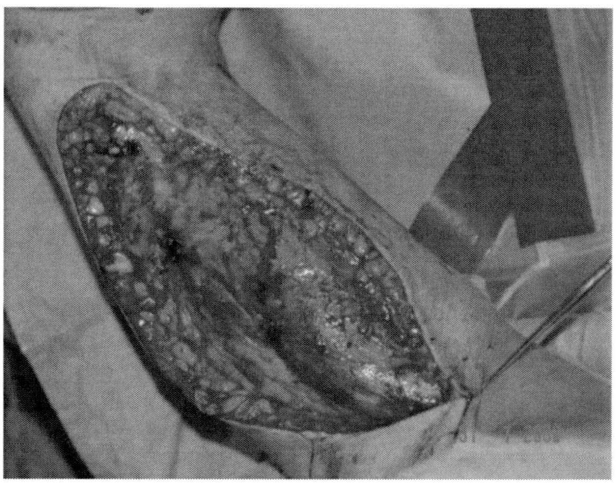

Figure 8. Brachioplasty: flap closure.

Post-Operative Care

Discharge is usually allowed within 2-3 days post-op. Elastic tubular bandages are worn for about 1 month post-op. Drugs and devices preventing pathological scars are strongly suggested, because hypertrophies and keloids are frequent in this area.

Complications

General complications are represented by scar hypertrophies/keloids (40%), edema (15%), seromas (10%), wound dehiscence (5%).

Specific rare complications include:

1) Compression of ulnar nerve (0,3%) with acute pain and hand motor deficiencies; the symptoms must be promptly recognized and solved by partial suture releasing and sequential delayed closure (1 stitch/day within 1 week);
2) Section of cutaneous branches of the anterior medial brachial nerve (0,8%), lasting in small areas of anesthesia (2-3 cm^2.).

Conclusions

As clearly evidenced by the images (Figure 9-12), this technique confers a natural arm shape and profile, reproducing the inferior concavity proximal to elbow. These results, compared with average ones published in literature, appear better. Linear scar is long, seldom of high quality, but often well hidden within medial bicipital groove and not visible in the frontal view as well as in the back one.

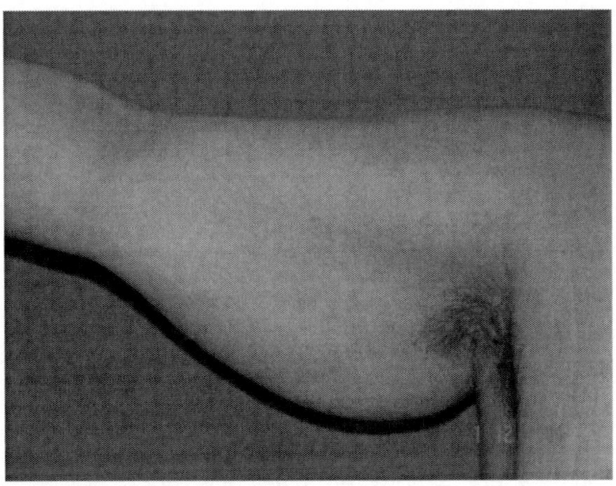

Figure 9. Brachioplasty: case 1 (♀ aa. 28, gastric by-pass) Pre-op.

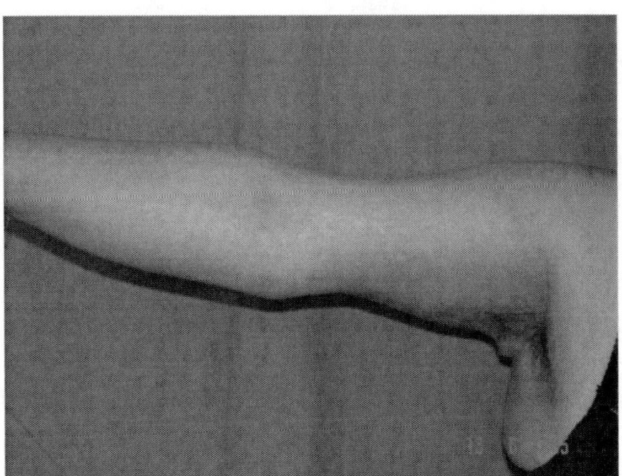

Figure 10. Brachioplasty: case 1 Post-op.

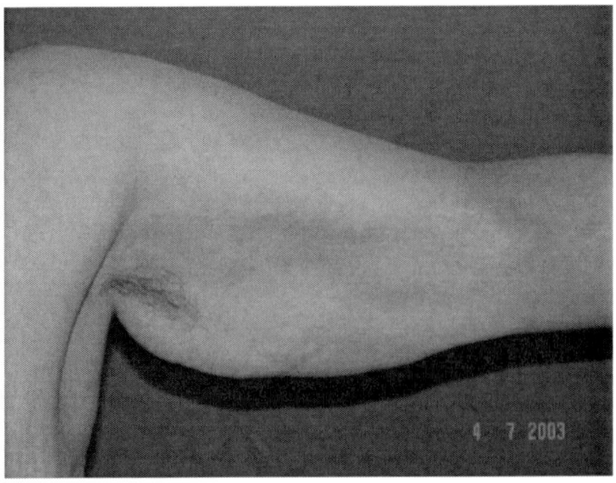

Figure 11. Brachioplasty: case 2 (♀ aa. 46, B. P. D.) Pre-op.

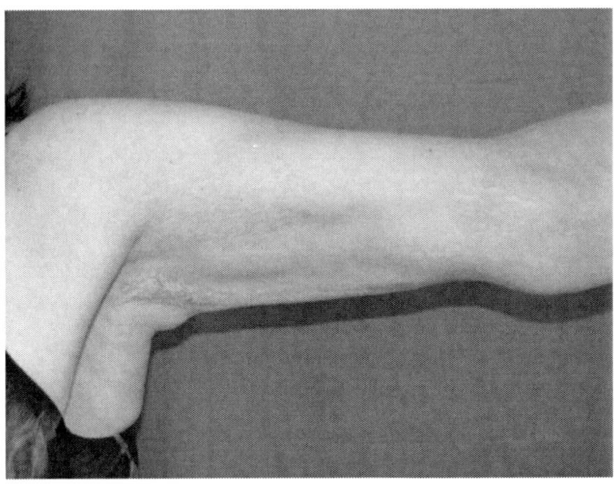

Figure 12. Brachioplasty: case 2 Post-op.

The respect of sensitive cutaneaous branches lets good preservation of touch within medial arm face.

Breast

Breast deformities in post-BS patients are different and more challenging than those from non-BS patients. The histological alterations confer the highest clinical consequences to this area: highest degrees of true ptosis [15], deflated and flattened glands, totally inelastic covering tissues. Hypertrophic breasts, needing further reduction, are quite rare.

Therefore, the main problems to be corrected on a M. W. L. breast are two:

1) Ptosis
2) Volume loss

Both problems need peculiar resolutions, due to peculiar characteristics.

Ptosis can be surgically *minor* or *severe*: we usually put a borderline around 6 cm. of ptosis correction. If the difference between the pre-operative nipple-areola complex (N. A. C.) position and the post-operative projected new position is less than this measure, a scar spearing technique is suitable. Beyond this measure, more extended scars are needed.

Volume loss is proportional to body weight loss. The amount of residual gland determines surgical choices. If the volume left is considered enough, from both the patient and surgeon, a gland reshaping should be performed. Volume evaluation must be subjective, as no granted procedure or device exists up to date. If a volume increase is considered advisable, a mammary implant is necessary. No dedicated prosthesis has never been conceived for the peculiar problems of a M. W. L. breast, and the existing implants cannot be considered adequate for these patients, because of their weight (hundreds of grams) pulling down loose M. W. L. tissues for an early ptosis recurrence: an ideal implant should be developed on an ultralight technology to carry out a weightless device ("feather" prosthesis) weighing only few grams. For these reasons, nowadays, the final choice should be, as far as possible, reshaping without implants.

Surgical Strategies

The choice strategy should follow this scheme:

	Suitable Volume	**Lacking Volume**
Minor Ptosis (N. A. C. correction < cm. 6)	"Round block"	"Round block" + mammary implants
Severe Ptosis (N. A. C. correction > cm. 6)	"L technique" + self prosthesis	"L technique" + mammary implants

As stated above, the choices **2** and **4** are controversial. However, while choice **2** occurs in a less ptotic breast (which means less deformed, less stressed, less loose and flabby) and can be considered suitable, choice **4** is at high risk of early aesthetical complications (i. e. deformities, ptosis recurrence). That's why it is advisable to stress as much as possible the indications of choice **3**, and to limit choice **4**.

N. A. C. correct vertical position is determined at the medial point of arm length: this point is usually placed at 19-21 cm. from sternal notch. The horizontal position stands at 9-11 cm. from medio-sternal line.

Surgical Techniques

Round Block

This technique was first described by Louis Benelli [16] in late '80s and represents a milestone in mammary plastic surgery, because of the great scar spearing. It is based on an "egg" shaped periareolar skin excision, a wide undermining allowing a wide access to the gland, which can be easily reshaped: the final circular dermic suture ("round block") completes the procedure. Only a periareolar scar is left.

The "round block" technique has two limits:

1) it is well suited for small breasts and minor ptosis;
2) it flattens the breast and reduces N. A. C. anterior projection.

Because of this limits, clinical experience through the years has suggested the use of this procedure for minor ptosis associated with a mammary implant. In M. W. L. breasts the controversy is evident: the need of a scar-spearing technique on one side, the need to reduce implants utilize on the other. At the present time, there is no escape from this compromise, and a careful case-by-case evaluation is needed.

The technical changes to the original procedure, applied and suggested in M. W. L. breasts are the following:

a) complete undermining of glandular upper pole (both front and rear aspects) to let breast lifting and anchorage to fascia, muscle and/or rib periostium (at least three stitches of threaded non-absorbable 0 or 1 suture); lower pole is left undetached, to guarantee blood perfusion (only 1-2 cm. periareolar are undermined).
b) if implants are needed, upside-down retroglandular undermining [17], taking great care to leave inframammary fold and 1-2 cm. of gland undetached. The implant is topside-bottom inserted with a "mailbox posting" action; inframammary fold should act like a barrier to prevent implant ptosis. The upper ⅓ of the implant is placed beneath pectoralis major muscle, with "dual-plane" technique.
c) the type of implant needed (round vs. anatomical) basically depends on the kind of aesthetical defect: major upper pole defects need round implants, major lower pole defects need anatomical implants. Patient's preferences are a primary factor in the decision [18].
d) periareolar suture is always performed with "interlocking" technique smartly conceived by Hammond [19].

L Technique

This technique was first described by De Longis [20], and represents one modern evolution of the great family of "vertical techniques", all descending from original Arié [21] technique.

As the majority of vertical techniques, L technique utilizes a superior pedicle to support N. A. C. and has been thought to suspend breast, either reducing or emphasizing volume. All vertical techniques have the great advantage to increase N. A. C. projection.

When N. A. C. is programmed to be lifted more then6 cm., the L technique is suggested. In M. W. L. breasts, once more, is advisable to comply with the need of volume emphasizing, restricting as much as possible implants insertion. To do this, "auto-prosthesis" appears to be a good compromise.

M. W. L. major ptotic breasts usually have 3 problems:

1) N. A. C. ptosis;
2) inframammary fold ptosis;
3) lack of projection (flattened shape).

Volume is not necessarily a problem, seldom is lacking or exceeding, often can be considered suitable. L technique with auto-prosthesis corrects all three above problems and simulates a volume increasing.

The technical key-points are the following:

a) auto-prosthesis is a flap drawn, de-epithelialized and sculptured on an inferior pedicle (6-8 cm. base, depending on breast width); the upper edge of the flap is incised and detached from upper pedicled N. A. C. flap, and undermined up to pectoralism. m. fascia;
b) auto-prosthesis is strongly anchored at 3rd rib periostium (at least three stitches of threaded non-absorbable 0 or 1 suture); this procedure lets inframammary fold **real** lifting and fixing;
c) if an implant is unavoidable, auto-prosthesis cannot be performed and all the mammary glandular tissue must be harvested on a superior pedicle; the implant is bottom side – top inserted, and the flap closed on it. This procedure doesn't prevent ptosis recurrence, doesn't lift inframammary fold, and adds implant weight: that's why should be avoided, if possible.

Post-Operative Care

Suction drains are maintained 1-2 days post-op. Drippings are very simple and light and maintained for almost 1 week. No compression is performed. A dedicated shaping bra is worn for 1 month day and night and further 2 weeks night-time only.

Breast reaches its final shape within 60-90 days. Scars cannot be considered stable before 6 months/1 year.

Complications

General complications are represented by scar dystrophies (13,2%), hematomas (8,7%), wound dehiscence (3,1%).

Considering ptosis recurrence as N. A. C. sliding >2 cm., 1 year post-op, its incidence is:

Round block	3,2%
Round block + implant	27,6%
L technique + self-prosthesis	13,3%
L technique + implant	75%

Best shapes (patient and surgeon compliance) are obtained with **2** and **3** techniques.

Conclusions

Results obtained by applying the strategy algorithm shown above are usually good (Figure 13-20), the choices **1/2** and **3** appear to be the more frequently applied and better fitted to cover the majority of M. W. L. breast defects. Choice **4** needs experienced hands and, anyway, has a high complication rate. In the future, the birth and the rise of new mammary implant concepts and technologies could completely change this algorithm.

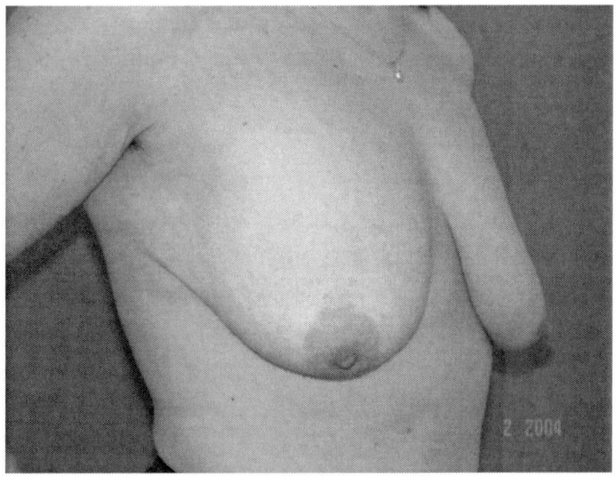

Figure 13. Mastoplasty: Round-block (aa. 37, Intragastric balloon) Pre-op.

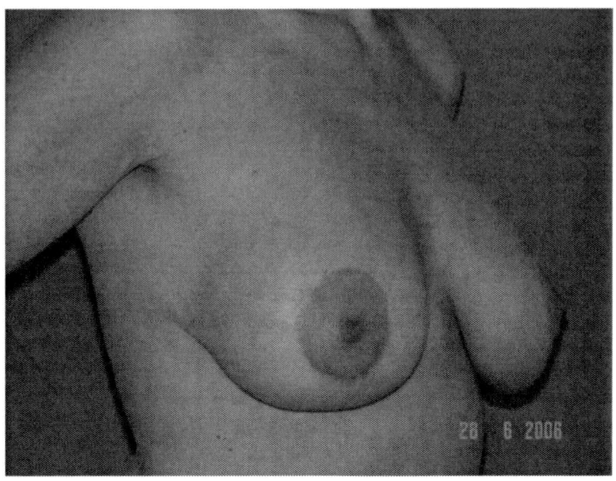

Figure 14. Mastoplasty: Round-block Post-op.

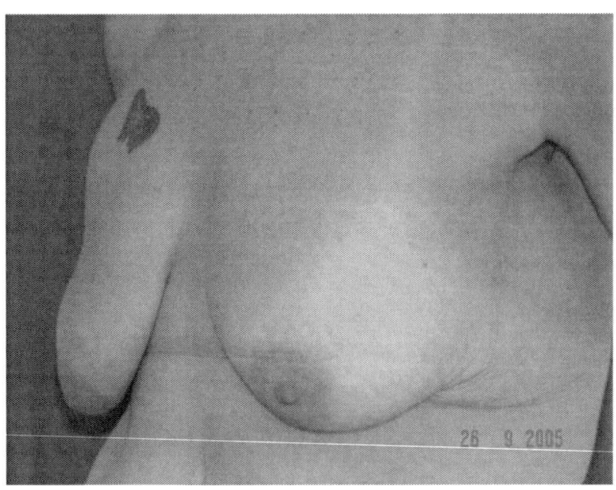

Figure 15. Mastoplasty: Round-block + prosthesis (aa. 32, BPD) Pre-op.

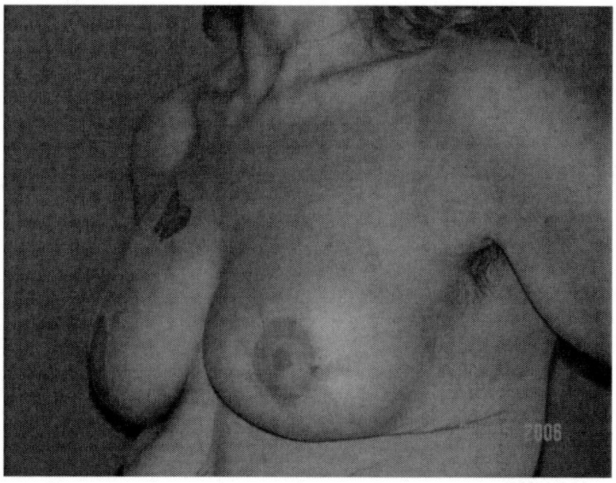

Figure 16. Mastoplasty: Round-block + prosthesis Post-op.

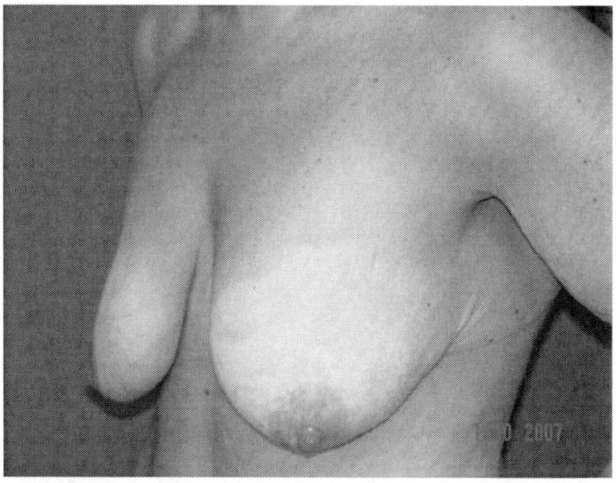

Figure 17. Mastoplasty: L technique + autoprosthesis (aa. 35, gastric by-pass) Pre-op.

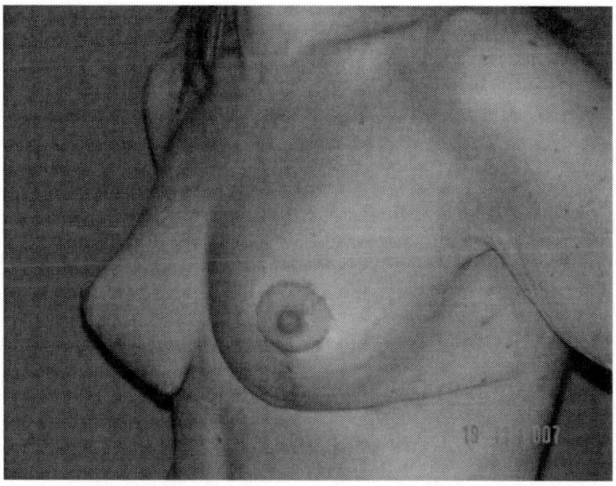

Figure 18. Mastoplasty: L technique + autoprosthesis Post-op.

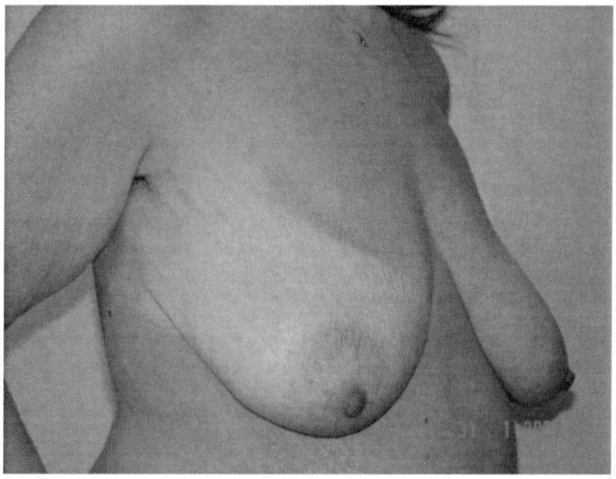

Figure 19. Mastoplasty: L technique + prosthesis (aa. 40, laparoscopic BPD) Pre-op.

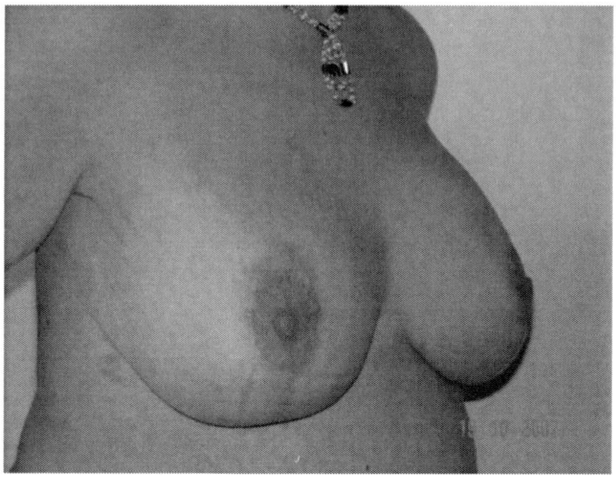

Figure 20. Mastoplasty: L technique + prosthesis Post-op.

Torso

Torso deformities in post-BS patients are mainly confined in an area extending anteriorly (Figure 21) from navel line cranially until a virtual line passing through groin folds caudally. Posteriorly runs from cranial edges of trochanteric eminences to infragluteal folds (Figure 22). Posterior area extension (65%) is major than anterior one (35%).

The main evaluation to be done in this area is whether the defect is confined on the plane of the abdominal wall (2 dimensions), or it is extended to all the torso area (3 dimensions). In the first case abdominoplasty is indicated, in the second one (the so called "Sharpei profile") torsoplasty is the solution. The key point is anterior-superior iliac spine: any defect extending laterally beyond this point should be treated with a torsoplasty, because a simple abdominoplasty could give an unsuccessful result [22]. At the same time, it must be kept in mind that liposuction has very limited indications in post-BS patients, and that torsoplasty is one of the most patient health challenging procedure in BC. So, if a clear indication cannot be identified, BC of torso area has to be discouraged.

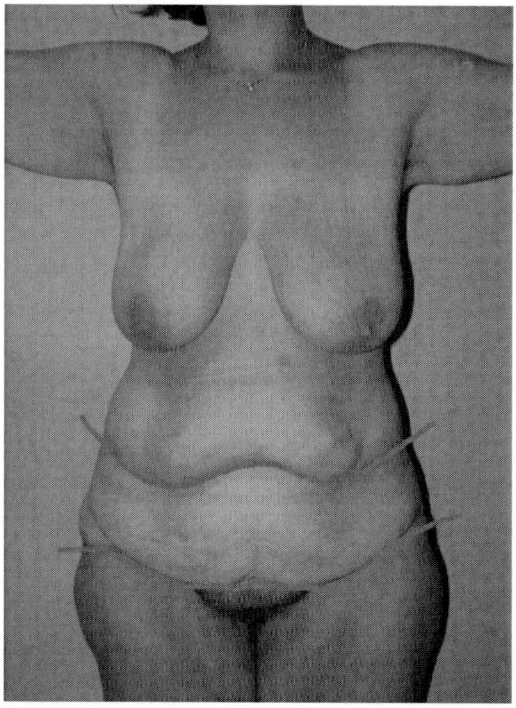

Figure 21. Torso area, Frontal view.

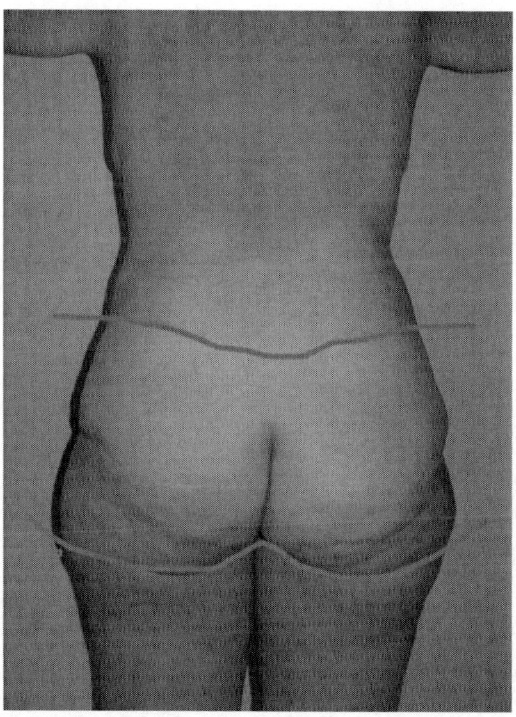

Figure 22. Torso area, back view.

Abdominoplasty

As a result of the above-described anatomosurgical modifications and of the high percentage of potential complications, the right abdominoplasty technique for this kind of patient should be quick and safe. Therefore, the "vest over pants" technique described by Planas [23, 24] with an inverted V excision, seems to be the safest to preserve a good abdominal wall blood perfusion. Two technical variations are suggested:

1) Drawing of the upper line of incision is made with patient standing, simulating the "vest over pants" movement and drawing the lower line. As patient will lie down the operating table, all the draws will move upwards, underlining a frequent error: making drawings with patient lying determines cuts in the wrong places (Figure 23-24). As in all BC, drawings must be made with patient standing.
2) Once lines of excision are well identified, it is advisable to start with lower incision, to perform the whole undermining and finally to cut the exceeding tissue: often the extensive BS scars limit abdominal wall elasticity and it is safer to finally check the amount of excision.

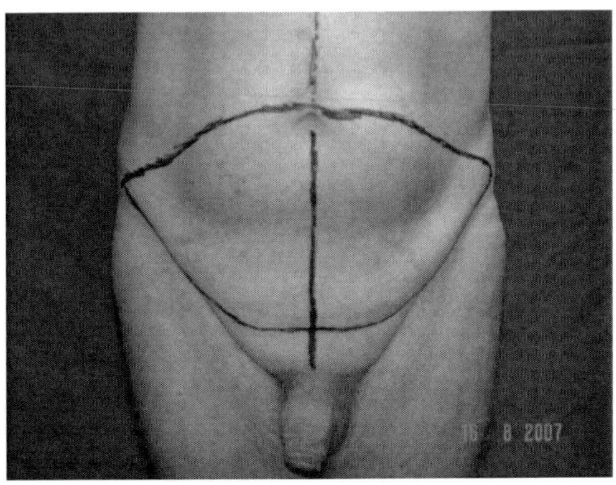

Figure 23. Abdominoplasty: drawings on standing position.

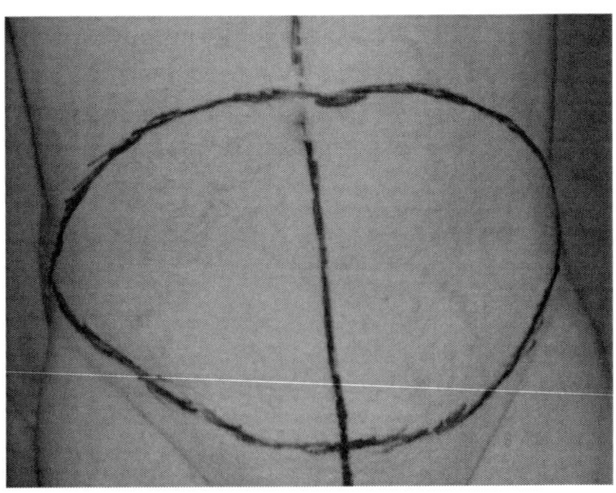

Figure 24. Abdominoplasty: same drawings (Figure 23) on lying position.

If performed on the right cases, abdominoplasty provides nice improvements, mainly on the lateral view of the abdominal wall (Figure 25-28).

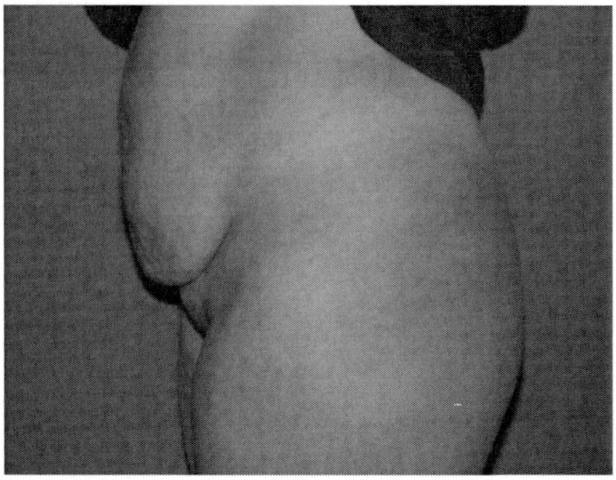

Figure 25. Abdominoplasty: case 1 (♀ aa. 38, BPD) Pre-op.

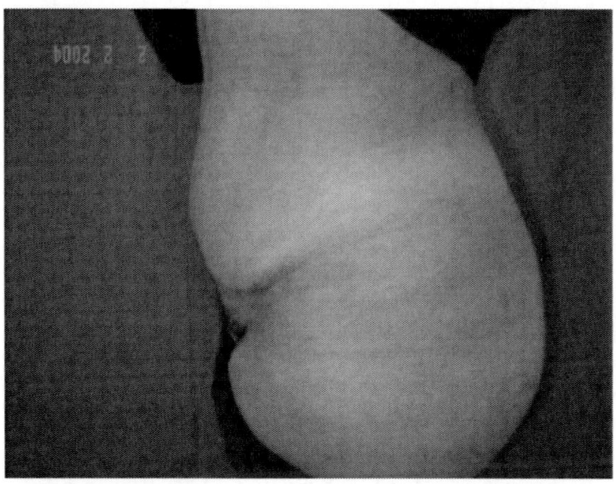

Figure 26. Abdominoplasty: case 1 Post-op.

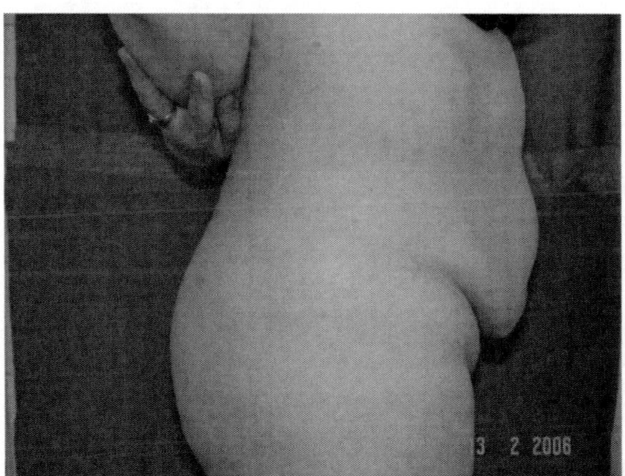

Figure 27. Abdominoplasty: case 2 (♀ aa. 42, BPD) Pre-op.

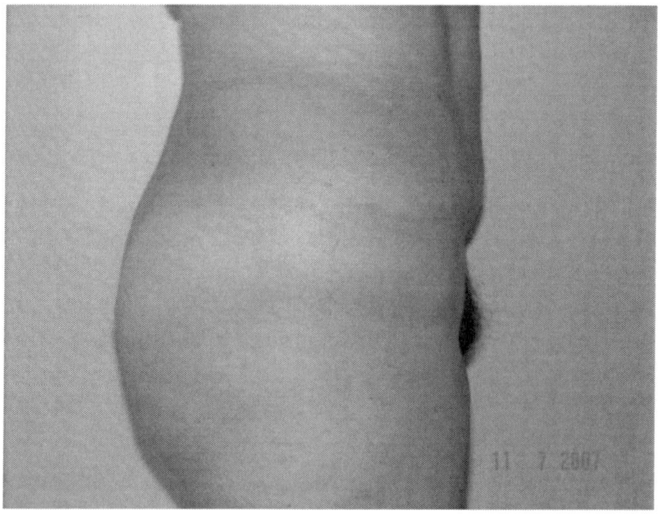

Figure 28. Abdominoplasty: case 2 Post-op.

Torsoplasty

Various techniques have been described to treat the M. W. L. "sharpei" profile [25, 26], all aiming to remove the redundant tissue in the belt area and to suspend the caudal districts, that means reshaping and lifting. Anyway torsoplasty can be considered the most invasive but at the same time the most aesthetically improving BC procedure.

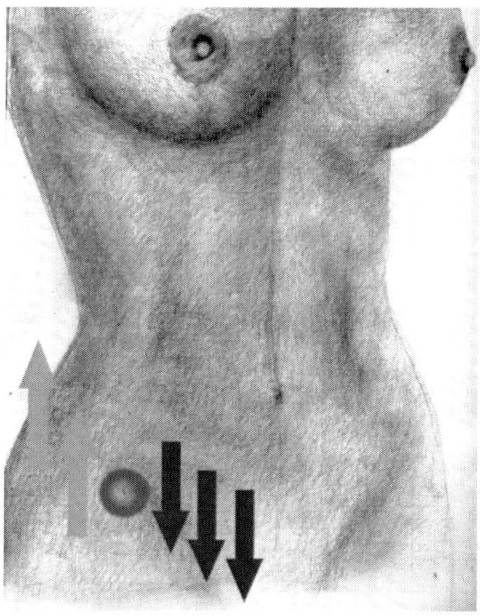

Figure 29. Traction Forces vectors scheme in torsoplasty.

The abdominal wall needs to be corrected with a "sliding down" movement of the exceeding tissue; on other hands, flanks and back need to be lifted and suspended with a "caudal-cranial" movement. We can represent the forces of the surgical correction with vectors and realize that an inversion of these vectors takes place on the anterior-superior iliac spine (rotation point) (Figure 29): posteriorly vectors are caudal-cranial oriented; anteriorly are cranial-caudal oriented.

Drawings

Drawings are performed the day before surgery with patient standing.

Posteriorly the upper point of intergluteal fold is marked (inferior edge of excision) (Figure30). This point is usually programmed to be lifted about 7-10 cm: with manual simulation, the upper point is marked (upper edge of excision).

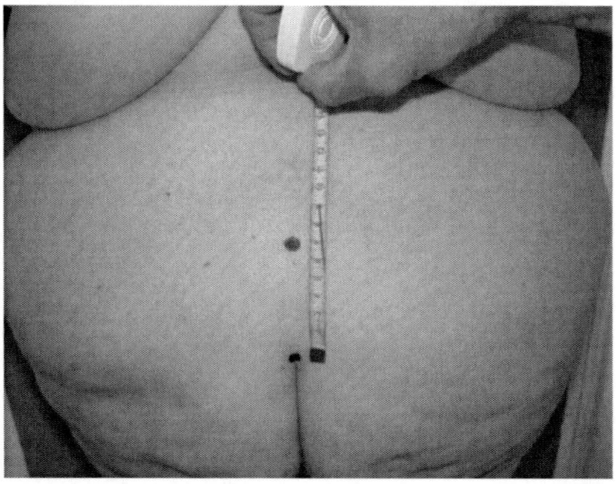

Figure 30. Torsoplasty: back keypoints drawings.

The amount of posterior and lateral tissue to be lifted must now be determined: caudal tissue is folded and tensioned with caudal-cranial movements, and superior and inferior edges of excision are marked (Figure31). All points are joined drawing lines of dorsal excisions (Figure 32). Within these areas, 3-4 cm. laterally the median line, two "dermal-adipose" elliptical islands (10-12 cm. wide, 6-8 cm. high) are measured and drawn: they will be utilized for buttocks emphasizing (Figure33).

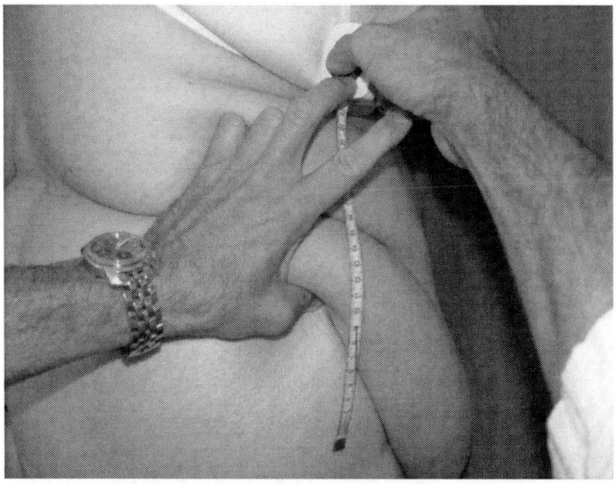

Figure 31. Torsoplasty: lateral excess tissue evaluation.

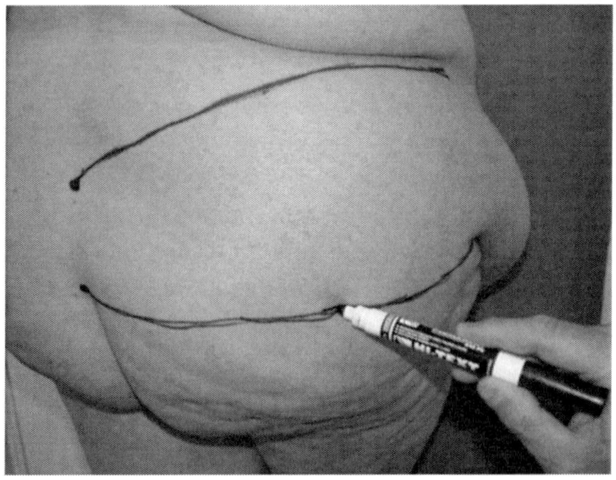

Figure 32. Torsoplasty: lateral excess tissue drawings.

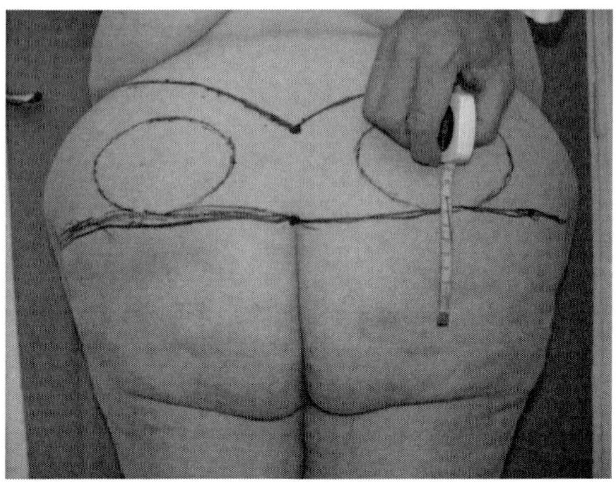

Figure 33. Torsoplasty: buttocks emphasizing island Flaps markings.

Anteriorly, with a mastoplasty–like handling, we determine the upper line of excision. Lower line is the same of a standard abdominoplasty (Figure34).

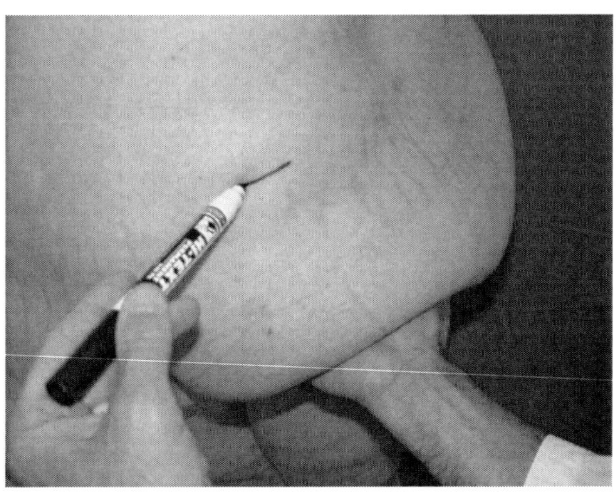

Figure 34. Torsoplasty: Frontal excess tissue drawing.

Surgical Technique

The operation is conducted in a prone-supine sequence.

In the prone position all the incisions are performed and all the exceeding tissue removed, while dermal-adipose islands are isolated and de-epithelialized (Figure35); then sutured and fixed deep into previously undermined buttocks (Figure36). Any other undermining, specifically in the pre-trochanteric areas, is greatly limited or avoided. Two suction drains are placed, all the back sutures completed and the patient is twisted.

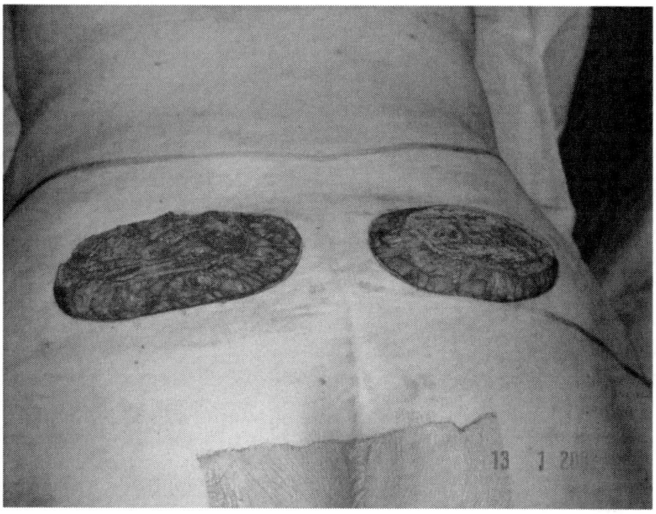

Figure 35. Torsoplasty: de-epithelialized island Flaps.

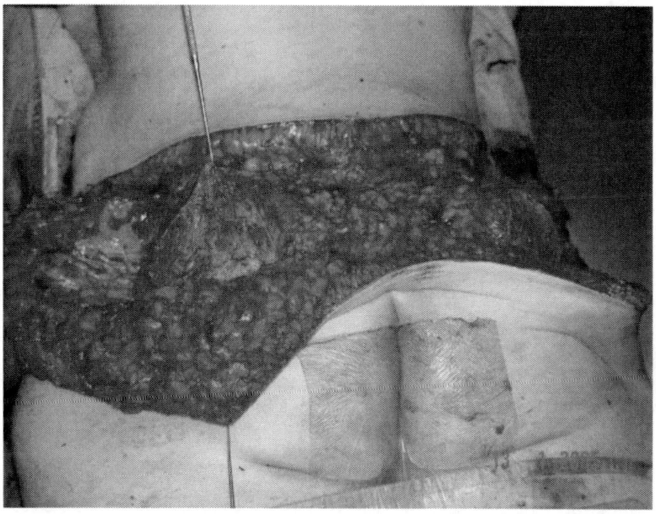

Figure 36. Torsoplasty: island Flaps deepened into undermined buttocks.

In the supine position, back incisions fading on the flanks are extended and completed, performing a traditional abdominoplasty, seldom associating the superficial fascial flap suggested by Wieslander [27] (Figure37) in order to prevent and reduce the amount of trophic complications. Two suction drains are inserted and all the sutures completed.

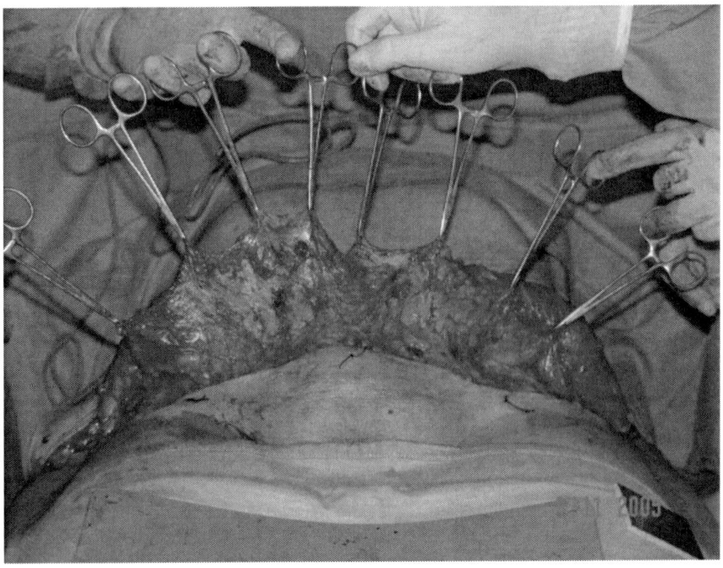

Figure 37. Wieslander superficial Fascial Flap.

The exceeding tissue is usually cut and removed into little pieces, and any piece is gently squeezed before cutting it: this procedure, rather than "en-bloc" excision, seems to reduce blood losses.

Drapings are performed with non adhesive wound dressings and compressive bands.

Post-Operative Care

When the total amount of excised tissue is over 10-12 kg., one or two days of intensive care recovery could be necessary. Usually all drains are removed within 6-8 days. Recovery lasts about 7-10 days.

Compression is removed after one week and a girdle worn day and night for one month, plus a further two weeks night-time only. If a small fat excess should remain in pre-trocantheric areas, a minor liposuction can be performed between 6 months and one year after (if no further body-contouring of thighs is scheduled).

Complications

Hematomas (5,4%) and seromas (3,8%) have dropped thanks to various preventing tricks and procedures.

The high incidence of abdominal wall complications [28, 29] (skin dehiscence and necrosis) (Figure 38), up to 45-50%, in this particular group of patients compared with non-BS patients and the review of anatomical studies [30, 31] has suggested to increase the research of causes by arteriographic study of the epigastric vessels. In five studied cases, no reliable modifications have been found. Therefore, without any other explanation, the only certain cause responsible for almost 70% of trophic complications following abdominoplasty is the presence of previous scars. In more recent BS cases operated by the laparoscopic approach (with very short abdominal scars), the percentage of complications has significantly decreased [32].

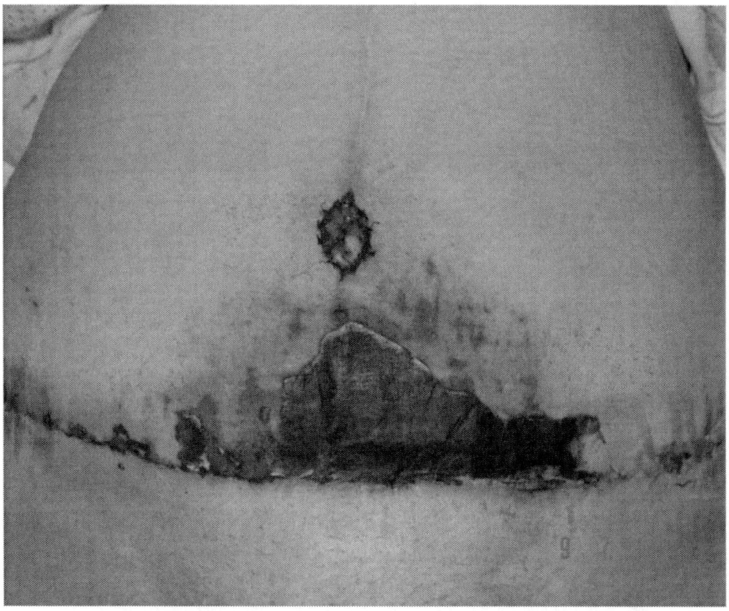

Figure 38. Abdominal wall complication (necrosis, 15th day post-op).

Conclusions

All patients achieve a nearly ideal torso contour (Figure 39-46), addressing very effectively all functional and aesthetical concerns of M. W. L. patients. This BC surgery is, without a doubt, highly challenging for both surgeon and patient: adequate learning curves, careful patient selections and education are essential in reaching a good outcome.

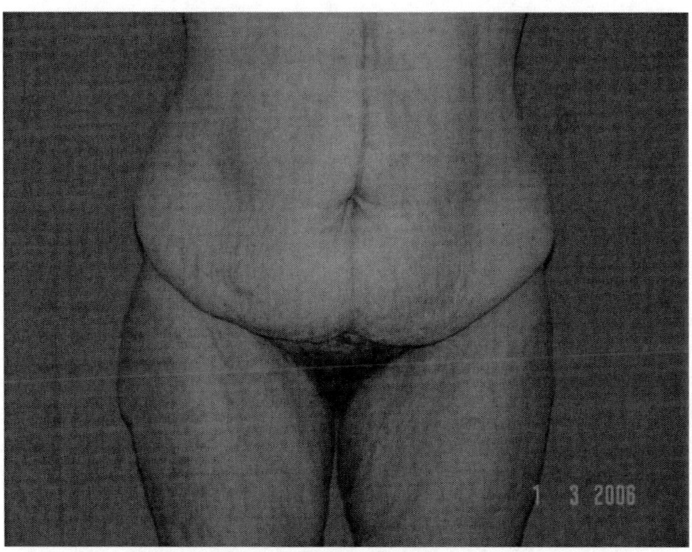

Figure 39. Torsoplasty case (♀ aa. 56, BPD): Pre-op Frontal view.

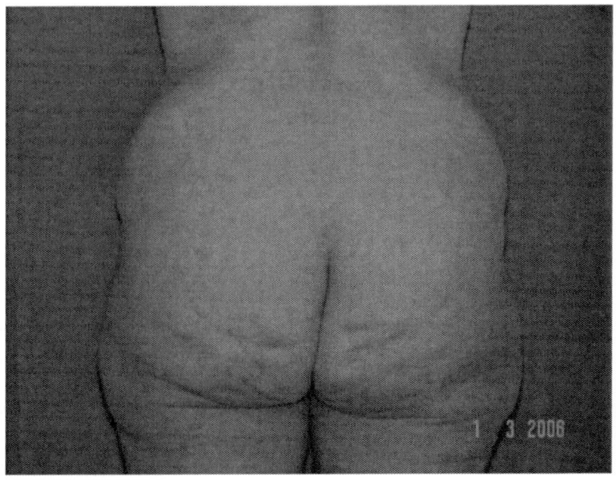

Figure 40. Torsoplasty case: Pre-op back view.

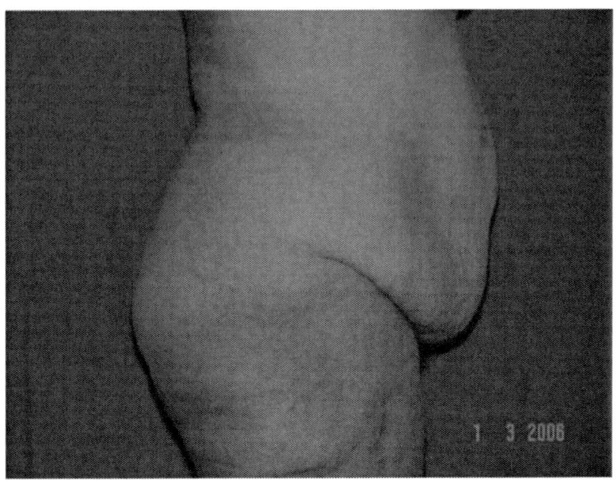

Figure 41. Torsoplasty case: Pre-op right view.

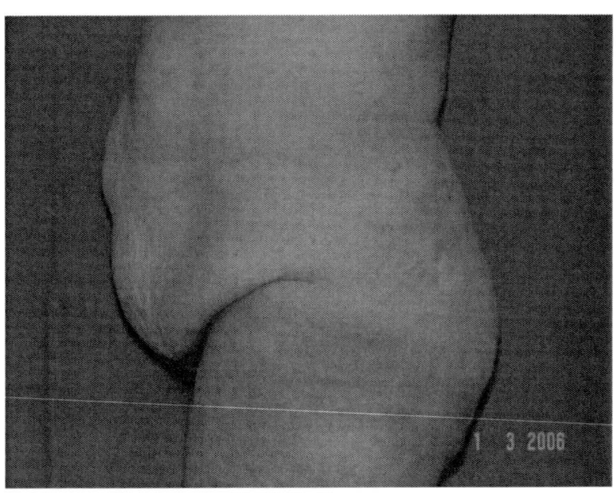

Figure 42. Torsoplasty case: Pre-op left view.

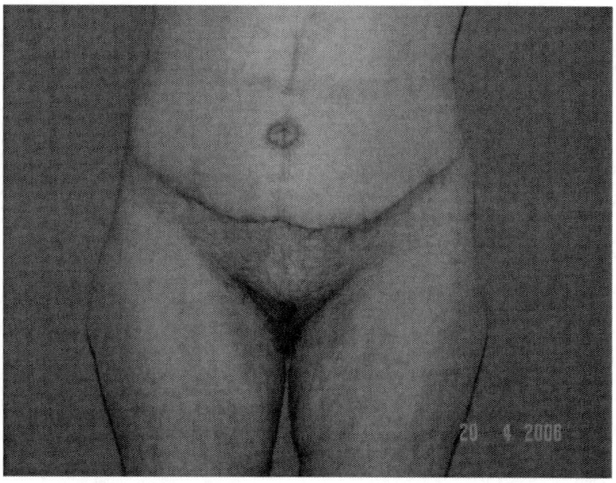

Figure 43. Torsoplasty case: Post-op Frontal view.

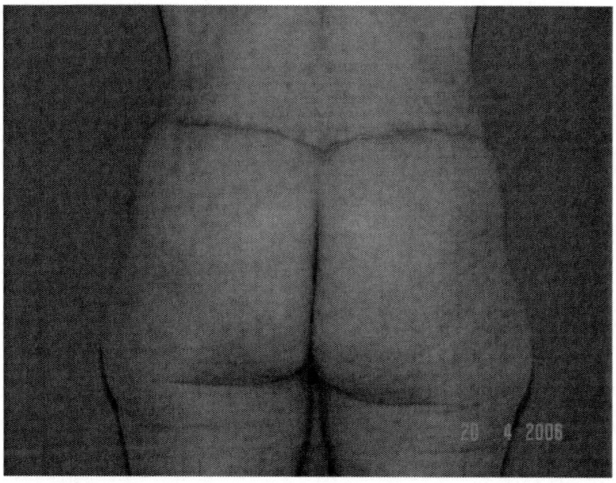

Figure 44. Torsoplasty case: Post-op back view.

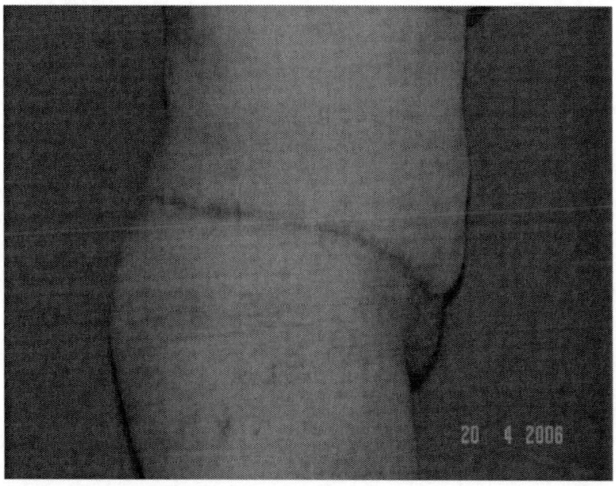

Figure 45. Torsoplasty case: Post-op right view.

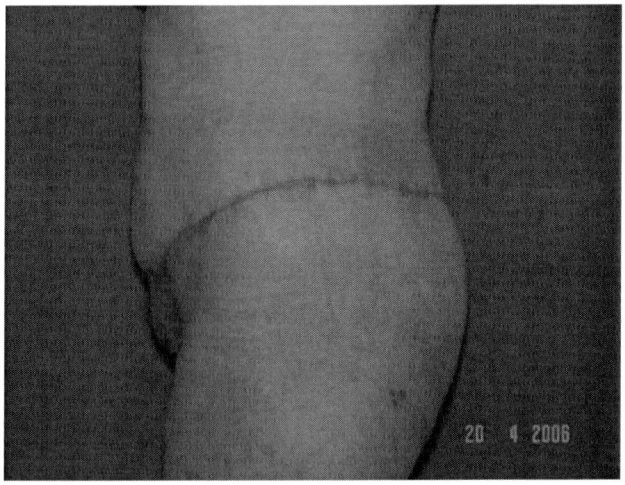

Figure 46. Torsoplasty case: Post-op left view.

Legs

The leg aesthetical problems in post-BS patients are mainly confined in the thigh and more or less resume the general problem of all M. W. L. patients: sagginess of body coverage. The loss of skin elasticity and of fat volume usually causes flabbiness of medial and/or lateral areas of the thighs.

Except classic lipodystrophy caused by general fat deposits, thigh BC can be very useful after BS. M. W. L. patients don't accept the skin excess located at inner and lateral aspects of the thighs, and the main demand for surgery is aesthetical improvement even if functional problems can be related too, like frictions and inflammations.

The lateral defects can be corrected with a body-lift [26] or a torsoplasty extended with a wide caudal undermining. Otherwise a *flankplasty* can be performed.

The inner thigh flabbiness requires specific surgical technique, the thigh lift. Depending on the different locations of the defects, the thigh lift can be conducted as:

Semicircular thigh lift
Circular thigh lift
Longitudinal thigh lift

Pursuing the aim of scar shortening, the suggestions of Le Louarn and Pascal [33] regarding excisions and suture are strongly advisable. To reduce possible lymphatic drainage complications and seromas, undermining must be avoided, choosing a full-thickness "en-block" removal of exceeding tissue.

Drawings

The preoperative drawing of the planned procedure is performed with patients standing and the legs 20-30 cm. abducted, paying great attention to symmetry. The upper line of incision is marked 1 cm above the inguinal fold, and 2 to 6 cm above the gluteal crease. A firm upward tension to the tissues to be lifted is applied, evaluating and marking the lower edge of excision.

Markings may be helped and guided by underwear traces so that the upper line of the drawing remains above the panty's lower edge.

If circular technique is needed, upper line continues from inguinal fold, turning back almost at greater trochanter height and joining back upper incision line.

If vertical technique is needed, the sequence described in Figures 47-51 is performed.

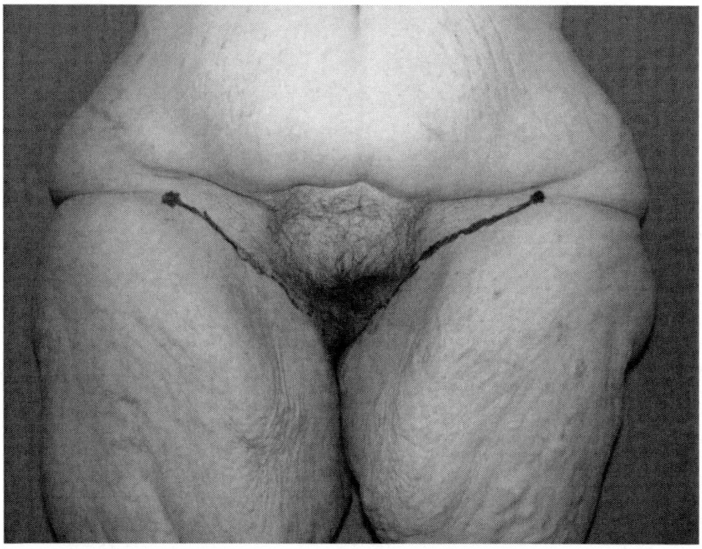

Figure 47. Thighplasty:Frontal upper markings.

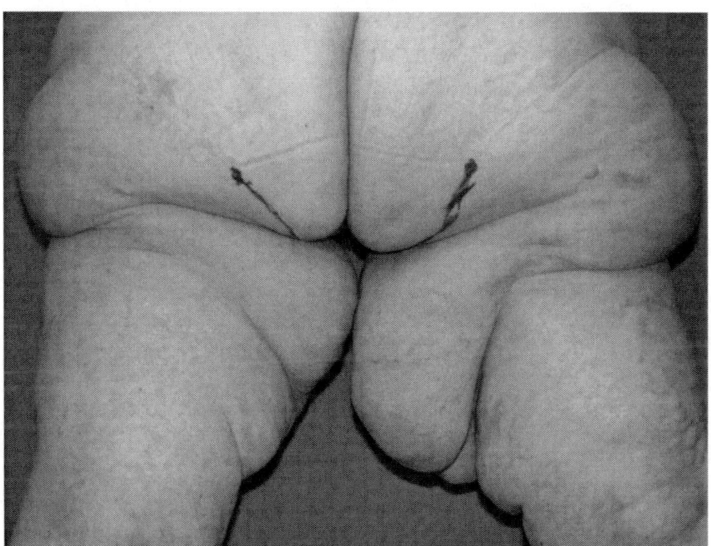

Figure 48. Thighplasty: back upper markings.

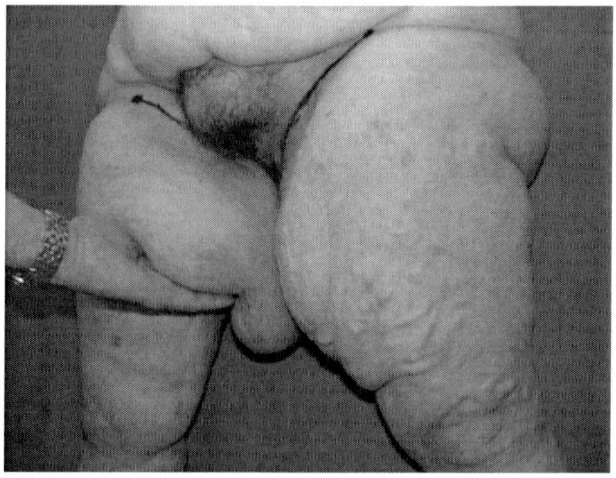

Figure 49. Thighplasty: excess tissue evaluation.

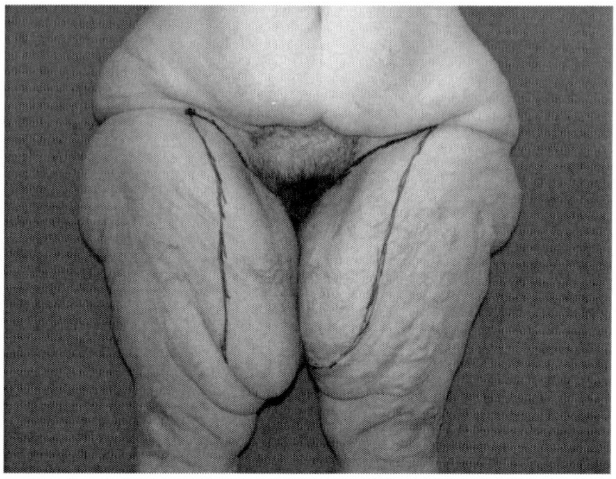

Figure 50. Thighplasty: Frontal markings completed.

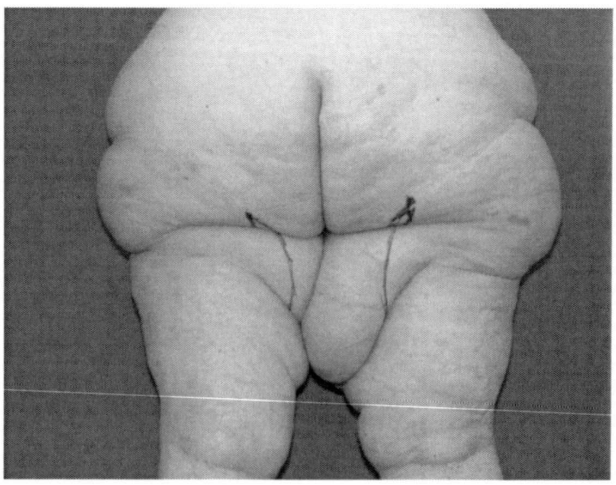

Figure 51. Thighplaty: Back markings completed.

Surgical Techniques

The *flankplasty*, as described by Baroudi [34], can be useful in few cases (Figures 52-53), but usually what can be corrected with it can be done with a torsoplasty as well. It is rare to find a post-BS patient with isolated lateral thigh defects.

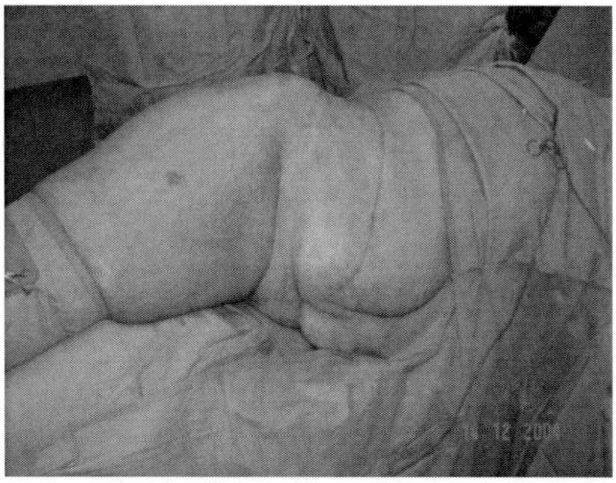

Figure 52. Flankplasty: Intra-op starting.

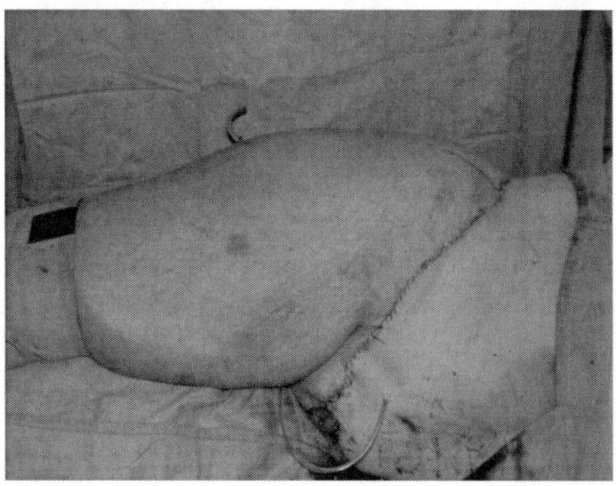

Figure 53. Flankplasty: Intra-op ending.

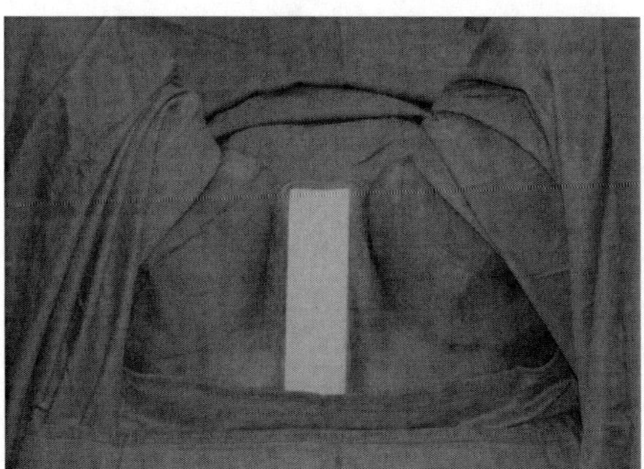

Figure 54. Thighplasty: Intra-op starting.

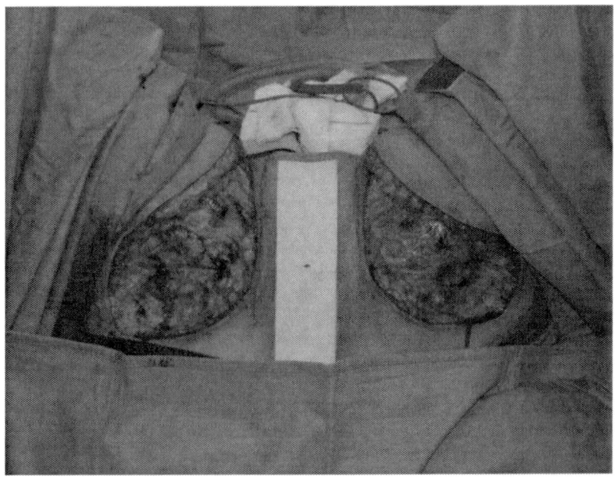

Figure 55. Thighplasty: excision completed.

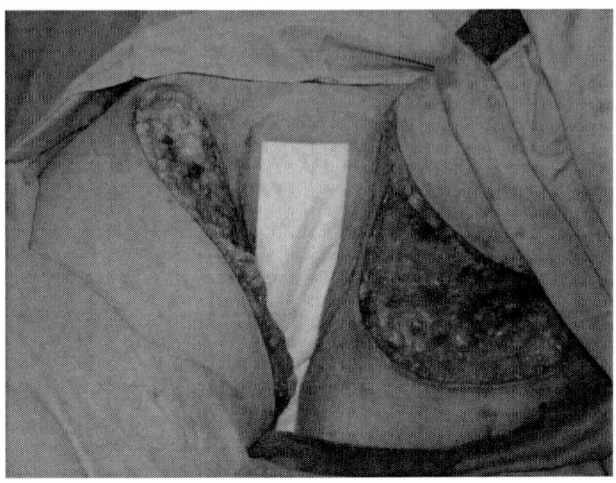

Figure 56. Thighplasty: right thigh suturing.

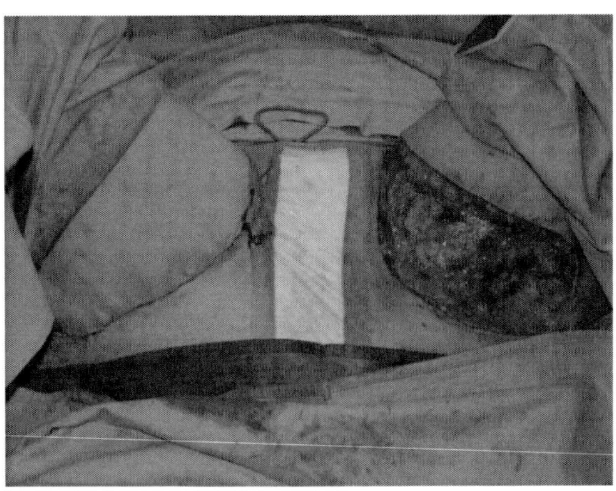

Figure 57. Thighplasty: right suture completed.

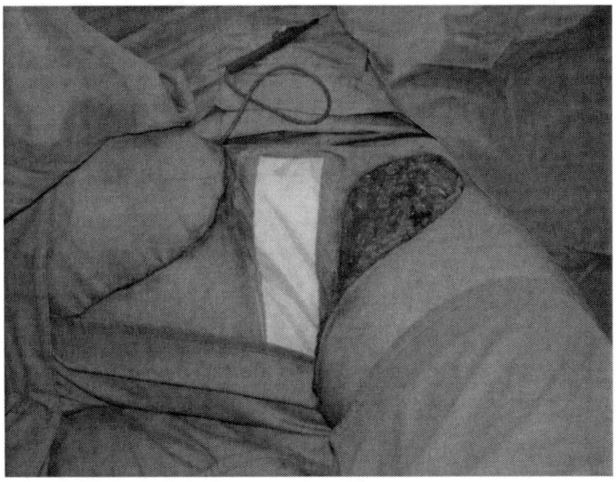

Figure 58. Thighplasty: left thigh suturing.

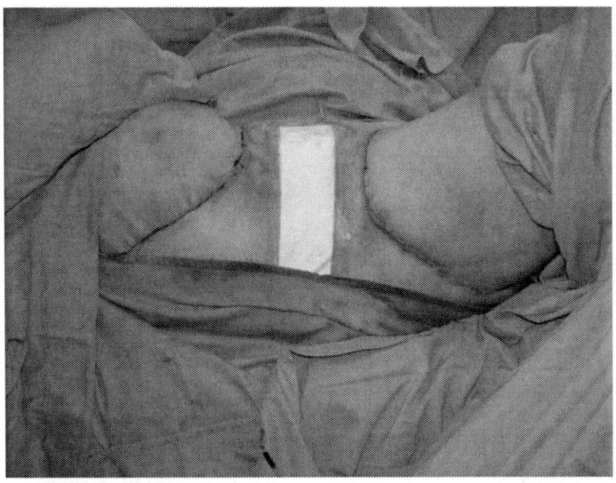

Figure 59. Thighplasty: Intra-op ending.

The *semicircular thigh lift* is based on the classical Pitanguy [35], Baroudi [36] and Lewis [37, 38] techniques.

Operation is performed in lithotomy position, alternatively adducting legs for the suturing time (Figures 54-59). The incisions cut skin and fat tissue straight down to the fascia, which is preserved. Removal of exceeding tissue is directly done on the fascia, with no undermining.

Firm and stable suspension is guaranteed by anchoring [33] the superficial fascia system and the dermis of inferior flap to the lateral band of Colles' fascia. This will successfully prevent the two major aesthetical complications: scar caudal displacement and early recurrence of the defect.

One drain per side is placed, and two layers suture performed to complete procedure.

Light draping is maintained for a few weeks. The use of elastic panty stockings is recommended for several weeks post-op.

The *circular thigh lift*, as Baroudi [36] explains, is necessary when redundant tissue extends to frontal and lateral aspects of the thighs, sagging down to the knees, and the semicircular technique is not enough. The operation is conducted first in prone position, then in lithotomy position.

The anterior incision is done 2 to 4 cm above the inguinal fold as far as possible medially and continued laterally inside underwear traces.

The only relevant technical difference with semicircular technique is lateral excision according to the amount of tissue to be dismissed, with no undermining.

The same type of suture, draping and wearing as for semicircular lift are performed.

The *longitudinal thigh lift* is rarely indicated and often avoided by surgeons and patients because of bad reputation of the results. Most deformities can effectively be reduced with the previous procedures, leaving hidden scars. Nevertheless, some post-BS cases need vertical(or longitudinal) reduction in order to obtain valuable results, even if bad and visible scars are expected, anyway better than skin excess. The suggested vertical excision is posteromedial, running straight to the popliteal region and ending as soon as the redundant tissue ends.

The main steps of the procedure are the same as for previous ones, performing no undermining as usual. Post-op management doesn't differ from other procedures.

Complications

General complications are represented by scar distrophies/keloids (22,7%), edema (14,2%), seromas (11,8%), lymphorrea (7,6%), wound dehiscence (2,9%).

Specific complications include vertical scar widening (37,1%), defect recurrence after 1 year (12,5%) and scar displacement (5%).

Conclusion

Although the characteristics of post-BS patients limit choices and chances, satisfying results are achieved not only as cosmetic correction but also in quality of life, because in this anatomical area functional improvements are mostly accomplished by BC (Figures 60-67).

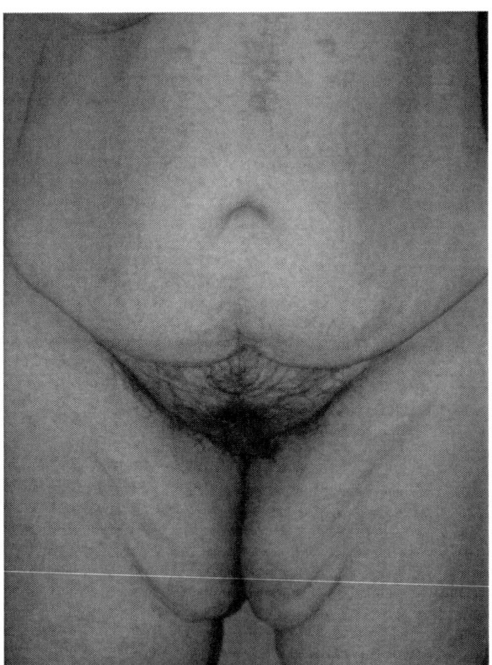

Figure 60. Thighplasty: case 1 (♀ aa. 45, BPD)semicircular, Pre-op.

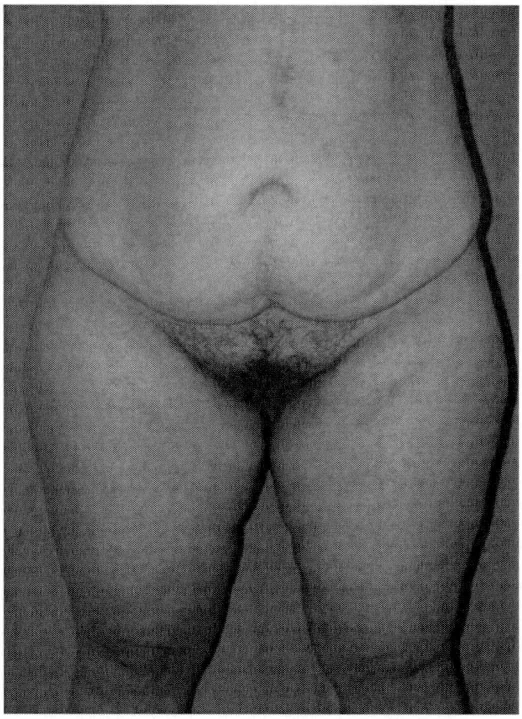

Figure 61. Thighplasty: case 1 Post-op.

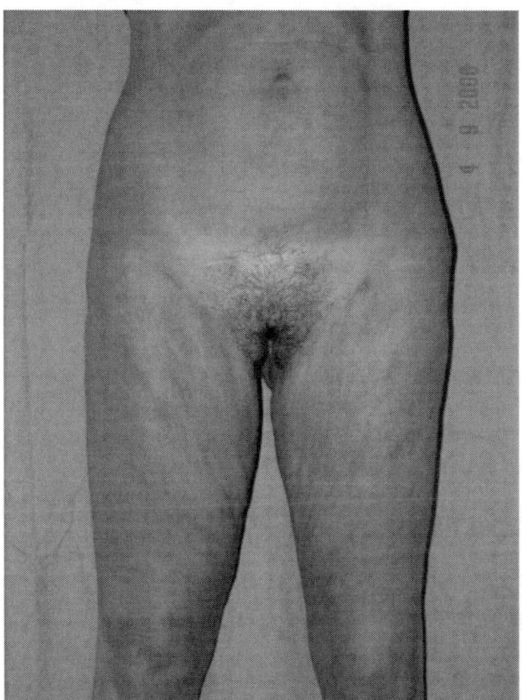

Figure 62. Thighplasty: case 2 (♀ aa. 38, BPD) semicircular, Pre-op.

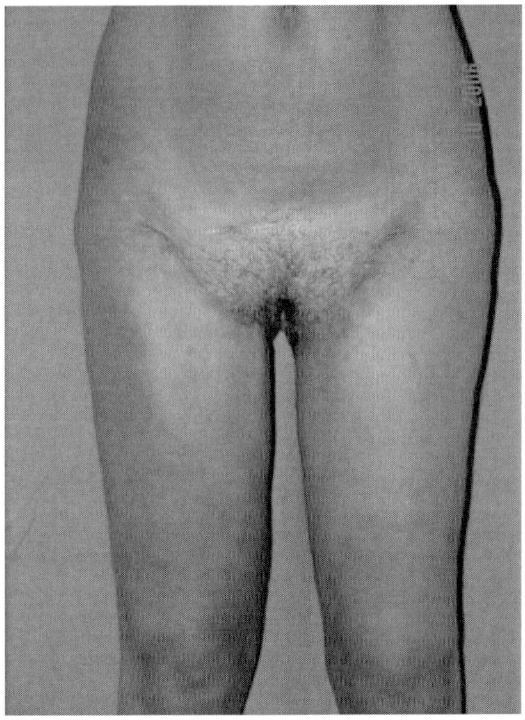

Figure 63. Thighplasty: case 2 Post-op.

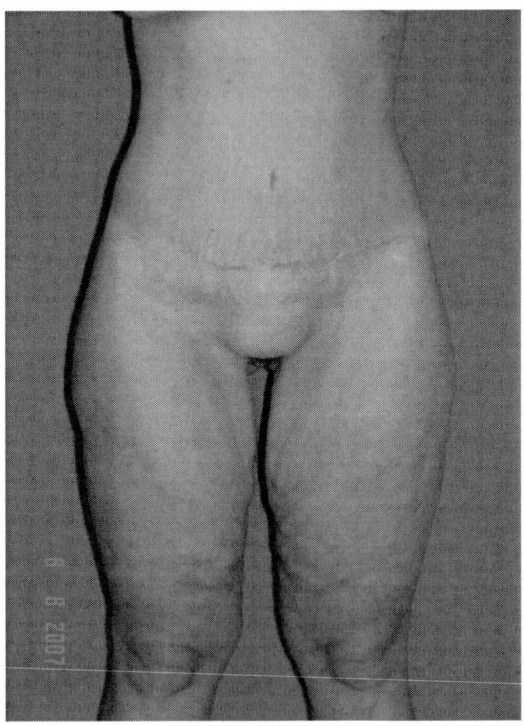

Figure 64. Thighplasty: case 3 (♀ aa. 31, BPD) longitudinal, Front Pre-op.

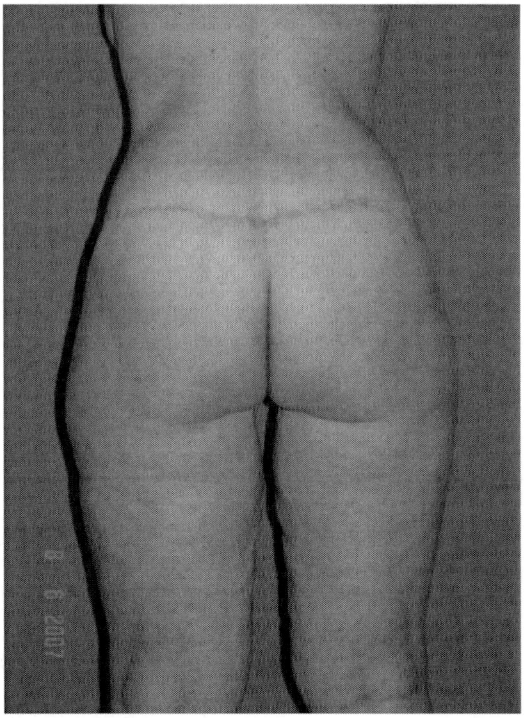

Figure 65. Thighplasty: case 3 back Pre-op.

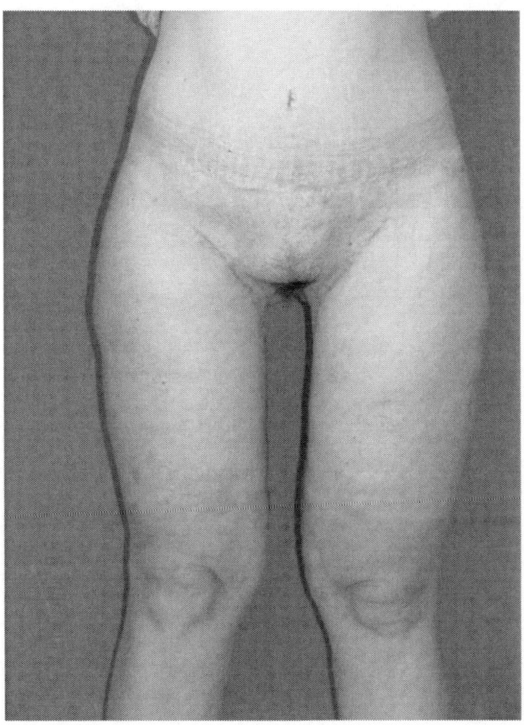

Figure 66. Thighplasty: case 3 Front Post-op.

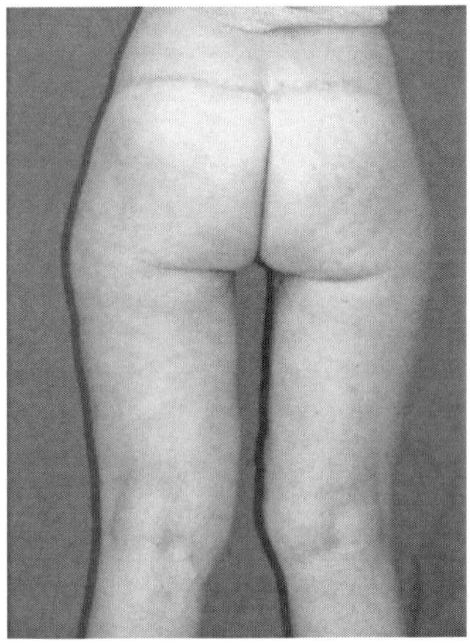

Figure 67. Thighplasty: case 3 back Post-op.

BUT

Indichi con una X la risposta più vicina alla sua esperienza attuale

		mai	raramente	qualche volta	spesso	molto spesso	sempre
1	Trascorro molto tempo davanti allo specchio	0	1	2	3	4	5
2	Non mi fido del mio aspetto: temo che cambi, all'improvviso	0	1	2	3	4	5
3	Mi piacciono gli abiti che nascondono le forme del mio corpo	0	1	2	3	4	5
4	Passo molto tempo pensando a certi difetti della mia immagine fisica	0	1	2	3	4	5
5	Quando mi spoglio evito di guardarmi	0	1	2	3	4	5
6	Penso che la mia vita cambierebbe profondamente se potessi correggere alcuni miei difetti estetici	0	1	2	3	4	5
7	Mangiare in presenza di altri mi provoca ansia	0	1	2	3	4	5
8	*Il pensiero di alcuni difetti del mio corpo mi tormenta tanto da impedirmi di stare con gli altri*	0	1	2	3	4	5
9	Ho il terrore di ingrassare	0	1	2	3	4	5
10	Faccio lunghi confronti fra il mio aspetto e quello degli altri	0	1	2	3	4	5
11	Se comincio a guardarmi mi è difficile smettere	0	1	2	3	4	5
12	Farei qualsiasi cosa per modificare certe parti del mio corpo	0	1	2	3	4	5
13	*Resto in casa ed evito di farmi vedere dagli altri*	0	1	2	3	4	5
14	Mi vergogno dei bisogni fisici del mio corpo	0	1	2	3	4	5
15	Mi sento derisa/o per il mio aspetto	0	1	2	3	4	5
16	Il pensiero di alcuni difetti del mio corpo mi tormenta tanto da impedirmi di studiare o di lavorare	0	1	2	3	4	5
17	Cerco nello specchio un'immagine di me che mi soddisfi e continuo a scrutarmi finché sono sicura/o di averla trovata	0	1	2	3	4	5
18	Mi sento più grassa/o di quello che dicono gli altri	0	1	2	3	4	5
19	Evito gli specchi	0	1	2	3	4	5
20	Ho l'impressione che la mia immagine cambi continuamente	0	1	2	3	4	5
21	Vorrei avere un corpo secco e duro	0	1	2	3	4	5
22	Sono insoddisfatta/o del mio aspetto	0	1	2	3	4	5
23	Il mio aspetto fisico è deludente rispetto alla mia immagine ideale	0	1	2	3	4	5
24	*Vorrei sottopormi a qualche intervento di chirurgia estetica*	0	1	2	3	4	5
25	Non sopporto l'idea di vivere con l'aspetto che ho	0	1	2	3	4	5
26	Mi guardo allo specchio e provo un senso di inquietudine e di estraneità	0	1	2	3	4	5
27	Temo che il mio corpo cambi contro la mia volontà in modi che non mi piacciono	0	1	2	3	4	5
28	Mi sento scollata/o dal mio corpo	0	1	2	3	4	5
29	*Ho la sensazione che il mio corpo non mi appartenga*	0	1	2	3	4	5
30	Il pensiero di alcuni difetti del mio corpo mi tormenta tanto da impedirmi di avere una vita sessuale	0	1	2	3	4	5
31	Mi osservo in quello che faccio e mi chiedo come appaio agli altri	0	1	2	3	4	5
32	Vorrei decidere io che aspetto avere	0	1	2	3	4	5
33	Mi sento diversa/o da come mi vedono gli altri	0	1	2	3	4	5
34	Mi vergogno del mio corpo	0	1	2	3	4	5

Università La Sapienza DSNPEE

M. Cuzzolaro, G. Vetrone, G.F. Marano Pagina 1 di 2

(A)

Figure 68. (Continued).

BUT

Indichi con una ✗ la risposta più vicina alla sua esperienza attuale

Del mio corpo, in particolare, detesto:

		mai	raramente	qualche volta	spesso	molto spesso	sempre
1	la statura	0	1	2	3	4	5
2	la forma della testa	0	1	2	3	4	5
3	la forma del viso	0	1	2	3	4	5
4	la pelle	0	1	2	3	4	5
5	i capelli	0	1	2	3	4	5
6	la fronte	0	1	2	3	4	5
7	le sopracciglia	0	1	2	3	4	5
8	gli occhi	0	1	2	3	4	5
9	il naso	0	1	2	3	4	5
10	le labbra	0	1	2	3	4	5
11	la bocca	0	1	2	3	4	5
12	i denti	0	1	2	3	4	5
13	le orecchie	0	1	2	3	4	5
14	il collo	0	1	2	3	4	5
15	il mento	0	1	2	3	4	5
16	i baffi	0	1	2	3	4	5
17	la barba	0	1	2	3	4	5
18	i peli	0	1	2	3	4	5
19	le spalle	0	1	2	3	4	5
20	le braccia	0	1	2	3	4	5
21	le mani	0	1	2	3	4	5
22	il torace	0	1	2	3	4	5
23	le mammelle	0	1	2	3	4	5
24	lo stomaco	0	1	2	3	4	5
25	il ventre	0	1	2	3	4	5
26	i genitali	0	1	2	3	4	5
27	le natiche	0	1	2	3	4	5
28	le anche	0	1	2	3	4	5
29	le cosce	0	1	2	3	4	5
30	le ginocchia	0	1	2	3	4	5
31	le gambe	0	1	2	3	4	5
32	le caviglie	0	1	2	3	4	5
33	i piedi	0	1	2	3	4	5
34	l'odore	0	1	2	3	4	5
35	i rumori	0	1	2	3	4	5
36	sudare	0	1	2	3	4	5
37	arrossire	0	1	2	3	4	5

M. Cuzzolaro, G. Vetrone, G.F. Marano — Pagina 2 di 2 — Università La Sapienza [illegible]

(B)

Figure 68. A) B. U. T. Frontpage, B) B. U. T. back page.

Outcome

Great "positive" thinking of these patients towards BC creates enormous expectations for improvement in quality of life (similar to the expectations which motivated these patients toward bariatric surgery) [39]. Of these operated patients, 99% declare themselves completely satisfied with the obtained results and go on to further body contouring. These kinds of results are not achievable by bariatric surgery alone and/or by eating behavior normalization, and have been tested with the Body Uneasiness Test (B. U. T.) [40] (Figure 68) on 5 different groups of these patients. On average, 2,5 operations have been performed on each patient.

The main points of patient satisfaction are: "body image" greatly improved, self-esteem recovery, improvement in life relationships, and sexual life resumption or improvement [41].

References

[1] Singh D., Forte A., Loerke C., Bell R., Thomson J. G. "P63: Prognostication of Body Contouring after Bariatric Surgery" –*Plast. Reconstr. Surg.* Abstract Supplement. 118(4) Supplement:144, September 15, 2006.

[2] O'Connell J. B. "Bariplastic Surgery" –*Plast. Reconstr. Surg.* 113(5):1530, April 15, 2004.

[3] Huemer G. M., Dunst K. "Massive Weight Loss after Bariatric Surgery: Friend or Foe?" –*Plast. Reconstr. Surg.* 114(6):1663-1664, November 2004.

[4] Baroudi R., Moraes M. "Philosophy, Technical Principles, Selection, and Indication in BodyContouring Surgery" –*Aesth. Plast. Surg.* 15:1-18, 1991.

[5] Folope V., Coëffier M., Déchelotte P. "Nutritional deficiencies associated with bariatric surgery" – *Gastroenterol. Clin. Biol.* 2007 Apr; 31(4):369-77.

[6] Shermak M. A., Chang D. C., Heller J. "Factors impacting thromboembolism after bariatric body contouring surgery" – *Plast. Reconstr. Surg.* 2007 Apr 15;119(5):1590-6.

[7] Guerrero-Santos J. "Brachioplasty" – *Aesth. Plast. Surg.* 1979; 3: 1-4.

[8] Strauch B,Greenspun D, Levine J et al. "A techniqueof brachioplasty" – *Plast. Reconstr. Surg.* 2004; 113: 1044-8.

[9] Bolivar de Souza Pinto E., Erazo P., Matsuda C. A. "Brachioplasty technique with the use of molds" – *Plast. Reconstr. Surg.* 105:1854, 2.

[10] Lockwood T. "Brachioplasty with superficial fascial system suspension" – *Plast. Reconstr. Surg.* 96:912, 1995.

[11] Goddio A. S. "A New Technique for Brachioplasty"–*Plast. Reconstr. Surg.* 84(1):85-91, July 1989.

[12] Mahjouri F. "A Technique in Brachioplasty" – *Plast. Reconstr. Surg.* 116(2):678-679, August 2005.

[13] Abramson D. L. "Minibrachioplasty: Minimizing Scars While Maximizing Results" – *Plast. Reconstr. Surg.* 114(6):1631-1634, November 2004.

[14] Teimourian B., Malekzadeh S. "Rejuvenation of the Upper Arm" – *Plast. Reconstr. Surg.* 102(2):545-551, August 1998.

[15] Brink R. "Management of true ptosis of the breast" – *Plast. Reconstr. Surg.* 91: 657, 1993.

[16] Benelli L. "A New PeriareolarMammaplasty: the "Round Block" Technique" – *Aesth. Plast. Surg.* 14:93-100, 1990.

[17] Migliori F. "Upside-Down Augmentation Mastopexy" – *Aesth. Plast. Surg.* 35:593-600, 2011.

[18] Càrdenas-Camarena L., Ramìrez-Macìas, R. "Augmentation/Mastopexy: How to Select and Perform the Proper Technique" – *Aesth. Plast. Surg.* 30:21-33, 2006.

[19] Hammond D. C., Khuthaila D. K., Kim J. "The Interlocking Gore-Tex Suture for Control of Areolar Diameter and Shape" – *Plast. Reconstr. Surg.* 119(3):804-809, March 2007.

[20] De Longis E. "Mammoplasty with an L-shaped limited scar and retropecto-raldermopexy" – *Aesth. Plast. Surg.* 10:171-175, 1986.

[21] Arié G. "Una nuevatéchnica de mastoplastia" – *Rev. Lat. Am. Cir. Plast.* 3:22, 1957.

[22] Matarasso A. "Liposuction as an Adjunct to a Full Abdominoplasty Revisited" – *Plast. Reconstr. Surg.* 106(5):1197-1202, October 2000.

[23] Planas J. "The "Vest Over Pants" abdominoplasty" – *Plast. Reconstr. Surg.* 61(5):694-700, May 1978.

[24] Planas J., Bisbal J., del Cacho C., Palacin J. M. "Further advantages of the "Vest over pants" abdominoplasty" – *Aesth. Plast. Surg.* 12:123-127, 1988.

[25] Lockwood T. E. "Lower body lift with superficial fascialsystem suspension" – *Plast. Reconstr. Surg.* 1993; 92: 1112-6.

[26] Pascal J. F., Le Louarn C. "Remodelling body-lift withhigh lateral tension" – *Aesth. Plast. Surg* 2002; 26:223-30.

[27] Wieslander J. B. "Preservation of fat under Scarpa's fascia in the lower abdomen reduces complications inabdominoplasties" - 10th Congress of the European Society of Plastic, Reconstructive and Aesthetic SurgeryE. S. P. R. A. S (Sept. 1st 2005).

[28] Nurkim M. V. et al. "Incidence of hematoma and seromain abdominoplasty with and without the use of drains" – Rev. Soc. Bras. *Cir. Plast.* 2002; 17: 69-74 (abstract).

[29] vanUchelen J. H., Werker P. M. N., Kon M. "Complications of abdominoplasty in 86 patients" – *Plast. Reconstr. Surg.* 2001; 107: 1869-73.

[30] Huger W. E. Jr. "The anatomic rationale for abdominal lipectomy" – *Ann. Surg.* 1979; 45: 612-7.

[31] Hester T. R. Jr., Nahai F., Beegle P. E. et al. "Blood supply of the abdomen revisited, with emphasis on the superficial inferior epigastric artery" – *Plast. Reconstr. Surg.* 1984; 47: 657-70.

[32] Scopinaro N., Marinari G. M., Camerini G. "Laparoscopic standard biliopancreatic diversion:technique and preliminary results" – *Obes. Surg.* 2002;12: 362-5.

[33] Le Louarn C., Pascal J. F. "The concentric medial thighlift" – *Aesth. Plast. Surg.* 2004; 28: 20-23.

[34] Baroudi R., Moraes M. "Philosophy, Technical Principles, Selection, and Indication in BodyContouring Surgery" – *Aesth. Plast. Surg.* 15:1-18, 1991.

[35] Pitanguy I. "Surgical reduction of the abdomen, thigh and buttocks" – *Surg. Clin. North. Am.* 51:479, 1971.

[36] Regnault P., Baroudi R., da SilveiraCarvalho C. G. (1979). "Correction of Lower Limb Lipodystrophy" –*Aesth. Plast. Surg.* 3:233-249.

[37] *Lewis J. R.* "An Atlas of Aesthetic Plastic Surgery" – 285-288 Little, Brown and Co., Boston,1973.

[38] Lewis J. R. "Correction of ptosis of the thighs: the thigh lift" – *Plast. Reconstr. Surg.* 37:494, 1966.

[39] Bolton M., Pruzinsky T., Cash T. et al. (2003). "Measuring outcomesin plastic surgery: body image and quality oflife in abdominoplasty patients" – *Plast. Reconstr. Surg.* ; 112: 619-25

[40] Pecori L., Serra Cervetti G. G., Marinari G. M., Migliori F., Adami G. F. "Attitudes of morbidly obese patients to weight loss and body image following bariatric surgery and body contouring" – *Obes. Surg.* 2007 Jan; 17(1) 68-73.

[41] Migliori F. et al. (2006). "Body contouring after biliopancreatic diversion" – *Obes. Surg.* Dec; 16(12): 1638-44.

In: Bariatric Surgery
Editor: Christos R. Iavazzo
ISBN: 978-1-62618-995-9

Chapter XIV

Bariatric Brachioplasty

Miguel Modolin, Wilson Cintra Jr. and Rodrigo Itocazo Rocha
Division of Plastic Surgery – Hospital das Clínicas –
University of Sao Paulo School of Medicine, Brazil

Introduction

Dysmorphism in the arms, following weight loss, is caused by the loss of fat content, limited skin retraction ability resulting from smaller amounts of collagen and elastin, and laxity due to distension of the superficial fascia.

Thus, the arms lose their cylindrical contour due to a skin fold that may extend from the elbow to the lateral thoracic wall, going beyond the axilla, thus characterizing a deformity known as "bat wing" (Figure 1).

This is treated surgically by brachioplasty to reduce volume thus enabling a wider range of motion, a more aesthetic looking arm contour, the use of sleeveless clothes and, ultimately, a better quality of life.

Surgical Technique

When the excess skin is restricted to the arm, it is resected by means of a fusiform excision in the medial aspect from the elbow which is combined with a transverse ellipse in the axilla thus defining the shape of a fish tail (Figure 3). If the excess skin extends to the thorax, the elliptical marking is prolonged to this region; in the axilla, a Z-plasty is performed. Resection is made above the superficial fascia.

Results

Despite the long scar, patients show great satisfaction because of the improvement in their quality of life through better hygienic care, wider range of motion, a more aesthetic looking arm contour, and the freedom to wear sleeveless clothes which was previously embarrassing because of their arm deformity.

Complications and Events

Complications are due to the failure to observe an accurate surgical technique, whereas events result from adverse biological factors. Events:

1. Edema and seroma;
2. Ecchymosis;
3. Keloid scar.

Complications:

1. Hematoma;
2. Dehiscence;
3. Limphorrhea and lymphocele;
4. Necrosis;
5. Hypertrophic scar;
6. Infection;
7. Paresthesia.

Bariatric Brachioplasty

Introduction

Bariatric surgeries, as a rule, lead to massive weight loss and marked changes in body contour, which assumes bizarre shapes.

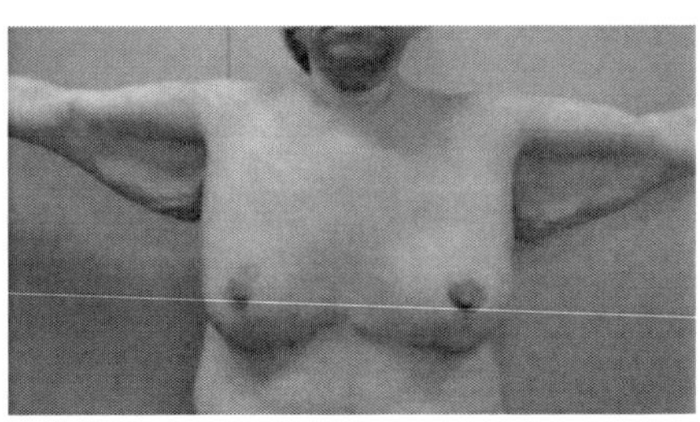

a

Figure 1. (Continued).

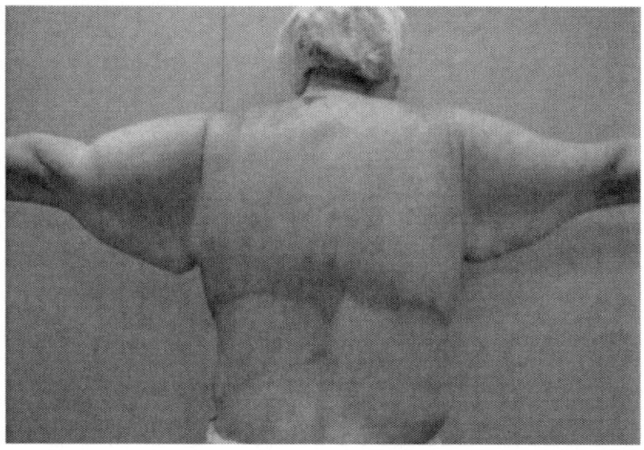

b

Figure 1. Severe brachial dysmorphy ("bat wing"). A. Anterior view. B. Posterior view.

This impacts the quality of life of the individuals affected by these deformities, known as dysmorphisms. Dysmorphism in the arms, following weight loss, is characterized by the loss of their cylindrical contour, due to a skin fold of varying size that may extend from the elbow to the axilla, or even beyond, reaching the lateral thoracic wall, thus defining a deformity known as "bat wing" (Figure 1). This is caused by the loss of fat content, limited skin retraction ability, and laxity due to distension of the superficial fascia.

Brachial dysmorphism is treated surgically by brachioplasty to restore a more aesthetic looking cylinder-shaped arm contour. Concomitantly, because the surgical procedure reduces volume, it enables a wider range of motion and the use of more comfortable clothes like sleeveless shirts in the summer.

Surgical Technique

In patients whose dysmorphism affects only the mid-portion of the arm, similar to a hammock, a fusiform excision of skin is sufficient. With the patient in the sitting position, an ellipse is medially marked 1 to 2 cm above and parallel to the brachial sulcus.

The posterior line is marked using a bidigital pinching maneuver, exercising care to avoid excessive tension, with the arm abducted to 90º and the elbow to 80º. It is crucial to make careful markings to avoid large resections that could lead to a difficult final wound closure and permanent damage such as transverse grooves or even a tourniquet effect in the distal portion of the upper limb. Both the anterior and posterior incisions converge toward the epicondyle of the humerus, and cephalad, toward the axilla, thus containing the excess skin to be resected (Figure 2). When the dysmorphic fold of the arm is larger, the ellipse is prolonged from the epicondyle to the anterior border of the axillary hair area, where another transverse ellipse is delimited and resected within the anterior and posterior axillary folds. The combination of these markings defines the "fish tail" resection (Figure 3). This strategy makes the resection of local dermal-cutaneous folds easier, since they usually require prolongation of the incision to the axilla; otherwise they may produce redundancies at the end of the scar known as "dog ear".

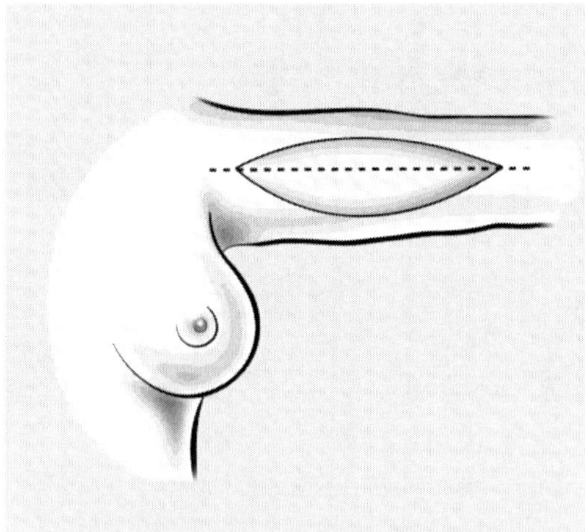

a

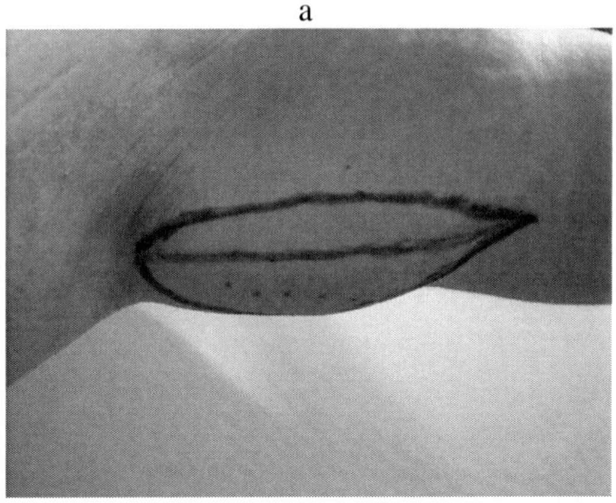

b

Figure 2. Fusiform technique. A. Drawing of the fusiform marking. B. Preoperative marking in a patient.

In patients whose deformity extends to the lateral thoracic wall, the elliptical marking is prolonged to this region containing the excess dermal-cutaneous fold. In the axilla, the wound closure line is decomposed using Z-plasty (Figure 4). The patient is placed lying in the supine position with his arms abducted upward, thus facilitating the surgical approach (Figure 5). In order to reduce the operative time, the procedure is performed by two teams simultaneously. The surgery is performed under general anesthesia and infiltration of the surgical area with saline solution containing epinephrine to minimize bleeding. Prophylactic antibiotic therapy with cephazolin is given during the anesthetic induction. Brachioplasty should be performed above the superficial fascia to avoid affecting the lymphatic vessels and nerves that run in the deeper plane. Plane closure is initiated after excision and careful hemostasis with electrocautery. In patients undergoing the axillary approach, the superficial fascia of the arm is fixed to the axillary fascia, thus promoting suspension of the posterior portion of the arm by means of an interrupted suture using 4-0 polyamide (Figure 6). This works as an arm sling that ensures tension of the tissues distended by obesity, which did not retract after weight loss. Wound closure in the deep subcutaneous plane, including the superficial fascia, is made with an interrupted suture using 4-0 polyamide.

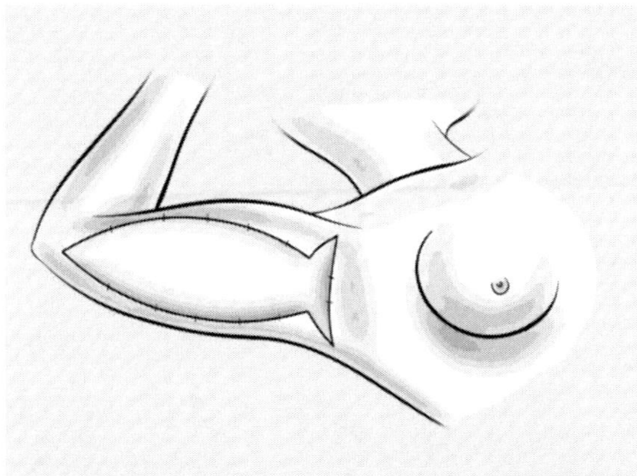

a

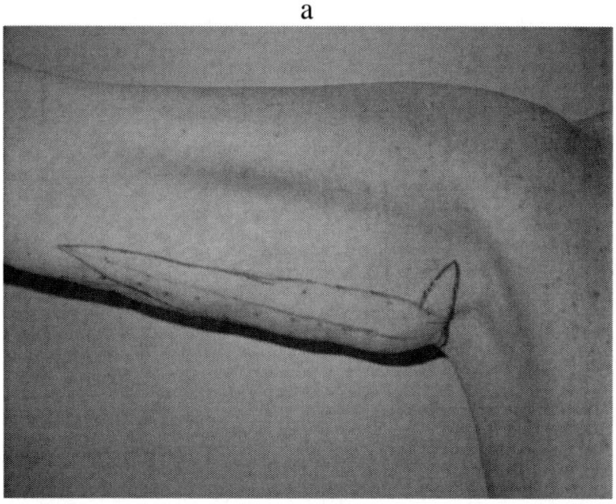

b

Figure 3. Double-ellipse technique. A. Drawing of the "fish tail" marking. B. Preoperative marking in a patient.

It is worth stressing that when over-resection occurs, closure of this plane – important for reestablishing the cylindrical shape of the arm – may determine transverse depressions that are difficult to correct. A running intradermal suture using 4-0 or 5-0 polyglecaprone is the final suture.

Following wound closure, Z-plasty should be performed in the middle of the axilla, in those cases in which the incision crossed it. It could be argued that this maneuver is unnecessary given that there is remaining skin; however, precisely because of it, Z-plasty is mandatory to define the axillary dome.

Another argument against Z-plasty is the transposition of a hairless area into a hair area and vice-versa. Nonetheless, we should consider that Z-plasty is performed in the middle of the axilla after considerable resection of hairy skin, making this transposition minimally perceptible, especially in female patients who are familiar with hair removal. Moreover, Z-plasty clearly prevents scar contracture (Figure 7).

Wound closure should be performed as fast as possible. In more extensive cases the temporary use of staples is recommended, later replaced by definitive suture. This reduces the edema, which can further make wound closure more difficult and frequently leads to ischemia in the wound area or to a tourniquet effect in the arm.

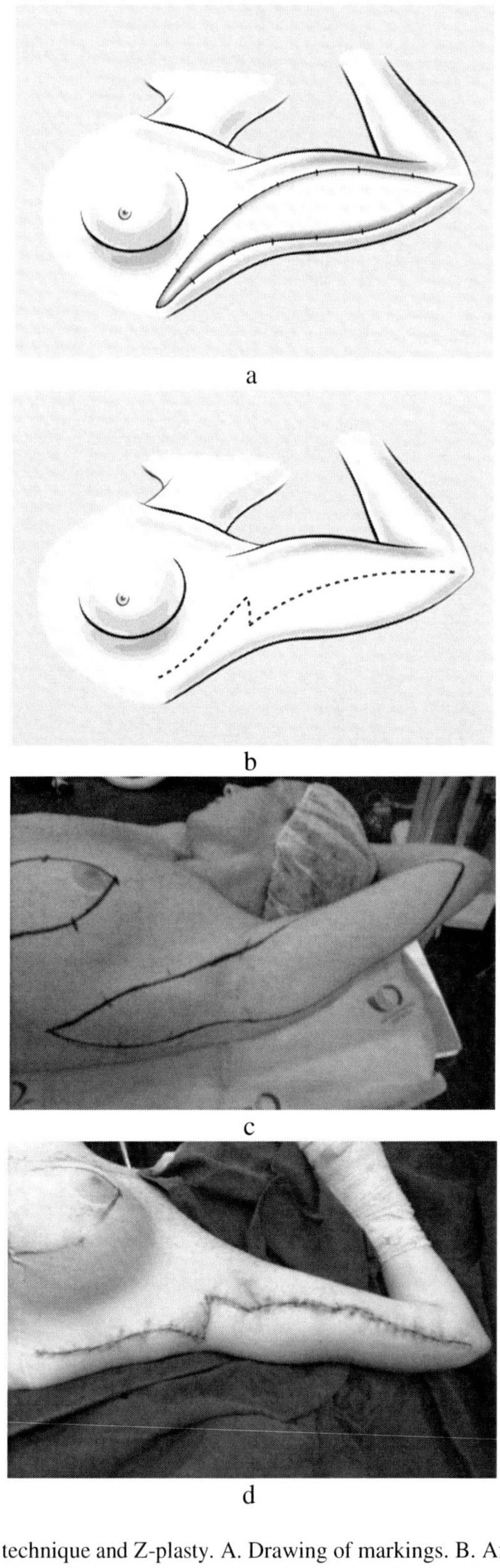

Figure 4. Prolonged ellipse technique and Z-plasty. A. Drawing of markings. B. After Z-plasty. C. Preoperative marking in a patient. D. Immediate postoperative period showing Z-plasty.

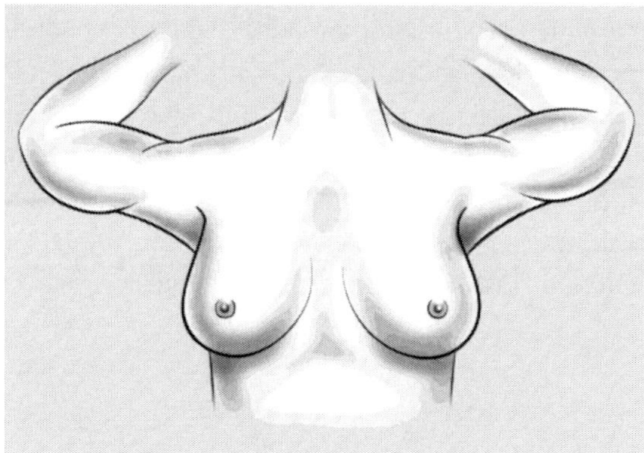

Figure 5. Drawing showing the intraoperative positioning of the upper limbs.

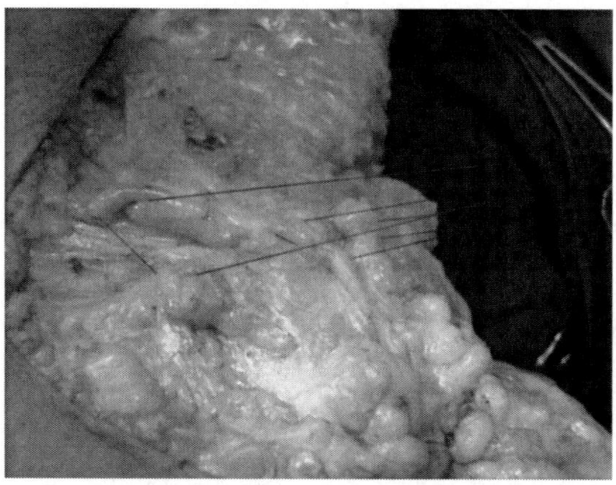

Figure 6. Fixation of the superficial fascia of the arm flaps to the axillary fascia.

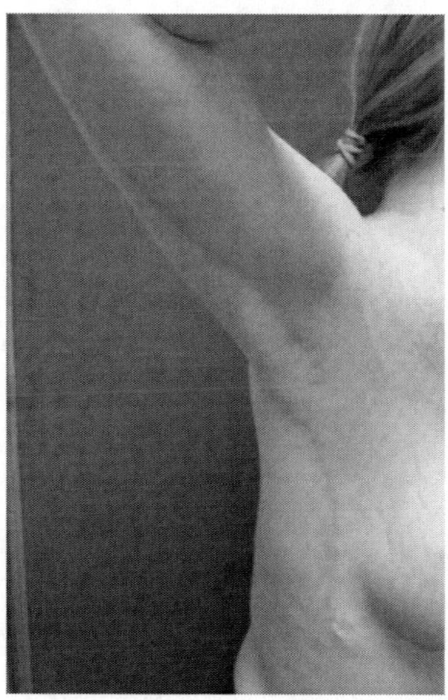

Figure 7. Good postoperative (1 year) scar appearance resulting from brachioplasty extended to the thorax.

The dressing is made with sterile micropore adhesive tape woven in a latticework pattern on the surgical wound protected by gauze greased with bactericidal ointment. Drains are not necessary since careful hemostasis is performed and the suture leaves no dead spaces. Compressive wrapping is not routinely used; however, the use of light compression meshes applied from the wrist to the thorax is recommended in larger resections. Meshes that compress only the arm should be avoided because their tourniquet effect may cause distal edema thus affecting the blood flow in the forearm and hand.

Results

Brachioplasty performed in patients after massive weight loss is extremely rewarding (Figures 8 and 9). A long scar is the price to pay for a rounder and more aesthetic looking arm contour. Nonetheless, former obese patients eligible for plastic surgeries receive thorough information regarding the scars that are to be expected; accordingly, they willingly accept those resulting from brachioplasty. It should be pointed out that the scar resulting from resection within the lines marked – as previously described – is located in the posterior portion of the arm.

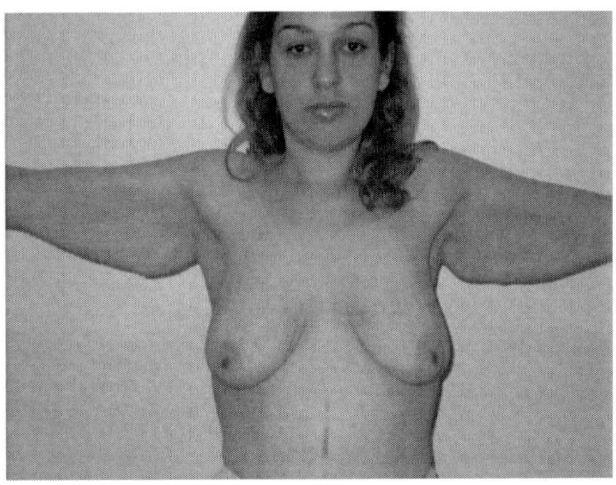

a

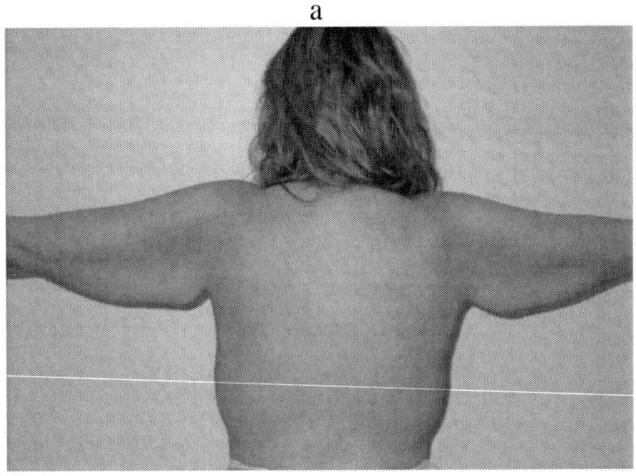

b

Figure 8. (Continued).

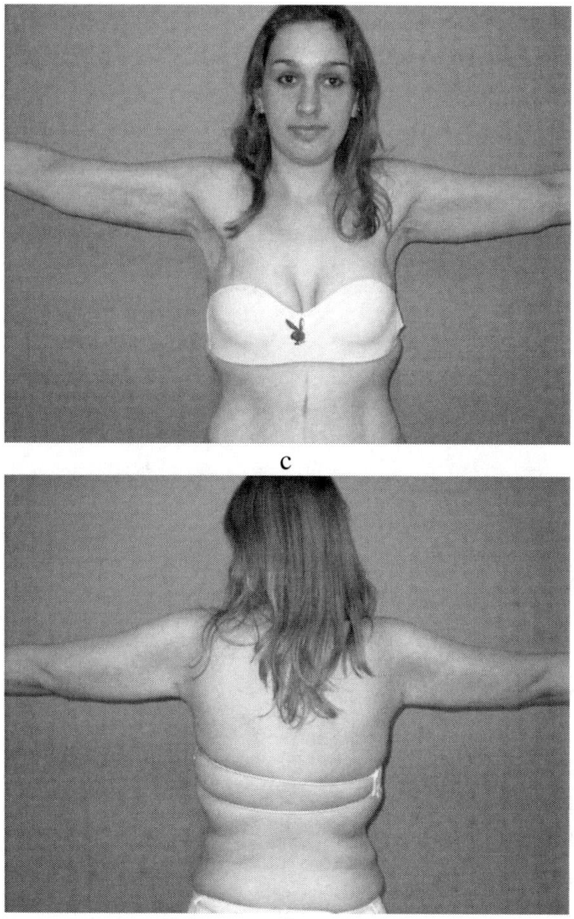

c

d

Figure 8. “Fish-tail” brachioplasty showing an improved arm contour. A-B. Preoperative period. C-D. Postoperative period.

Thus, it can hardly be noticed when the upper limb is adducted. Brachioplasty provides remarkable personal satisfaction since it improves the quality of life by allowing more effective hygiene and a wider range of motion of the upper limbs. In many aspects it is extremely rewarding for women since it allows them to wear sleeveless clothes, previously embarrassing because of their arm deformities.

Complications

When brachioplasty is performed by well-trained hands, complications are not very significant. On the other hand, even when well-performed, adverse biological factors may be present that do not depend on the technical accuracy. These are known as events, but are usually not severe and are easy to solve.

The most common are edema and seroma. Both result from surgical damage, and it should be pointed out that the greater the damage the more severe the events. Edema usually resolves within approximately 30 days, and is further improved by upper limb massage, also known as lymphatic drainage. Seroma is caused by a local accumulation of post-traumatic inflammatory exudate. As a rule, drainage sessions under strict asepsis will solve the problem. Naturally, ecchymosis may also be listed as an event following manipulation and surgical damage; therefore, soft and delicate maneuvers are recommended to prevent them.

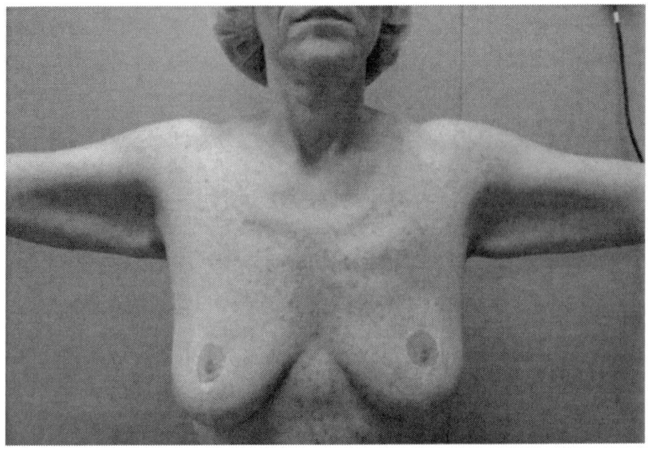

a

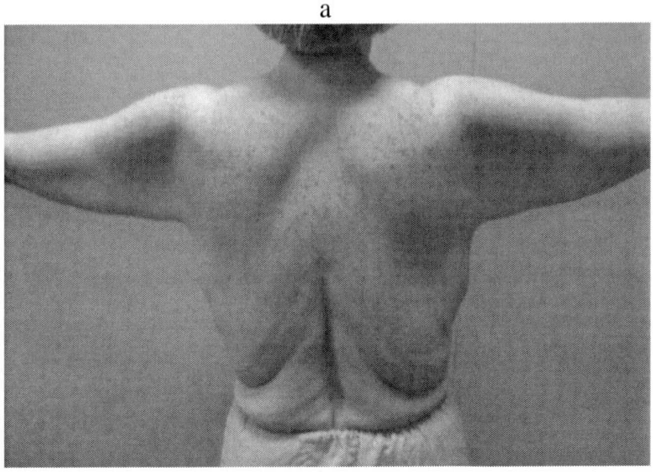

b

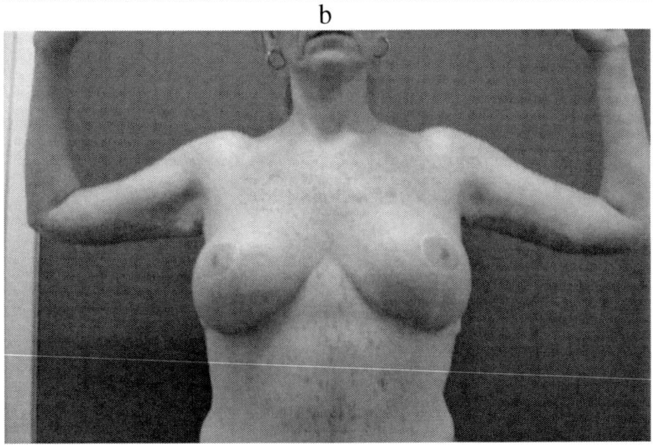

c

Figure 9. (Continued).

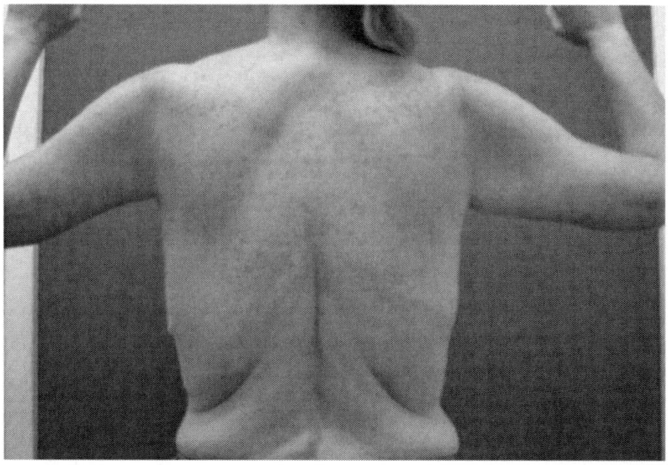

d

Figure 9. Brachioplasty using the extended ellipse technique. A-B. Preoperative period. C-D. Postoperative period.

The hematomas which result from failure to observe careful hemostasis techniques are more severe. When detected early, they should be drained; recurrence imposes surgical exploration to identify the bleeding vessel and proceed to correct hemostasis. When left inadequately treated, hematomas may lead to solid cysts that cause unattractive elevations in the arm and are sometimes accompanied by pain, because of the compressive effect on subjacent surfaces.

Dehiscence is a complication resulting from tension on the suture, as seen in over-resections. Fortunately, dehiscences are partial and sometimes occur even without suture tension. To understand this complication, it is important to remember that the skin in the medial aspect of the arm is extremely thin. The suture may not stand the tension of post-traumatic edema, causing the wound to break open. A partial dehiscence heals by second intention in a short period of time, provided it is cleansed periodically, i. e., two to three times a day. Larger dehiscences require skin grafts.

Lymphorrhea is a very disagreeable complication. Exeresis made in a deeper plane below the superficial fascia may lead to damage of lymphatic vessels and subsequent lymphorrhea. Lymph leakage always occurs through the most distal portion of the incision, close to the epicondyle. Lymphorhea starts within the first days of the postoperative period and spontaneously disappears within 30 days. On rare occasions, this lymphorrhea may accumulate, thus forming a cyst called lymphocele. This complication requires puncture and drainage sessions; however, the best option is surgical removal of the cyst, maintaining suction drainage for two to three days.

Infection is an uncommon event, thanks to prophylactic measures. Some of these may include exhaustive and thorough preoperative cleansing of the entire upper limb using antiseptic soaps and plenty of water, a procedure that should be repeated several times. Axillary hair removal should be performed after cleansing, approximately 30 minutes prior to surgery. Hair removal by means of creams or wax are contraindicated, because these products can occlude the hair follicle ostium, thus leading to formation of cysts within which bacterial colonization will occur; this may infect the site and result in infection. Local infections may determine dehiscence or abscess formation. In the most severe cases, surgical debridement is indicated. Use of antibiotics is vital and should target pathogens, as determined by culture and antibiogram tests. Infections more frequently occur in the axilla; they usually affect small areas and resolve with cleansing and proper antibiotic therapy.

Skin necrosis may occur, whether due to excessive tension or to infection. In these situations, the necrotic area is of varying size. Nonetheless, it requires careful resection, but resection of tissues of doubtful vitality should be avoided, even if this may result in an additional debridement procedure. In smaller areas, wound healing occurs by second intention, whereas in larger areas, skin grafting is mandatory on the raw area that remains after debridement. In both cases, the outcome is poor because the aesthetic appearance is affected.

Despite its size, the scar resulting from brachioplasty is well accepted by the patients. This scar may be deformed by hypertrophy or, in more severe cases, it may turn into a keloid scar.

Hypertrophic scars may result from suture tension. However, we should remember that incisions are made contrary to the relaxed skin tension lines of the arm, thus favoring hypertrophic wound healing. This is why scar massage with triamcinolone creams and the use of silicone sheeting are recommended, even when this event is only remotely suspected. Once the hypertrophic scar has formed, a scar resection may be performed 6 months to 1 year later, followed by the use of triamcinolone creams plus silicone sheeting. A keloid scar is genetically related and more common in individuals with black or yellow skin color. It is a pathological wound healing that looks very unsightly and has symptoms of pain and itching. To date, the best approach is resection followed by radiation therapy.

If deeper planes of dissection are reached, neurological changes may occur, the most common of which are sensory changes in the anteromedial aspect of the forearm. This can also result from the excessive and inadvertent use of electrocautery that leads to damage of the anteromedial cutaneous nerve of the forearm. The nerve may also be lodged in the deep plane closure, and this leads to severe pain. In the first situation, sensitivity is reestablished spontaneously after 4 to 6 months. In the second, an additional surgical approach is necessary to remove the nodule lodging the nerve.

References

[1] Aly A., Pace D., Cram A. Brachioplasty in the patient with massive weight loss. *Aesth. Surg. J.,* 26(1): 76-84, 2006.

[2] Baroudi R. Dermolipectomy of the upper arm. *Clin. Plast. Surg.,* 2:485, 1975.

[3] Baroudi R. Braquioplastia in Baroudi R; Cirurgia do Contorno Corporal. Ed. Indexa, Rio de Janeiro, Brasil, pág. 60-84, 2009.

[4] Hurwitz DJ., Holland SW. The L brachioplasty: an innovative approach to correct excess tissue of the upper arm, axilla and lateral chest. Plast Reconstr Surg. 117(2): 403-11; *discussion,* 412-3, 2006.

[5] Lockwood T. Brachioplasty with superficial fascial system suspension. *Plast. Reconstr. Surg.,* 96(4): 912-20, 1995.

[6] Modolin M., Cintra Jr W., Faintuch J., Silva M M., Moraes Luciana B., Gemperli R., Ferreira MC: Improved double-fuse technique for post-bariatric brachioplasty. *Rev. Col. Bras. Cir.,* 38(4): 217-222, 2011.

[7] Orpheu SC., Coltro PS., Scopel GP., Gomez DS., Rodrigues CJ., Modolin ML. et al.: Collagen and elastic content of abdominal skin after surgical weight loss. *Obes. Sur.,* 20(4):480-6, 2010.

[8] Pitanguy I. Correction of lipodysthophy of the lateral thoracic aspect and inner of the arm and elbow in dermosenescence. *Clin. Plast. Surg.,* 2(3): 477-83, 1975.

[9] Regnault P. Brachioplasty, Axilloplasty and Pre-axilloplasty. *Aesth. Plast. Surg.,* 7:31-36, 1983.

[10] Samra S., Sawh-Martinez R., Liu YJ., Samra F., Persing JA: Optimal placement of brachioplasty scar: a survey evaluation. *Plast. Reconstr. Surg.,* 126(suppl 4S):77 (Abstract), 2010.

[11] Strauch B., Greenspun D., Levine J., Baum T: A technique of brachioplasty. Plast Reconstr Surg. 113(3): 1044-8, *discussion,* 1049, 2004.

[12] Symbas JD., Losken A: An outcome analysis of brachioplasty techniques following massive weight loss. *Ann. Plast. Surg.,* 64(5): 588-91, 2010.

In: Bariatric Surgery
Editor: Christos R. Iavazzo
ISBN: 978-1-62618-995-9

Chapter XV

Pregnancy Complications after Bariatric Surgery Procedures

Christos Iavazzo
Iaso Maternity Hospital, Athens, Greece

Abstract

Introduction: The application of bariatric surgery has recently spread among obese women including women of reproductive age. This chapter aims to clarify the role of bariatric surgery in gestational diabetes, hypertensive disorders during pregnancy , as well as neonate's development and birth weight. Moreover, the diet, monitoring and complications of such women during pregnancy are also discussed. A question is also raised whether conception should be postponed or not for at least 18 months after bariatric operation to avoid complications concerning both mother and fetus mainly associated with nutritional deficiencies due to the anatomical and physiological changes of such operations.

Introduction

The World Health Organization characterizes obesity a global health problem with a higher prevalence in women than men. The USA National Institute of Health recommends bariatric surgery for obese patients with a body mass index (BMI) of at least 40 kgr/m^2 and/or patients with a BMI 35 kgr/m^2 with coexisting commorbidity such as diabetes mellitus or sleep apnea [1]. In the UK, between 2000–2003 approximately 35% of the women who died in pregnancy, childbirth, or in the postpartum period were obese, while 30% of mothers who had a stillbirth or neonatal death were obese [2]. Moreover, it is known that obese women have elevated risk of preterm labour, miscarriage and fetal chromosomal anomalies, as well as macrosomia [3]. Thromboembolism, gestational diabetes, pregnancy-induced hypertension, and preeclampsia are also more common entities in those women [4]. They also have a greater incidence of dysfunctional labour, caesarian section and postpartum hemorrhage, as well as associated perioperative morbidity [4].

Bariatric surgery is the most effective treatment for obesity, resulting in considerable weight loss and improvement in many comorbidities [5]. The total number of bariatric surgery operations has increased during the last decade among obese women of reproductive age. Women aged 18-45 account for 83% of all bariatric surgery procedures [6]. There is increasing evidence to suggest that weight loss after bariatric surgery can improve maternal and perinatal outcomes. The most widely applied procedures of bariatric surgery are the laparoscopic gastric banding and the Roux-en-Y operation. Women who conceive after bariatric surgery usually seem to have uncomplicated pregnancies, but special attention is required to some complications that can occur after these procedures. Physicians must have concerns regarding the safety of pregnancy after bariatric surgery as the number of bariatric surgeries being performed in women is increased.

The aim of this chapter is to discuss the related problems during pregnancy in women who have undergone bariatric surgery.

Discussion

A careful review of the literature suggests that the optimum way to reduce obesity-associated morbidity is by weight reduction before pregnancy [7]. Bariatric surgery is a popular, safe and effective treatment for obesity. Weight reduction has been shown to change the hormonal imbalance of the oligomennorheic, hyperinsulinemic and hyperandrogenemic obese woman leading to an improved menstrual regularity, ovulation, and an increased fecundity by normal or IVF procedures [8, 9]. In a prospective study of 17 obese patients with PCOS, a decreased hirsutism and blood levels of androgens, as well as menstrual regularity were found in all women after bariatric surgery [10].

Bariatric surgery results in many anatomic and physiologic changes in the abdomen and consequently affects future pregnancies causing perinatal complications associated with nutritional deficiencies. Common complications encountered are iron, follate, calcium, vitamin A, vitamin B12 and vitamin K deficiencies that are causatively related with gestational complications [11, 12]. It was shown that women with history of bariatric surgery had iron deficiency in 80% of the pregnancies, vitamin D in 46,7%, vitamin A in 20%, vitamin E in 13,3% and vitamin B12 in 26,7% (13). Obese women having undergone a bariatric operation before pregnancy usually face anemia problems, for this reason iron and multivitamin supplements should be prescribed in such women [14]. Less common complications during pregnancy are hyperemesis, intestinal hernias, strangulation of upper jejunum [15], hypoxic hepatitis [16]. Fetal cerebral hemorrhage caused by vitamin K deficiency [17] and neural tube defects due to follate deficiency [18] are also serious fetal complications presented in the literature.

Although, it is suggested that women should delay pregnancy for at least one postoperative year, in a recent review by Karmon et al. it was suggested that future studies should examine the safety of earlier postoperatively programmed pregnancies [19]. Sheiner et al. showed that women who conceived the first postoperative year had no significant differences in hypertensive disorders (15. 4% in the early vs 11. 2% in the late postoperative pregnancy; P = . 392); diabetes mellitus (11. 5% vs 7. 3%; P = . 392); perinatal outcomes, such as congenital malformations (1. 9% vs 1. 3%; P = . 485); or bariatric complications (6. 7% vs7. 0%; P = . 392) [20] Moreover,, our findings support such a proposal [21]. The weight loss and marked reduction in food intake following bariatric surgery does not lead to growth or development problems for the neonate [22], however weight stabilization is strongly recommended after bariatric surgery, before a pregnancy occurs [23]. Obstetricians should cooperate with surgeons in order to achieve a close postoperative monitoring and control of weight gain and appropriate nourishment [24].

According to recent reports gestational complications were less common between women who underwent bariatric surgery. Ducarme et al. showed that among obese women, the incidence of adverse outcomes was less in those who underwent gastric banding than in those who did not [25]. In a recent review [26], it has been shown that pregnancy after Roux-en-Y gastric bypass is safe with an incidence of perinatal complications similar to that of non obese patients and lower than that of obese patients who had not undergone bariatric surgery. Furthermore, in another study no differences in neonatal outcomes were found in pregnant women after bariatric surgery [27].

More analytically, in a recent review, Magdaleno et al. showed an improved fertility and a reduced risk of gestational diabetes, pregnancy-induced hypertension and preeclampsia, macrosomia in pregnant women after bariatric surgery. However, the incidence of IUGR and SGA infants were found to be elevated. In this study, no conclusions concerning the risk for cesarean delivery and the best surgery-to-conception interval could be drawn [28]. Belogolovkin et al. in a retrospective cohort study showed that non-obese mothers with bariatric surgery history were more likely to have anemia, chronic hypertension, endocrine disorders, and SGA infants, whereas obese mothers without prior bariatric surgery were at greater risk of having gestational diabetes, chronic hypertension, macrosomic infants, as well as prolonged hospital stay compared to non-obese mother without prior bariatric surgery [29]. Weintraub et al. in a retrospective study showed a significant reduction in gestational diabetes rates (17. 3% versus 11. 0%; P = 0. 009) and hypertensive disorders in pregnancy (23. 6% versus 11. 2%; P = 0. 001) of women with a prior history of bariatric surgery [12]. Similarly, another study showed that such women had substantially lower rates of preeclampsia and eclampsia (odds ratio 0. 20, 95% confidence interval 0. 09 to 0. 44), chronic hypertension complicating pregnancy (0. 39, 0. 20 to 0. 74), and gestational hypertension (0. 16, 0. 07 to 0. 37), even after adjustment for age, multiple pregnancy, surgical procedure, and preexisting diabetes [30). In different studies, a reduction of fetal macrosomia was shown in pregnant women with bariatric surgery especially after Roux-en-Y gastric [12, 31]. However, such procedures could cause nutritional deficiencies which might be the cause of an increased rate of IUGR or SGA infants in post-bariatric surgery patients compared with controls [25, 31]. The time period between bariatric surgery and pregnancy has not been shown to affect birth weight. Regarding miscarriage rates, a decline of 33. 3% to 7. 8% was shown in women with a history of bariatric surgery [9], while no such correlation was found for preterm labor rates in women with or without bariatric surgery matched for BMI [32, 33]. Similar perinatal mortality rate, as well as congenital malformations rates were found comparing all pregnancies of patients with and without previous bariatric surgery [34]. Gastric banding is well tolerated during pregnancy [35]. Total dysphagia, severe epigastric pain vomiting after the first trimester of pregnancy and IUGR fetuses are the more serious complications in women after gastric banding surgery [36]. Similarly, Guelinckx et al. also found an increased risk of IUGR embryos [11].

Stone et al. tried to investigate what happened in women who underwent bariatric surgery but remained obese [37]. Those women had higher rates of cesarean section (63. 5% vs. 36. 0%, p=0. 010) and development of pregnancy-related hypertension (36. 5% vs. 8. 0%, p=0. 001) compared to non-obese women while no difference was mentioned in development of gestational diabetes, gestational age at delivery, neonatal intensive care unit admission, or nursery days [37].

Regarding the different types of bariatric surgery, no difference in the affect on pregnancy outcome were found. More specifically, in a retrospective study including 449 deliveries (of which laparoscopic gastric banding (LAGB; n = 202), silastic ring vertical gastroplasty (SRVG; n = 136), and vertical-banded gastroplasty (VBG; n = 56)-and Roux-en-Y gastric bypass (RGB, n=55), no significant differences were noted between the groups regarding BMI before the bariatric surgery or prepregnancy BMI, while patients following LAGB had significantly higher BMI before delivery (36. 8 +/- 5. 9 kg compared to the SRVG 33. 4 +/- 6. 0, VBG 34. 2 +/- 5. 4, and RGB 34. 9 +/- 6. 8 groups; p < 0. 001). Following LAGB, patients had higher weight gain during pregnancy (13. 1 +/- 9. 6 kg) compared to the SRVG (8. 8 +/- 7. 4), VBG (8. 5 +/- 8. 0), and RGB (11. 6 +/- 9. 6; p < 0. 001) groups. The interval between operation and pregnancy was shorter in the LAGB group (22. 8 months) compared to the SRVG (41. 0) and the VBG (42. 1) groups and was significantly higher in the RGB group (57. 4; p < 0. 001). Birth weight was significantly higher among newborns of patients following RBG (3,332. 8 +/- 475. 5 g) compared to the restrictive procedures (3,104. 3 +/- 578. 7 in the LAGB, 3,086. 7 +/- 533. 1 in the SRVG, and 3,199. 2 +/- 427. 2 in the VBG groups). It should also be noticed that no significant differences in low birth weight (<2,500 g) or macrosomia (>4,000 g), or low Apgar scores or perinatal mortality were noted between the groups [20]. Facchiano et al. compared laparoscopic adjustable gastric banding and laparoscopic Roux-en-Y gastric bypass in a series of morbidly obese women with respect to maternal and neonatal outcomes [38]. The results of the two groups were comparable regarding age, parity, gravidity, interval from surgery to conception, weight and BMI at conception, weight and weight gain during pregnancy, weight and BMI at 2 weeks after pregnancy, complications during pregnancy, gestational age, method of delivery, fetal birth weight, and fetal outcome while only the preoperative weight and BMI were greater in the laparoscopic Roux-en-Y gastric bypass group. A higher frequency of cesarean deliveries was found in both groups [38]. Future studies with larger numbers of participants should be encouraged in order to reach safer conclusions regarding interactions between bariatric surgery and pregnancy. An interesting perspective would be to compare the nutritional state of newborns of pregnant women who did and did not undergo bariatric surgery or to compare the outcome between women who conceived earlier to those who conceived later after surgery.

Conclusion

The number of bariatric surgeries performed in obese women has increased the last decade. It is believed that conception after bariatric surgery should be postponed for 18 months because the time of weight loss should not be the same with the time of pregnancy's elevated nutritional needs. During pregnancy, daily multivitamin consumption and close supervision are suggested in order to avoid gestational complications related with nutritional deficiencies. Most women after bariatric surgery have successful pregnancy outcomes with minimum complications regarding gestational diabetes and hypertension or lower birth weight.

Further studies are required regarding the long-term maternal outcomes in pregnancies after bariatric surgery as well as the effect on the offspring. A multidisciplinary team management including cooperation between obstetrician, general surgeon, endocrinologist, gastrentrologist, and dietologist is proposed.

References

[1] Malcolm K. Robinson, Editorial, Surgical treatment of obesity -- weighing the facts. *N. Engl. J. Med.,* 361:520, July 30, 2009.

[2] Perinatal Mortality, 2005. Confidential Enquiry into Maternal and Child Health. CEMACH, 2007.

[3] Nohr EA, Bech BH, Davies MJ, Frydenberg M, Henriksen TB, Olsen J. Pre pregnancy obesity and fetal death: a study within the Danish national birth cohort. *Obstetrics and Gynecology,*2005;106:250–259. [PubMed].

[4] Chu SY, Kim SY, Schmid CH, et al. Maternal obesity and risk of cesarean delivery: a meta-analysis. *Obesity Reviews,*2007;8(5):385–394.

[5] Buchwald H, Avidor Y, Braunwald E, Jensen MD, Pories W, Fahrbach K, et al. Bariatric surgery: a systematic review and meta-analysis. *JAMA,* 2004;292:1724-37.

[6] Maggard MA, Yermilov I, Li Z, Maglione M, Newberry S, Suttorp M, et al. Pregnancy and fertility following bariatric surgery: a systematic review. *JAMA,* 2008;300:2286-96.

[7] Grundy MA, Woodcock S, Attwood SE. The surgical management of obesity in young women: consideration of the mother's and baby's health before, during, and after pregnancy. *Surg. Endosc.,* 2008 Oct;22(10):2107-16.

[8] Nelson SM, Fleming R. Obesity and reproduction: impact and interventions. Current Opinion in Obstetrics and Gynecology,2007;19(4):384–389.

[9] Bilenka B, Ben-Shlomo I, Cozacov C, Gold CH, Zohar S. Fertility, miscarriage and pregnancy after vertical banded gastroplasty operation for morbid obesity. **Acta**Obstetricia et GynecologicaScandinavica,1995;74(1):42–44.

[10] Escobar-Morreale HF, Botella-Carretero JI, Álvarez-Blasco F, Sancho J, San Millán JL. The polycystic ovary syndrome associated with morbid obesity may resolve after weight loss induced by bariatric surgery. Journal of Clinical Endocrinology and Metabolism, 2005;90(12):6364–6369.

[11] Guelinckx I, Devlieger R, Vansant G. Reproductive outcome after bariatric surgery: a critical review. Hum. Reprod. Update, 2009 Mar-Apr;15(2):189-201.

[12] Weintraub AY, Levy A, Levi I, Mazor M, Wiznitzer A, Sheiner E. Effect of bariatric surgery on pregnancy outcome. *Int. J. Gynaecol. Obstet.,*2008 Dec;103(3):246-51.

[13] González Navarro I, Pereira Cunill JL, Serrano Aguayo P, Morales Conde S, MartosMartínez JM, García Luna PP. Maternal and fetal outcomes in pregnancy following bariatric surgery. *Nutr. Hosp.,* 2011 Mar-Apr;26(2):376-83.

[14] Love AL, Billett HH. Obesity, bariatric surgery, and iron deficiency: true, true, true and related. *Am. J. Hematol.,* 2008 May;83(5):403-9.

[15] Wang CB, Hsieh CC, Chen CH, Lin YH, Lee CY, Tseng CJ. Strangulation of upper jejunum in subsequent pregnancy following gastric bypass surgery. *Taiwan J. Obstet. Gynecol.,* 2007 Sep;46(3):267-71.

[16] Kummer N, Cackovic M, Paidas M, Funai E. Hypoxic hepatitis in a pregnant patient: a complication of gastric bypass surgery. *Am. J. Perinatol.,* 2008 Sep;25(8):469-71.

[17] Van Mieghem T, Van Schoubroeck D, Depiere M, Debeer A, Hanssens M. Fetal cerebral hemorrhage caused by vitamin K deficiency after complicated bariatric surgery. *Obstet. Gynecol.,* 2008 Aug;112(2 Pt 2):434-6.

[18] Moliterno JA, DiLuna ML, Sood S, Roberts KE, Duncan CC. Gastric bypass: a risk factor for neural tube defects? Case report. *J. Neurosurg. Pediatr.,* 2008 May;1(5):406-9.

[19] Karmon A, Sheiner E. Pregnancy after bariatric surgery: a comprehensive review. Arch. Gynecol. Obstet., 2008 May;277(5):381-8.

[20] Sheiner E, Edri A, Balaban E, Levi I, Aricha-Tamir B. Pregnancy outcome of patients who conceive during or after the first year following bariatric surgery. *Am. J. Obstet. Gynecol.,* 2011 Jan;204(1):50. e1-6.

[21] Iavazzo C, Ntziora F, Rousos I, Paschalinopoulos D. Complications in pregnancy after bariatric surgery. *Arch. Gynecol. Obstet.,* 2010 Aug;282(2):225-7.

[22] Sapre N, Munting K, Pandita A, Stubbs R. Pregnancy following gastric bypass surgery: what is the expected course and outcome? *N. Z. Med. J.,* 2009 Nov 20;122(1306):33-42.

[23] Bienstman-Pailleux J, Gaucherand P. Laparoscopic adjustable gastric banding and pregnancy. *J. Gynecol. Obstet. Biol. Reprod. (Paris),*2007 Dec;36(8):770-6.

[24] Karmon A, Sheiner E. Timing of gestation after bariatric surgery: should women delay pregnancy for at least 1 postoperative year?Am. J. Perinatol.,2008 Jun;25(6):331-3.

[25] Ducarme G, Revaux A, Rodrigues A, Aissaoui F, Pharisien I, Uzan M. Obstetric outcome following laparoscopic adjustable gastric banding. *Int. J. Gynaecol. Obstet.,*2007 Sep;98(3):244-7.

[26] Patel JA, Patel NA, Thomas RL, Nelms JK, Colella JJ. Pregnancy outcomes after laparoscopic Roux-en-Y gastric bypass. *Surg. Obes. Relat. Dis.,* 2008 Jan-Feb;4(1):39-45.

[27] Maggard MA, Yermilov I, Li Z, Maglione M, Newberry S, Suttorp M, Hilton L, Santry HP, Morton JM, Livingston EH, Shekelle PG. Pregnancy and fertility following bariatric surgery: a systematic review. *JAMA,*2008 Nov 19;300(19):2286-96.

[28] Magdaleno R Jr, Pereira BG, Chaim EA, Turato ER. Pregnancy after bariatric surgery: a current view of maternal, obstetrical and perinatal challenges. *Arch. Gynecol. Obstet.,* 2011 Dec 29.

[29] Belogolovkin V, Salihu HM, Weldeselasse H, Biroscak BJ, August EM, Mbah AK, Alio AP. Impact of prior bariatric surgery on maternal and fetal outcomes among obese and non-obese mothers. *Arch. Gynecol. Obstet.,*. 2011 Nov 6.

[30] Bennett WL, Gilson MM, Jamshidi R, et al. Impact of bariatric surgery on hypertensive disorders in pregnancy: retrospective analysis of insurance claims data. *British Medical Journal,*2010;340:p. c1662.

[31] Patel JA, Patel NA, Thomas RL, Nelms JK, Colella JJ. Pregnancy outcomes after laparoscopic Roux-en-Y gastric bypass. *Surgery for Obesity and Related Diseases*, 2008;4(1):39–45.

[32] Richards DS, Miller DK, Goodman GN. Pregnancy after gastric bypass for morbid obesity. *Journal of Reproductive Medicine for the Obstetrician and Gynecologist,* 1987;32(3):172–176.

[33] Dixon JB, Dixon ME, O'Brien PE. Birth outcomes in obese women after laparoscopic adjustable gastric banding. *Obstetrics and Gynecology,*2005;106(5):965–972.

[34] Sheiner E, Levy A, Silverberg D, et al. Pregnancy after bariatric surgery is not associated with adverse perinatal outcome. American Journal of Obstetrics and Gynecology,2004;190(5):1335–1340.

[35] Vejux N, Campan P, Agostini A. Pregnancy after gastric banding: maternal tolerance, obstetrical and neonatal outcomes. *Gynecol. Obstet. Fertil.,* 2007 Nov;35(11):1143-7.

[36] Jasaitis Y, Sergent F, Bridoux V, Paquet M, Marpeau L, Ténière P. Management of pregnancies after adjustable gastric banding. *J. Gynecol. Obstet. Biol. Reprod (Paris),*2007 Dec;36(8):764-9.

[37] Stone RA, Huffman J, Istwan N, Desch C, Rhea D, Stanziano G, Joy S. Pregnancy outcomes following bariatric surgery. *J. Womens Health (Larchmt),* 2011 Sep;20(9):1363-6.

[38] Facchiano E, Iannelli A, Santulli P, Mandelbrot L, Msika S. Pregnancy after laparoscopic bariatric surgery: comparative study of adjustable gastric banding and Roux-en-Y gastric bypass. *Surg. Obes. Relat. Dis.,* 2011 Jun 24.

In: Bariatric Surgery
Editor: Christos R. Iavazzo
ISBN: 978-1-62618-995-9

Chapter XVI

Pelvic Floor Disorders and Bariatric Surgery

Christos Iavazzo
Iaso, Maternity Hospital, Athens, Greece

Abstract

This chapter presents the role of bariatric surgery operations in the improvement of the pelvic floor disorders that many obese patients mainly women are facing.

Introduction

Obesity is a state of excessive body weight and adipose tissue mass. A proper diagnosis of obesity would require the so called body mass index (BMI), which is defined as weight/height2 (kg/m2) or assessment of body fatness by the dual energy x-ray absorptionmetry. The cut-off point for obesity is a BMI =30 kg/m2 [1]. According to the World Health Organization [1], obesity is classified as class I for a BMI between 30 and 34. 9 kg/m2, class II for a BMI between 35 and 39. 9 kg/m2, and class III for a BMI ≥ 40 kg/m2 [1]. Current data estimate that there are 300 million obese adults worldwide living especially in the developed countries [1, 2]. A rise was also noticed in the younger population (18 to 29 years) and especially in women. The impact of obesity on quality of life is broad causing pelvic floor disorders among other conditions.

Pelvic floor disorders (urinary or faecal incontinence and pelvic organ prolapse) are common conditions affecting many obese women today. The exact prevalence of pelvic floor disorders in the general population is approximately 11%, but it should be higher in obese women [3]. In the different studies, pelvic floor disorders affect between 2% and 42% of women, depending on the definition of the condition and the study population [4-6].

Chronically increased abdominal pressure is the main mechanism causing the development of pelvic floor disorders as it overts structural damage or neurologic dysfunction predisposing to prolapse and incontinence [7-10]. Animal studies showed an association between obesity and urinary incontinence by evaluating urethral sphincter incontinence, urethral length or tone [11]. Elevated abdominal and intravesical pressures are also found in patients with increased sagittal abdominal diameter and elevated BMI [7], while significant weight loss improves stress urinary incontinence [12, 13]. The etiology of pelvic floor disorders also includes either the direct injury and denervation to the pelvic floor musculature or defects in the supporting system of the endopelvic fascia and ligaments [14]. Some studies suggest that neurogenic disease caused by obesity might lead to pelvic floor disorders [11]. For example, a study proposed that the risk for abnormal median nerve conduction was 3. 5-fold greater in obese workers [15], while a higher incidence of lumbar disk herniation is also found in obese patients [16]. Conditions such as menopausal status, chronic constipation, chronic cough, and heavy lifting major predisposing factors [17].

It was shown that although signs of pelvic organ prolapse are frequently observed, the condition seldom causes symptoms especially in younger ages [18]. However, vaginal or uterine descent at or through the introitus can become symptomatic. Symptoms may also include a sensation of vaginal fullness or pressure, sacral back pain with standing, vaginal spotting from ulceration of the protruding cervix or vagina, coital difficulty, lower abdominal discomfort, and voiding and defecatory difficulties [18].

Since weight is a modifiable risk factor for incontinence, weight reduction may be an effective treatment . Studies of weight loss have examined its effects and explored the pathophysiologic mechanisms of improvement in pelvic floor disorders. The aim of our study is to clarify the role of bariatric surgery procedures in improvement of pelvic floor disorders and quality of life of obese women.

Discussion

More than 90 percent of morbidly obese women experience some degree of pelvic floor disorders, and 50 percent of these women report that symptoms adversely impact quality of their life [19]. In these women, obesity was found to be strongly correlated in predicting pelvic floor disorders in the same extent as obstetric history [19]. An association between obesity and urinary incontinence exists, while the association between obesity and other pelvic floor disorders is less clear.

However, Chen et al. showed the presence of any pelvic floor disorder in 75% of the obese patients compared with 44% in non-obese (P <. 0001) [20]. More obese patients experienced stress urinary incontinence, urge urinary incontinence, and anal incontinence, but not pelvic organ prolapse. The severity of those symptoms were higher in more obese patients [20].

A number of studies have shown improvements in urinary incontinence after bariatric surgery [8, 13, 21, 22]. Evidence indicates that massive weight loss (45 to 50 kg) improves incontinence in morbidly obese women after bariatic surgery [12, 13]. Fifty per cent reductions in incontinence frequency were observed among women who lost as little as 5% to 10% of baseline weight. Women who achieved a weight loss of 5% or greater had at least a

50% reduction in incontinence frequency (p =0. 03) [23]. It is reported that an average weight loss of 69% of excess body weight could lead to significant changes in sagittal abdominal diameter (32 to 20 cm, P < 0. 0001) and intravesical pressure (17 to 10 cmH_2O, P < 0. 001) [22]. In another study, a weight loss greater than 50% leads to a reduction in stress urinary incontinence from 61 to 11. 6% (P < 0. 001) [12]. Similar studies reported improvement in urodynamic parameters after bariatric surgery operations [8, 13]. Greater weight loss was associated with greater improvement of incontinence; as from the patients who lost more than 18 BMI points, 71% regained urinary continence [24].

The role of obesity in faecal incontinence is less well defined. The prevalence of faecal incontinence in the general population is reported to be 2 to 9% [5, 25]. Obesity appears to be correlated with higher rates of faecal incontinence and diarrhoea.

However, in morbidly obese patients undergoing evaluation for bariatric surgery, the prevalence of anal incontinence was notable at 32%, while incontinence of liquid stool was 21. 1% and solid stool was 8. 8% [26].

The effects of bariatric surgery on these conditions are not well defined. A systematic review showed that faecal incontinence improved after Roux-en-Y gastric bypass in studies with preoperative data, while the effects of bariatric surgery on diarrhoea were unclear [27]. It should be mentioned that one of the major disadvantages of the biliopancreatic diversion with duodenal switch operation is diarrhea. Although duodenal switch is associated with more bowel episodes than gastric bypass, the difference is not statistically significant. More specifically, bowel habits were found to be similar in patients who achieved 50% estimated body weight loss with duodenal switch surgery or gastric bypass [28]. Surgically induced weight loss has a beneficial effect on symptoms of pelvic floor disorders in morbidly obese women.

In a questionnary based study, it was shown that the prevalence of pelvic floor disorders symptoms improved from 87% before surgery to 65% after surgery [29]. There was also a significant reduction in total mean distress scores after surgery, which was attributed mainly to the significant decrease in urinary symptoms.

Moreover, reductions in the scores were noted for the other pelvic floor disorders, while quality of life total scores also improved. Age, parity, history of complicated delivery, percent excess body weight loss, BMI, type of weight loss procedure and presence of diabetes mellitus and hypertension had no predictive value for postoperative outcomes in the same study [29]. Cuichi et al. evaluated clinically and instrumentally pelvic floor disorders before and after bariatric surgery in obese women and found that a clear association exists between BMI and urinary incontinence [30]. Weight loss after bariatric surgery resulted in improved urinary incontinence, fecal incontinence, and symptoms of pelvic organ prolapse. [30]. After a mean BMI reduction of 10 kg/m(2), the prevalence of pelvic floor disorders decreased to 48% (P = . 02), with a significant improvement in quality of life. The prevalence of urinary incontinence decreased from 61% to 9. 2% (P = . 0001) and was associated with the decrease in postoperative BMI (P = . 04) (30). On the other hand, according to McDermott et al. the prevalence of pelvic floor disorders did not improve greatly after surgery. More specifically, even with significant weight loss (BMI, 43. 7 kg/m(2) to BMI, 29 kg/m(2); P<0. 001), there was no significant difference in the prevalence of pelvic floor symptoms before and after surgery (94% to 81%, P=0. 2) the first postoperative year [31]. However, significant weight loss improved the degree of bother and quality of life related to these symptoms as it was shown by PFDI-20 and PFIQ-7 scores [31].

Conclusion

Bariatric surgery can lead to significantly weight reduction of obese women. This method also acts as a treatment for the pelvic floor disorders that those women face by offering improvement in incontinence and quality of life.

References

[1] World Health Organization Obesity and Overweight. Http://www. who. int /dietphysicalactivity/publications/facts/obesity/en/
[2] Mokdad AH, Ford ES, Bowman BA, et al. Prevalence of obesity, diabetes, and obesity-related health risk factors, 2001. *JAMA,* 2003 Jan 1;289(1):76–9.
[3] Olsen AL, Smith VJ, Bergstrom JO, Colling JC, Clark AL. Epidemiology of surgically managed pelvic organ prolapse and urinary incontinence. Obstet. Gynecol. Apr., 1997;89(4):501-6.
[4] Melville JH, Katon W, Delaney K, et al. Urinary incontinence in US women: a population-based study. *Arch. Intern. Med.,* 2005 Mar 14;165(5):537–42.
[5] Kalantar JS, Howell S, Talley NJ. Prevalence of faecal incontinence and associated risk factors; an underdiagnosed problem in the Australian community? *Med. J. Aust.,* 2002 Jan 21;176(2):54–7.
[6] Morrill M, Lukacz ES, Lawrence JM, et al. Seeking healthcare for pelvic floor disorders: a population-based study. *Am. J. Obstet. Gynecol.,* 2007 Jul;197(1):86. e1–6.
[7] Noblett KL, Jensen JK, Ostergard DR. The relationship of body mass index to intra-abdominal pressure as measured by multichannel cystometry. *Int. Urogynecol. J. Pelvic. Floor Dysfunct.,* 1997;8(6):323–6.
[8] Lara MD, Kothari SN, Sugerman HJ. Surgical management of obesity: a review of the evidence relating to the health benefits and risks. *Treat. Endocrinol.,* 2005;4(1):55–64.
[9] Bouldin MJ, Ross LA, Sumrall CD, et al. The effect of obesity surgery on obesity comorbidity. *Am. J. Med. Sci.,* 2006;331(4):183–93.
[10] Lambert DM, Marceau S, Forse RA. Intra-abdominal pressure in the obese. *Obes. Surg.,* 2005 Oct;15(9):1225–32.
[11] Cummings JM, Rodning CB. Urinary stress incontinence among obese women: review of pathophysiology therapy. *Int. Urogynecol. J.,* 2000;11:41–4.
[12] Deitel M, Stone E, Kassam HA, et al. Gynecologic-obstetric changes after loss of massive excess weight following bariatric surgery. *J. Am. Coll. Nutr.,* 1988 Apr;7(2):147–53.
[13] Bump RC, Sugerman HJ, Fantl JA, et al. Obesity and lower urinary tract function in women: effect of surgically induced weight loss. *Am. J. Obstet. Gynecol.,* 1992 Aug;167(2):392–7.
[14] Bidmead J, Cardozo LD: Pelvic floor changes in the older women. *Br. I. Urol.,* 1998; 82(Suppl 1):18-25.
[15] Nathan PA, Keniston RC, Myers LD, et al. Obesity as a risk factor for slowing of sensory conduction of the median nerve in industry. A cross-sectional and longitudinal study involving 429 workers. *J. Occup. Med.,* 1992;34:379–83.

[16] Heliovaara M. Body height, obesity, and risk of herniated lumbar intervertebral disc. *Spine,* 1987;12:469–72.

[17] Lin SY, Tee YT, Ng SC, Chang H, Lin PP, Chen GD: Changes in the extracellular matrix in the anterior vagina of women with or without prolapse. *Int. Urogynecol. J. Pelvic. Floor Dysfunct.,* 2007; 18:43-8

[18] Baden WF, Walker TA. Genesis of the vaginal profile: a correlated classification of vaginal relaxation. *Clin. Obstet. Gynecol.* Dec., 1972;15(4):1048-54.

[19] Wasserberg N, Haney M, Petrone P, Ritter M, Emami C, Rosca J, Siegmund K, Kaufman HS. Morbid obesity adversely impacts pelvic floor function in females seeking attention for weight loss surgery. *Dis. Colon. Rectum.,* 2007 Dec;50(12):2096-103.

[20] Chen CC, Gatmaitan P, Koepp S, Barber MD, Chand B, Schauer PR, Brethauer SA. Obesity is associated with increased prevalence and severity of pelvic floor disorders in women considering bariatric surgery. *Surg. Obes. Relat. Dis.,* 2009 Jul-Aug;5(4):411-5.

[21] NIH Conference Gastrointestinal surgery for severe obesity. Consensus Development Conference Panel. *Ann. Intern. Med.,* 1991 Dec 15;115(12):956–61.

[22] Sugerman H, Windsor A, Bessos M, et al. Effects of surgically induced weight loss on urinary bladder pressure, sagittal abdominal diameter and obesity co-morbidity. *Int. J. Obes. Relat. Metab. Disord.,* 1998 Mar;22(3):230–5.

[23] Subak LL, Johnson C, Whitcomb E, et al. Does weight loss improve incontinence in moderately obese women? *Int. Urogynecol. J. Pelvic. Floor Dysfunct.,* 2002;13(1):40–3.

[24] Burgio KL, Richter HE, Clements RH, et al. Changes in urinary and fecal incontinence symptoms with weight loss surgery in morbidly obese women. *Obstet. Gynecol.,* 2007 Nov;110(5):1034–40.

[25] Nelson R, Norton N, Cautley E, et al. Community-based prevalence of anal incontinence. *JAMA,* 1995 Aug 16;274(7):559–61.

[26] Richter HE, Burgio KL, Clements RH, et al. Urinary and anal incontinence in morbidly obese women considering weight loss surgery. *Obstet. Gynecol.,* 2005;106:1272–7.

[27] Poylin V, Serrot FJ, Madoff RD, Ikrumuddin S, Mellgren A, Lowry AC, Melton GB. Obesity and bariatric surgery: a systematic review of associations with defecatory dysfunction. *Colorectal. Dis.,* 2011 Jun;13(6):e92-103.

[28] Wasserberg N, Hamoui N, Petrone P, Crookes PF, Kaufman HS. Bowel habits after gastric bypass versus the duodenal switch operation. *Obes. Surg.,* 2008 Dec;18(12):1563-6.

[29] Wasserberg N, Petrone P, Haney M, Crookes PF, Kaufman HS. Effect of surgically induced weight loss on pelvic floor disorders in morbidly obese women. *Ann. Surg.,* 2009 Jan;249(1):72-6.

[30] Cuicchi D, Lombardi R, Cariani S, Leuratti L, Lecce F, Cola B. Clinical and instrumental evaluation of pelvic floor disorders before and after bariatric surgery in obese women. *Surg. Obes. Relat. Dis.,* 2011 Aug 28.

[31] McDermott CD, Terry CL, Mattar SG, Hale DS. Female Pelvic Floor Symptoms Before and After Bariatric Surgery. *Obes. Surg.,* 2012 Jan 19.

In: Bariatric Surgery
Editor: Christos R. Iavazzo
ISBN: 978-1-62618-995-9

Chapter XVII

Bariatric Surgery: A Medicolegal Perspective

O. A. Khan*, K. M. Reddy and K. A. Hamdan
Department of Upper Gastrointestinal Surgery, St George's Hospital, London, UK
Digestive Diseases Department, Brighton and Sussex University Hospitals, Brighton, UK

Abstract

There has been a steady increase in the number of medicolegal claims following bariatric surgery. This is due to a number of factors including high patient expectation, the technical demands of surgery itself and the requirement for on-going lifelong follow-up. In order to avoid medicolegal pitfalls it is essential to have a robust consenting process; perform well-documented and technically proficient surgery and provide a comprehensive follow up strategy. In addition there is an increasing burden on the non-specialist surgeon to manage bariatric surgical emergencies. Although the medicolegal standard applied to such non-specialists is lower than that expected from a specialist unit, close collaboration with a specialist centre is strongly advised to prevent successful medicolegal claims.

Introduction

Despite advances in the peri-and post-operative management of bariatric surgical patients, bariatric procedures are still associated with a significant incidence of early post-operative and long term morbidity. As a consequence of this and other factors, there has been a steadily increasing rate of medical negligence claims in bariatric surgery - a fact which has reflected in steadily rising insurance premium for bariatric surgeons worldwide. In this chapter, we will explore some of the issues underlying bariatric surgical litigation, analysing

* Correspondence: Omar Khan, Department of Upper GI Surgery, St George's Healthcare NHS Trust, Blackshaw Road, London, SW17 0QT, Tel: 0044 208 725 3180.

the legal principles underpinning such claims as well as a potential medical legal pitfalls associated with bariatric surgery. This chapter will also attempt to define the role of the general surgeon and the medicolegal ramifications of looking after post-bariatric surgery patients who are admitted with complications. Given the wide variations in legal tradition and statutes and in individual jurisdictions, we have chosen to use template of English law in this chapter in order to illustrate the wider principles associated with bariatric medical legal claims.

Legal Principles

In most jurisdictions, with the exception of gross clinical negligence, the vast majority of clinical negligence claims comes under the purview of civil litigation. In English law, all clinical negligent cases are considered under the principles of tort law. For any clinical negligence case to be successful, the plaintiff must demonstrate that:

1) The doctor or hospital had a duty of care

2) This duty of care was breached

3) That this breach in turn materially contributed towards harm which was both foreseeable and quantifiable

4) But for the breach of duty, this harm could have been avoided.

With particular reference to bariatric surgery, the main areas of contention surrounding most medico-legal cases centre around the validity of the patient's consent; the performance of surgery itself and the management of the patient following surgery. With respect to question of what constitutes the valid and informed consent different jurisdictions apply different rules. For example many states in the USA, applied the so-called "prudent patient test" - in other words for consent to be valid, the patient would need to be given all material information necessary for a "prudent patient" to make an appropriate decision. By contrast, consent under English law has been governed by the so-called "Bolam principle"- namely that provided a body of medical practitioners would agree with the consenting process, it would be deemed to be of an acceptable standard.

Moreover this principle not only applies to consent, but all aspects of pre-, intra- and post-operative management. This approach of peer validation has been criticised as allowing too much leeway to medical practitioners and it should noted in the majority of legal jurisdictions do have higher standards which medical practitioners need to attain in order to prevent successful claims of negligence.

Bariatric Surgery and the Medicolegal Environment

Despite the general reduction in peri-operative morbidity and mortality following elective surgery seen in the Western world in the last 20 years, there has been an increase in the number of claims in the bariatric surgery. Indeed, in the United Kingdom, bariatric surgery is now classed one of the highest litigation risks by the major medical insurance companies. The reasons for this are multifactorial, but include:

1. Patient expectation- Bariatric patients have a high incidence of depression and psychological disorders as compared to the general population. This can lead to unrealistic expectations of what surgery can offered to them this consequence of this, these patients may have an increased tendency to seek legal redress should these expectations not be met. In addition, bariatric patients tend to be better informed about their operations than patients undergoing most other forms of surgery typically due to the high level of information and support groups available on the Internet. Finally in most countries with a predominantly state-funded health care system, there is often an underprovision of bariatric surgery in the publically-funded hospitals. As a consequence of this, a large number of patients are forced to pay these operations privately and as such tend to have a lower threshold for complaining should something go wrong.
2. Nature of surgery: Bariatric surgery is a relatively new, technically-demanding and rapidly developing branch of surgery. Although, there are now established fellowship programmes to allow junior surgeons to develop their skills under appropriate supervision and mentorship, a significant proportion of bariatric surgery is performed by surgeons whose primary training and experience is in resectional upper gastrointestinal surgery. Although a large number of these skills are transferable to bariatric surgery, some surgeons (particularly those trained in the era of open as opposed to laparoscopic surgery) may not have the training necessary to perform laparoscopic bariatric surgery to a high level. Similarly bariatric operations pose considerable challenges to anaesthetists, many of whom may not have the familiarity and experience to deal with particular medical issues associated with the morbidly obese. Finally many hospitals do not have the specialist equipment needed to deal with challenges of managing bariatric patients (eg CT scanners capable of coping with the weight of the morbidly obese).
3. Postoperative care: Unlike traditional resectional gastrointestinal surgery where the vast majority of clinical input occurs in the immediate postoperative period, bariatric patients tend to require continued longer-term follow-up and supervision. For example patients with gastric bands require multiple band adjustments whilst patients undergoing gastric bypass and duodenal switch require multivitamin supplementation for life and regular monitoring of their micronutrient levels. In addition, a significant number of patients represent with emergency complications related to their bariatric procedures many years following their original surgery, a subject that will be discussed later in this chapter. For example patients with gastric bands may present with acute band slippage whilst gastric bypass patients may present with intestinal

obstruction secondary to internal hernia. The management of these conditions can be a source of medicolegal claims, particularly as the late diagnoses of these problems can result in significant long-term ongoing morbidity. Finally, a significant portion of patients regain weight in the longer term following surgery and this can be a source of dissatisfaction and potential litigation.

Burden of Medical Legal Claim in Bariatric Surgery

Despite the obvious importance of medicolegal claims in bariatric surgery, there is surprising little in medical literature on this subject. In the largest study on this topic, Cotta et al. [1] reviewed the case notes of 100 consecutive bariatric lawsuits. The most common adverse events initiating litigation were leaks followed by intra-abdominal abscess, bowel obstruction, major airway events, organ injury and pulmonary embolism. In terms of clinical outcomes, 32 patients had a documented intra-operative complication and 72 required additional surgery. A total of 53 of the patients died and 28 had a full recovery with remainder having minor or major disability. Analysis by a medical malpractice lawyer found potential negligence in 28% of cases - the most common cause of negligence being delay in diagnosis of a complication or misinterpretation of vital signs.

Interestingly, surgeons with a low level of experience (i.e. less than one year of experience in bariatric surgery) were most likely to be involved in lawsuits. It should be noted that this analysis was performed on cases performed between 1997 and 2005 and as such included a significant number of operations which are which are no longer routinely undertaken such as vertical banded gastroplasty and open gastric bypass. In addition, none of the patients in the cohort underwent gastric band insertion which again probably reflects the timeframe during which this study was conducted. In a similar study Bruguera et al. [2] reviewed the case files of 49 medicolegal bariatric cases presented to the Professional Liability Department of the Catalonian Medical Colleges Council from 1992 to 2009. In 47% of the cases the patients died, 21% made a complete recovery and the remainder had some residual impairment. The most frequent causes of death were peritonitis due to suture dehiscence (48%), and respiratory complications Malpractice was considered to have occurred in 20% of cases and interestingly in 6% of cases the surgeons were convicted in criminal court of criminal negligence.

In both of these studies, the finding of negligence was typically based on the failure to detect complications in a timely fashion as supposed to the complications themselves. It should also be noted that both studies focused on early postoperative complications associated with bariatric surgery and did not analyse litigation associated with late complications following surgery.

Avoiding Medicolegal Pitfalls in Bariatric Surgery

Given the rising burden of the medicolegal claims, the obvious question for any bariatric surgeon is how these can be avoided. Although there are no hard and fast rules on this subject, the following principles should be useful in reducing and mitigating medicolegal claims following surgery:

1. Consenting: It is critical that bariatric patients undergo a fully informed consenting process. This consists of pre-operative counseling preferably by the operating surgeon as to the risks and benefits of bariatric surgery. Although individual patient's medical co-morbidities must be taken into consideration in counseling patients as to the risks of surgery, the following generic risks should be emphasised:
   a) Laparoscopic gastric band insertion- In terms of the significant and serious risks of this procedure, these include bleeding, deep vein thrombosis and pulmonary embolism and collateral injury to the surrounding structures during port insertion. The patient should be made aware that the band will require multiple adjustments and be counseled as to the risks of infection of the band, tubing and the port site as well as the risk of the band tubing fracturing or disconnecting leading to a loss of fluid and hence restriction in the band. Finally, the patient must be aware of the long term risks of band slippage and erosion necessitating revision surgery.
   b) Laparoscopic sleeve gastrectomy- The risks of this procedure include bleeding, infection, collateral injury to the surrounding structures and staple line leakage. Overall, the mortality rate from this procedure estimated to be 1 in 1000. The procedure is irreversible and there is at present limited long-term data on the outcomes in terms of weight regain.
   c) Laparoscopic gastric bypass- The immediate postoperative risks of this procedure include bleeding, infection, deep vein thrombosis and pulmonary embolism and anastomotic leak. The overall mortality rate for this procedure is approximately 1 in 200. In addition, the patients need to be aware that there is a long term risk of internal herniation and they will require vitamin supplementation and regular blood test monitoring for life.

All patients should be counseled that there is a significant chance of weight regain after any bariatric procedure and their expected weight loss will be determined by a number of factors including the technical performance of the operation and the patient's willingness to alter their behaviour in terms of the dietary intake following surgery. All patients should also be warned that they will have a significant risk of loose overhanging skin after surgery which may require plastic surgical intervention.

Following surgical consultation patients should be discussed in a multidisciplinary team environment with the involvement of dietitians, psychologists, anaesthetists and physicians. The purpose of the multidisciplinary team involvement is to assess suitability of the patient for bariatric surgery and also in conjunction with the patient to decide which bariatric operation best suits each individual patient. The patient should also be given a written summary of the risks and benefits of each of the bariatric operations and allowed a cooling period prior to surgery to allow them to take stock of their options before written consent is reconfirmed.

2. Technical performance of the operation: There is surprisingly little in the literature on what constitutes an appropriate medicolegal standard in the performance of surgery. Clearly gross technical errors (eg the attachment of the biliary limb to the gastric pouch during gastric bypass surgery – the so-called Roux en O) are indefensible but these are relatively rare. As previously discussed, the most common

cause of successful litigation is failure to detect and act on the complications in a timely manner. For example although a leak following gastric bypass surgery is not in itself an indicator of negligence, failure to detect and act upon this would be regard as a negligent error. This can be problematic as the signs of leak can be subtle and as such bariatric surgeons should have very low threshold for investigating patients whose clinical recovery appears to be delayed. In addition to surgical complications, it should be noted that bariatric patients often have significant co-morbidities which need to be optimally managed during their hospital stay. In particular, bariatric patients have a high risk of deep vein thrombosis and suitable thromboprophylaxis is an essential part of their care.

3. Post-discharge management: Following discharge from hospital, patients should be given written advice regarding their dietary intake in the immediate postoperative period and appropriate information regarding their vitamin supplementation. Although these patients should ideally be followed up for life by the bariatric team and this may not be logistically feasible, however if a patient is to be discharged it is incumbent on the bariatric surgeon to ensure that appropriate follow-up is arranged with their primary care physician.

Bariatric Medicolegal Issues for the Non-Specialist

There is an increasing burden of patients presenting to their primary care physician or emergency department requiring either routine follow-up or emergency management of complications related to bariatric surgery.

The reasons for this recent rise in the number of patients requiring clinical input from non-specialist, non-bariatric institutions are multifactorial and include:

1) As the number of patients who have had bariatric surgery grows, there is a growing pool of patients within the community susceptible to the potential long-term complications associated with bariatric surgery.
2) Given the specialist nature of bariatric surgery, there are relatively few bariatric centres and hence patients often have travel a long distance to have their surgery in these specialist hospitals. In addition, there is a large, well-advertised international market for bariatric operations and hence many patients do go abroad for their surgery. Both of these classes of patient are likely to access their local health services as opposed to their original institution.
3) Unlike patients undergoing resections for gastrointestinal cancer, bariatric patients are relatively young. As such there is a significant incidence of patient migration for work or personal reasons from the area where the original surgery was performed.
4) Sub-optimal follow-up by their bariatric surgical unit can result in patients presenting *in extremis* with for example metabolic complications following a failure to monitor and adjust vitamin supplementation after gastric bypass.

Typical emergency presentations related to bariatric surgery include early post-operative complications such as late anastomotic leak as well as long-term complications many years following surgery (eg gastric band slippage and internal herniation following Roux-en-Y gastric bypass surgery). These patients present a particular clinical problem for institutions administering emergency care. For start patients presenting as emergencies will typically will go to their local Emergency Department, and these hospitals may not have surgeons with familiarity in bariatric surgery nor experience in dealing with post-bariatric surgical emergencies. In addition, the facilities in such hospitals may not be able to cater for the special needs of morbidly obese patients. The question which then arises is- what is the minimum medicolegal standard of care that these hospitals need to provide to such emergency bariatric patients? Although these standards can vary from jurisdiction to jurisdiction, under English law, the hospital will be expected to provide a standard of care provided by a reasonably competent general surgeon in a non-specialist hospital, as opposed to the optimum standard of care which would be afforded by a specialist bariatric unit. An important principle is that these patients should be discussed at the earliest opportunity with a bariatric unit (ideally the institution where the surgery was originally performed) and, where possible and appropriate, early transfer of the patient should be arranged. However this should not delay treatment as the majority of complications after bariatric surgery tend to be general surgical complications (eg intestinal obstruction) and as such the management of these complications should be within the remit and capacity of a general surgeon covering the emergency take. Failure to recognise these problems early and intervene in a timely fashion is one of the most common causes of preventable, major long-term disability or death in bariatric surgical patients and hence such failures should be considered to be sub-standard provision of care.

Conclusion

Bariatric surgery is designed in conjunction with other behavioural modifications to improve the long-term functional outcome of patients. Unlike traditional resection of gastrointestinal surgery, bariatric surgery requires a different paradigm

with a truly multidisciplinary approach both pre- and post-operatively to improve the long-term functional outcomes of patients. This in turn creates a large number of medical legal pitfalls which, in ever more litigious society are likely to result in more legal claims. However with appropriate multidisciplinary involvement and robust protocols for the pre-, intra- and postoperative management of these patients these risks can be mitigated and reduced. Finally it should be noticed that we have so far focused exclusively on the medicolegal aspects of patients enrolled within a surgical programme. However, in countries such as the United Kingdom with a predominantly state-funded health care system, there is a growing problem with access to publically-funded bariatric surgery. For example in the United Kingdom, less than 1% of the patients who would benefit clinically from bariatric surgery are in fact funded for this operation. It is likely that this rationing of bariatric surgery will become a significant source of medicolegal claims in the future.

References

[1] Cottam D, Lord J, Dallal RM, Wolfe B, Higa K, McCauley K, Schauer P. Medicolegal analysis of 100 malpractice claims against bariatric surgeons. *Surg. Obes. Relat. Dis.*, 2007; 3: 60-66.

[2] Bruguera M, Delgado S, Viger M, Benet J, Bruguera R, Arimany J. Medicolegal analysis of legal claims in bariatric surgery. *Cir. Esp.*, 2012; 90: 254-9.

Index

#

A

B

C

D

E

F

G

H

I

P

Q

R

S

T

U

V

W

X

Y

Z